Communications
in Computer and Information Science   1856

Editorial Board Members

Rationale

The CCIS series is devoted to the publication of proceedings of computer science conferences. Its aim is to efficiently disseminate original research results in informatics in printed and electronic form. While the focus is on publication of peer-reviewed full papers presenting mature work, inclusion of reviewed short papers reporting on work in progress is welcome, too. Besides globally relevant meetings with internationally representative program committees guaranteeing a strict peer-reviewing and paper selection process, conferences run by societies or of high regional or national relevance are also considered for publication.

Topics

The topical scope of CCIS spans the entire spectrum of informatics ranging from foundational topics in the theory of computing to information and communications science and technology and a broad variety of interdisciplinary application fields.

Information for Volume Editors and Authors

Publication in CCIS is free of charge. No royalties are paid, however, we offer registered conference participants temporary free access to the online version of the conference proceedings on SpringerLink (http://link.springer.com) by means of an http referrer from the conference website and/or a number of complimentary printed copies, as specified in the official acceptance email of the event.

CCIS proceedings can be published in time for distribution at conferences or as post-proceedings, and delivered in the form of printed books and/or electronically as USBs and/or e-content licenses for accessing proceedings at SpringerLink. Furthermore, CCIS proceedings are included in the CCIS electronic book series hosted in the SpringerLink digital library at http://link.springer.com/bookseries/7899. Conferences publishing in CCIS are allowed to use Online Conference Service (OCS) for managing the whole proceedings lifecycle (from submission and reviewing to preparing for publication) free of charge.

Publication process

The language of publication is exclusively English. Authors publishing in CCIS have to sign the Springer CCIS copyright transfer form, however, they are free to use their material published in CCIS for substantially changed, more elaborate subsequent publications elsewhere. For the preparation of the camera-ready papers/files, authors have to strictly adhere to the Springer CCIS Authors' Instructions and are strongly encouraged to use the CCIS LaTeX style files or templates.

Abstracting/Indexing

CCIS is abstracted/indexed in DBLP, Google Scholar, EI-Compendex, Mathematical Reviews, SCImago, Scopus. CCIS volumes are also submitted for the inclusion in ISI Proceedings.

How to start

To start the evaluation of your proposal for inclusion in the CCIS series, please send an e-mail to ccis@springer.com.

Leszek A. Maciaszek · Maurice D. Mulvenna ·
Martina Ziefle
Editors

Information and Communication Technologies for Ageing Well and e-Health

7th International Conference, ICT4AWE 2021
Virtual Event, April 24–26, 2021, and 8th International
Conference, ICT4AWE 2022, Virtual Event, April 23–25, 2022
Revised Selected Papers

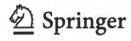 Springer

Editors
Leszek A. Maciaszek
Wrocław University of Economics Institute
of Business Informatics
Wrocław, Poland

Macquarie University
Sydney, Australia

Martina Ziefle
RWTH Aachen University
Aachen, Germany

Maurice D. Mulvenna
University of Ulster
Newtownabbey, UK

ISSN 1865-0929 ISSN 1865-0937 (electronic)
Communications in Computer and Information Science
ISBN 978-3-031-37495-1 ISBN 978-3-031-37496-8 (eBook)
https://doi.org/10.1007/978-3-031-37496-8

This Springer imprint is published by the registered company Springer Nature Switzerland AG
The registered company address is: Gewerbestrasse 11, 6330 Cham, Switzerland

Preface

The present book includes extended and revised versions of a set of selected papers from the International Conference on Information and Communication Technologies for Ageing Well and e-Health (ICT4AWE 2021 and 2022), which were exceptionally held as online events, due to COVID-19.

ICT4AWE 2021 received 33 paper submissions from 23 countries, of which 15% were included in this book. ICT4AWE 2022 received 50 paper submissions from 24 countries, of which 32% were included in this book.

The papers were selected by the event chairs and their selection is based on a number of quality criteria that include the classifications and comments provided by the program committee members, the session chairs' assessment and also the program chairs' general assessment of all papers included in the technical program. The authors of selected papers were then invited to submit a revised and extended version of their papers having at least 30% innovative material.

The International Conference on Information and Communication Technologies for Ageing Well and e-Health fosters close exchange and collaboration in the field of digital assistive technologies in the health care domain. The conference aims to be a meeting point for those that study age and health-related quality of life and apply information and communication technologies to help people stay healthier, more independent and active at work or in their community. ICT4AWE facilitates the exchange of information and dissemination of best practices, innovation and technical improvements in the fields of age and health care, education, psychology, social coordination and ambient assisted living. From e-Health to intelligent systems and ICT devices, the conference is a vibrant discussion and collaboration platform for all those that work in research and development or in companies involved in promoting the quality of life and well-being of people, by providing room for research and industrial presentations, demos and project descriptions.

The papers selected to be included in this book contribute to the understanding of relevant trends of current research on Information and Communication Technologies for Ageing Well and e-Health, including: Decision Support Systems, Home Care Monitoring Systems, Systems to Encourage Healthy Lifestyles, Diagnostic Support, Acceptance of Ambient Technology, Internet of Things and Smart Devices for Independent Living, Mobile Health Monitoring, Psychological Dimension of Aging Population, Privacy and Ethical Issues, Open Data and Health Information, Inclusive Design, Human Communication and Behavioural Studies of Senior Citizens, Health Information Systems, Game-Based Approaches towards Health Awareness, Electronic Health Records, Case Studies in eHealth and Autonomy and Active Ageing.

We would like to thank all the authors for their contributions and also the reviewers who have helped to ensure the quality of this publication.

April 2022   Leszek Maciaszek
                                                  Maurice Mulvenna
                                                  Martina Ziefle

Organization

Conference Chair

Leszek Maciaszek   Wrocław University of Economics Institute of Business Informatics, Poland and Macquarie University, Australia

Program Co-chairs

Martina Ziefle   RTWH Aachen University, Germany
Maurice Mulvenna   Ulster University, UK

Program Committee

Served in 2021

Amit Nanavati	IBM Research, India
Andrea Vitaletti	Sapienza University of Rome, Italy
Annica Kristoffersson	Mälardalen University, Sweden
Antonio Lanatà	University of Florence, Italy
Asta Thoroddsen	University of Iceland, Iceland
Bert-Jan van Beijnum	University of Twente, The Netherlands
Dympna O'Sullivan	TU Dublin, Ireland
Javier Gomez	Universidad Autónoma de Madrid, Spain
Kathleen McCoy	University of Delaware, USA
Mehdi Adda	Université du Québec à Rimouski, Canada
Philipp Brauner	RWTH Aachen University, Germany
Roberto Hornero	University of Valladolid, Spain
Sami Shaban	United Arab Emirates University, UAE
Sandra Baldassarri	University of Zaragoza, Spain
Xiaomu Zhou	Northeastern University, USA

Served in 2022

Andrea Tales	Swansea University, UK
Bo Xie	University of Texas at Austin, USA
Gillian Cameron	Inspire Workplaces & Ulster University, UK
Judith Sixsmith	University of Dundee, UK
Michael O'Grady	University College Dublin, Ireland
Rémi Bastide	University of Toulouse, France

Served in 2021 and 2022

Åsa Smedberg	Stockholm University, Sweden
Andreas Schrader	Universität zu Lübeck, Germany
David Fuschi	Coventry University, UK
Eila Järvenpää	Aalto University, Finland
Elvis Mazzoni	University of Bologna, Italy
Evi Zouganeli	Oslo Metropolitan University, Norway
Georg Duftschmid	Medical University of Vienna, Austria
George Xylomenos	Athens University of Economics and Business, Greece
Heikki Lyytinen	University of Jyväskylä, Finland
Jaakko Hakulinen	Tampere University, Finland
Jane Bringolf	Centre for Universal Design Australia Ltd, Australia
Jitae Shin	Sungkyunkwan University, South Korea
Josep Silva	Universitat Politècnica de València, Spain
Karsten Berns	TU Kaiserslautern, Germany
Laurent Billonnet	University of Limoges, France
Marco Porta	Università degli Studi di Pavia, Italy
Mario Ciampi	National Research Council of Italy, Italy
Marko Perisa	University of Zagreb, Croatia
Maurice Mars	University of KwaZulu-Natal, South Africa
Meng Wong	National Institute of Education, Singapore
Mikel Larrea	Universidad del País Vasco, Spain
Oh-Soon Shin	Soongsil University, South Korea
Paula Forbes	University of Abertay, UK
Raul Montoliu	Universidad Jaume I, Spain
René Meier	Lucerne University of Applied Sciences, Switzerland
Renato Bulcão-Neto	Federal University of Goiás, Brazil
Stefano Federici	University of Perugia, Italy
Susanna Spinsante	Università Politecnica delle Marche, Italy

Taro Sugihara	Tokyo Institute of Technology, Japan
Telmo Silva	University of Aveiro, Portugal
Ulrich Reimer	Eastern Switzerland University of Applied Sciences, Switzerland
Yao Chang	Chung Yuan Christian University, Taiwan, Republic of China

Additional Reviewers

Served in 2022

Edith Maier	Eastern Switzerland University of Applied Sciences, Switzerland
Ernesto Veiga	Federal University of Goiás, Brazil

Invited Speakers

2021

Eling D. de Bruin	ETH Zürich, Switzerland and Karolinska Institute, Sweden
Bo Xie	University of Texas at Austin, USA
Alex Mihailidis	University of Toronto, Canada
Sunil Agrawal	Columbia University, USA

2022

Sabine Koch	Karolinska Institutet, Sweden
Arlene J. Astell	University of Toronto, Canada
Ray Jones	University of Plymouth, UK
Jesse Hoey	University of Waterloo, Canada

Contents

Telemedicine and Independent Living

Digital Health and e-health

Aging Well - Social and Human Sciences Perspective

Turntable: The Co-creation of a Digital Solution Supporting Older Adults in Active Aging

Benedek Szakonyi[1]([✉]) [iD], István Vassányi[1] [iD], Angelika Mantur-Vierendeel[2] [iD],
Daniela Loi[3] [iD], Guilherme Correia[4] [iD], and Bojan Blažica[5] [iD]

[1] Medical Informatics Research and Development Centre, University of Pannonia, Veszprém,
Hungary
{szakonyi.benedek,vassanyi.istvan}@mik.uni-pannon.hu
[2] EuroFIR AISBL, Brussels, Belgium
am@eurofir.org
[3] Department of Electrical and Electronic Engineering, University of Cagliari, Cagliari, Italy
daniela.loi@unica.it
[4] Laboratory for Automation and Systems, Instituto Pedro Nunes, Coimbra, Portugal
gcorreia@ipn.pt
[5] Jožef Stefan Institute, Ljubljana, Slovenia
bojan.blazica@ijs.si

Abstract. The Turntable Solution addresses the challenges around activity, vitality, and social interactions for older adults – people aged 60 or over – by using a gardening oriented mobile device-based approach. This paper presents the findings of co-creation sessions introducing the Turntable Solution, its main concepts and initial functionality. The sessions were held in Belgium, Italy, Portugal and Slovenia with five participants each, where the mobile solution's features were discussed. The lifestyles of potential users, their general perception and acceptance of mobile technology and their experience with using existing and planned features were surveyed in hands-on trials using mock-ups and prototypes. Results showed that while the place of living (country) has a notable effect on how the Solution is perceived, it was generally accepted and favoured. Even though less technologically proficient users tend to like mobile solutions less, mainly due to their (previous) negative experiences, such bias can be effectively negated by providing proper user experience. Moreover, their willingness to try such solutions was increased as they found the Turntable App features - gardening hints, nutritional guidance, and social interactions – interesting and useful.

Keywords: Older adults · Co-creation · Digital services · Well-being · Gardening · Health · Turntable

1 Introduction

1.1 Background

Age-related physical and cognitive decline is usually accelerated as people become less active and more sedentary as they age. Challenges related to eating healthily and maintaining social activity arise more frequently [1]. Falls become more frequent and

L. A. Maciaszek et al. (Eds.): ICT4AWE 2021/2022, CCIS 1856, pp. 3–16, 2023.
https://doi.org/10.1007/978-3-031-37496-8_1

4	B. Szakonyi et al.

dangerous as muscle mass, strength, and power decline. Even everyday tasks appear to be more intimidating than before. The resulting inclination of avoiding risky situations (e.g. by not leaving the house) worsens physical conditions and causes social isolation (as people stop visiting each other). These worsening conditions also contribute to developing chronic diseases, the leading causes of healthcare expenditure in modern societies – making this problem significant not just for individuals but also for the global population.

Good nutrition, physical activity and social interaction were found to highly impact both actual and perceived quality of life for older adults [2–4]. So helping individuals to prepare healthy meals (achieving a balanced diet) and live an active lifestyle through recreational social activities is crucial. For assisting older adults in sustaining (or re-adopting) such healthy habits, maintaining motivation and providing support is vital [5].

One potential activity addressing physical, cognitive and social aspects all at once is (leisure) gardening [6]. Increasing evidence can be found in recent scientific literature about home and community gardening having numerous physical, health and restoration benefits [7–9]. Their positive effects include improved self-perception related to ageing [10], and even the risk of premature death can be lowered [11, 12]. As people generally like spending time in nature, gardening can be a good motivator in solutions assisting users to achieve lifestyle changes and healthy living.

Using digital solutions could be an effective way for making such interventions more successful. The widespread use of smartphones, tablets, and other similar devices provides a powerful basis for exploiting the advantages of Information Technology. The ease of accessing and sharing information, communication without difficulties, the computational power to solve complex problems. Of course, a common question related to this topic is how well older adults can utilize these solutions or use them at all. On one hand, participation in modern societies relies more and more on having basic digital skills, even for older adults [13]. This implies that the number of people struggling with using digital devices should decline as years go by. On the other hand, providing well-designed applications for older adults can also support them in developing and maintaining these much-needed skills, not just in healthy living.

1.2 The Turntable Project

Based on these concepts, a platform promoting active ageing among older adults is being developed in the Turntable AAL project [14], which also aims to help older users prolong their autonomous and independent lives. As a first stage of the project, co-creation sessions were held in four European Member States (Portugal, Italy, Belgium and Slovenia) to investigate target users' gardening habits and needs and discuss and test possible features of a gardening-oriented mobile solution. This paper reports the findings of these co-creation sessions, and a brief introduction of the solution's main components and features is included.

1.3   Previous Work

The first data analysis results of the co-creation sessions were published at the ICT4AWE 2021 conference [14]. This paper provides additional research data, further data analysis results, and more details about the main components used.

2   Related Work

Already in 2013, a literature review [15] has found ample evidence for gardening (horticultural activities) having positive effects on the lives of older adults, including overall quality of life, health, physical and cognitive ability, and socialization. Other reviews publish since then, examining the findings of more recent works, have also confirmed these positive effects [7–9]. The similar results of their reviewed studies, with participants from multiple different countries (China, Hong Kong, Iran, Japan, Netherlands, Norway, South Korea, Taiwan, UK, USA), suggest that the positive effects of gardening can be perceived by older adults regardless of their cultural background. Reports from Australia [16] and Singapore [17] also confirm this. So gardening is a potent basis for solutions addressing older adults' difficulties in achieving healthy living globally.

The advances in assistive technologies for older adults increase the number of available options. There are generic smart living solutions in the form of wearable devices [18], programs for cognitive stimulation [19], applications used by home care organizations [20] and more. While useful, these solutions generally focus on only one or two aspects needed to achieve healthy living, not all at once (or at least as much as possible).

Lekjaroen et al. introduced a so-called IoT Planting solution as an initial gardening based solution, allowing users to monitor soil moisture, temperature, light via an Android application. They found that older adults have both the willingness and skills to use such solutions [21]. However, the functionality offered can be considered somewhat limited, as it is more like a remote-controlled plant manager than a solution aiding users in active gardening. It also lacks one of the key domains of gardening, the sociality and skill-sharing aspect [22].

Based on co-design workshops, Wherton et al. [23] identified four main aspects that assisted living applications should consider: providing social support, raising awareness and sharing knowledge, offering sufficient customization and adaptation, and ensuring effective coordination of care services.

Both newly created and existing solutions can greatly benefit from having potential users testing already available solutions (e.g. fitness applications [24]), as their feedback can ensure more effective development. Including older adults in the design process of digital solutions allows identifying the potential barriers, such as data privacy and management, technology literacy, the accessibility of technology, and the need for co-design itself [25]. Moreover, involving individuals with special needs (physical or mental health conditions) in co-design sessions reveals specific requirements that should be addressed – such as advanced emotional support and crisis support, along with the general need to be well informed and motivated [26].

Accordingly, the Turntable project aims to develop a solution covering all key aspects of gardening, to provide an effective tool for achieving healthy living, with the inclusion of older adults in the process.

3 Digital Services Included

Five already existing components with thousands of registered users serve as the foundations for the development of the Turntable Solution. These components are *OPEN, Tomappo, Lifely, IntegrAAL Social Engine* and *MARIA*. Throughout the project, the main goal is to integrate these components into one single solution and tailor that to provide all necessary features required to match user expectations.

The *OPEN* nutrition app serves as a dietary assessment and personalized meal logging and planning tool. It aims to help users pay more attention to their eating and physical activity habits and provide a basis for planning changes and setting goals. Currently, it is available only as a web-based platform for clinical nutrition, as a food composition database to identify the key nutritional elements (carbohydrates, fats, protein) of different foods and meals prepared (also concerning the different food preparation methods). It can compute the dietary reference intake, which helps planning the diet for the following days and weeks. It supports creating "recipes" to facilitate easier logging of frequently consumed items, along with some pre-recorded meals.

The *Tomappo* application, available on Android and the web, helps users manage their gardens and grow their own vegetables. It guides users through a whole gardening season with daily advice, from initial steps such as soil preparation and where and what to plant (i.e. garden planning), through "everyday nurturing" tasks, and up to the harvest. Garden planning includes watching out for the good and bad neighbors of plants, estimating the suitable distance to keep between the plants, giving the correct amount of seed or plantings based on the size of the given garden and the intended yield. It also supports using crop rotation. Its seed exchange feature encourages users to connect with other fellow gardeners to exchange not just seeds or seedlings, but also experience, and it aims to facilitate social interaction (Figs. 1 and 2).

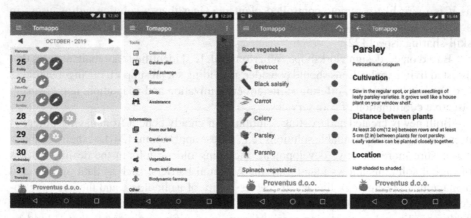

Fig. 1. The main screens of the Tomappo Application.

Lifely Agrumino is a gardening device comprising a wireless sensor monitoring temperature, light water reservoir and soil humidity. The device is installed in the user's garden and uses a mobile application to manage it. Apart from providing "raw data", it

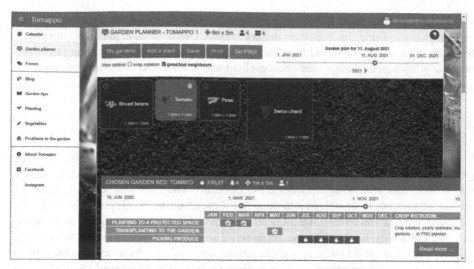

Fig. 2. The Tomappo garden planner in a web browser.

also allows users to set the type of the plant it is attached to. This helps users interpret the measured values (e.g. "the plant needs more sunlight, and much less water") (Fig. 3).

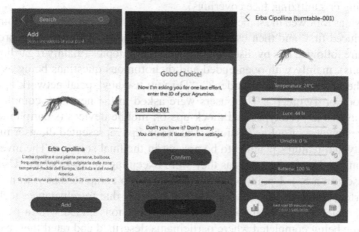

Fig. 3. The main screens of the Lifely application.

The *IntegrAAL Social Engine* (*ISE*), working in the background, is aimed to build a user profile that can monitor user behavioral patterns and detect unusual changes, to trigger an alert or other action when non-conformant trends or events are detected.

MARIA is a region-specific multi-audio device for voice recognition. It allows voice interaction for sensors and services used by users in their own houses.

The idea behind the integration process is that a single application could be created to combine and exploit the various features of the standalone components. To allow users to do everyday tasks such as designing their garden based on their food preferences (by extracting the information from their dietary logs). Or vice versa, to plan their next meal based on what can be harvested from their garden. To learn or share gardening tips with old or new friends, exchange seeds, request help with chores, etc. All in order to promote and support achieving an active and healthy lifestyle.

4   Co-creation Sessions

User-oriented co-creation sessions with five participants each were organized in Belgium, Italy, Portugal and Slovenia. The 20 participants' (11 female, 9 male) mean age was 67.35 years with a standard deviation of 5.285. The topics to be asked and covered (scenarios) were organized into three sessions, resulting in 60 sittings in total. The inclusion criteria were being aged 60 or over, having an interest in gardening activities and the ability to give informed consent. The exclusion criterion was having any impairments that would interfere with executing the sessions. As necessary, the ethical approvals required to perform the sessions were acquired and managed locally in each participating country.

As the co-creation sessions took place between the end of June and the middle of July 2020, public health measures related to Covid-19 had to be implemented. The multiple group sessions planned initially were replaced with remote sessions or one-on-one sittings where all necessary precautions were adhered to (e.g. social distancing, hand washing or sanitizing, face coverings).

All sessions followed the same structure. The project goals and the main components were introduced first, and then users could ask any questions they had. A pre-session questionnaire followed this by discussing more general topics (mainly regarding participants' habits), mainly with open-ended and dichotomous questions being asked (e.g. "What is the main reason you garden?", "Do you use any social network application like Facebook or Twitter?"). Then users were asked in the next task completion part to test the available prototypes and mock-ups on mobile devices (smartphone, tablet) or computers in case of online sessions. The mock-ups represented the user interfaces, functionality and features planned to be present in the final solution. The investigators present monitored users' progress as they were executing the tasks given. User results were assessed on a 5 + 1 point scale (1 – user tried to complete but with no result at all, 5 – perfect solution, 0 – the user did not even try due to reluctance, technical or any other problems) and by free-text reports. All sessions ended with a post-session questionnaire being completed where participants described and rated their experience (concerning both conceptual and accessibility aspects). This rating procedure primarily consisted of 5-point Likert scale questions (1 being the most negative, 5 the most positive response). The exact questionnaires used in pre- and post-session interviews are provided in Appendices A1, A2 and A3, the tasks (user manuals on what to do) in B1, B2 and B3, respectively.

The questions asked during the first session related to gardening habits and information technology proficiency. The task completion consisted of testing the features of the standalone OPEN, Tomappo and Lifely components in their current development status (e.g. logging a meal in the nutrition app, planning a garden, setting up a sensor for a plant). Then users were asked to rate their experience with each application separately. Their ideas were also asked about possible features of ISE and MARIA (e.g. "Would you like to have a function that alerts your friends if something was unusual in your activity?", "Do you find voice more useful than buttons to manage Turntable?").

Social interaction and activity were addressed in the second session. User habits related to contacting family and friends were discussed, such as frequency (e.g., calling once a week) and means of making contact (e.g., via mobile, landline or online calls/messages). A mock-up representing the so-called Dashboard component was used during the testing phase. This component is intended for managing other application users (e.g., adding friends, messaging others), social interaction and editing personal settings (e.g., visibility of personal information, components' access to users' data). Finally, users were asked to rate their experience with the features tested, similarly to the first session.

Future Integrated features of the platform and its possibilities were in the focus of the third session. Users' ideas and expectations were asked on how they imagined using such a system, what data should be shared between components, and how they should work together. The users tested and rated possible workflows during the testing phase (e.g., importing sensor data into the garden planner, having OPEN plan a meal based on the content of the garden managed in Tomappo).

The data received during the sessions were anonymized locally in each country to protect sensitive personal data before being forwarded to the partner executing the data analysis.

5 Data Analysis

5.1 Data Preparation

The first data processing step was the quality assessment of the data provided, as finding some inaccurate, incorrect or missing items is almost inevitable in data collection processes. In this case, the reasons behind these were technical or coding anomalies (e.g., the text report contradicts the numerical values provided regarding the number of assists needed for a user to complete the task) or simply human error (interviewer mistakes). Such mistakes were corrected where possible, while missing values were replaced if related answers could be used.

As another frequently used data analysis step, the key numerical and textual variables were transformed (categorized) into nominal variables wherever possible to obtain meaningful results, based on a priori classes or actual data ranges and distributions. Task- and user-level descriptors and satisfaction indices were also introduced. Conclusions were drawn based on majority opinions from the individually evaluated free-text answers.

Eight user-level descriptors were defined from the data received. These were age, gender, country, average completion time and scoring parameters (shown in Table 1). Two categories were defined for the age, one for those above the average age (68 years) and the other for the rest. Three groups of scoring parameters were defined: task scores given by investigators (rating completion success of given users and tasks); the component scores (component-wise average of task scores); and the average user scores (the average of task scores). The "task assists" variable was defined as the number of occasions when the user requested assistance in completing a given task (values were derived manually using text logs of the tasks).

Table 1. The defined nominal variables for user-level statistics [14].

Variable name	Multiplicity	No. of classes	Note
Age	For each user	2	Younger, older
Gender	For each user	2	Male, Female
Country	For each user	4	Country no. 1, 2,3 and 4
Completion time	For each user	3	The average time needed to complete a session: low, middle, high
Task scores	For each user in each task	5	The score given by the manager: 1, 2, 3, 4, or 5
Component scores	For each user, avg. For each app	5	Component-wise average of task scores: 1, 2, 3, 4, or 5
User score	For each user	5	User-wise average of task scores: 1, 2, 3, 4, or 5
Task assists	For each user in each task	4	The number of occasions when the user requested assistance: 0, 1, 2 or 3

The average task completion time shows how much time the user needed to complete a session (all tasks in that session). Three classes were defined based on the average values of all participants: LOW (0–17 min), MIDDLE (18–26 min) and HIGH (more than 26 min) time need.

A total of nine variables were defined for task-level descriptive statistics: the minimum, maximum and average values for completion time, number of assists needed, and task-wise scores received.

The satisfaction indices were derived from post-session answers to represent the overall impressions of users about the features introduced. These indices range from 1 (did not like at all) to 5 (really liked). A total of 8 assessment categories/indices have been defined: 5 indices for the five main components, one index for the *Dashboard* mock-up, one for the *Integrated features* mock-up, and one as an *Overall* rating index (the weighted average of the other 7 indices). Indices were calculated separately for all users, and are shown in Table 2. The "source" questions and the user-wise indices and can be found in Appendices C1.

Table 2. The source data used in the attribute ranking analysis [14].

Country	Gender	Age	Time	Score	Satisfaction							
					T	A	O	I	M	D	In	Ov
BE	M	YOUNG	MID	MID	4	3	3,5	1	5	4	3	3,4
BE	M	YOUNG	LOW	LOW	3	4	2,5	1	3	5	3	3,1
BE	M	YOUNG	LOW	LOW	4	3	3	1	3	4	4	3,1
BE	F	YOUNG	MID	LOW	3	4	2,5	1,7	3	4	4	3,2
BE	F	YOUNG	LOW	LOW	4	3,5	3	1	4	4	4	3,4
IT	M	OLDER	HIGH	MID	4	5	3	3	3	5	4	3,9
IT	F	YOUNG	HIGH	MID	5	5	5	3	4	5	5	4,6
IT	M	YOUNG	HIGH	HIGH	3	5	3	3	3	5	4	3,7
IT	F	YOUNG	LOW	HIGH	4	5	3	1	4	5	4	3,7
IT	F	YOUNG	LOW	HIGH	4	4	3	2,3	4	4	4	3,6
PT	F	YOUNG	HIGH	HIGH	4	4	5	5	1	4	4	3,9
PT	M	OLDER	MID	LOW	5	4,5	4,5	5	5	3	4	4,4
PT	F	OLDER	HIGH	MID	4,5	4,5	4,5	5	1	4	4	3,9
PT	F	OLDER	MID	MID	4	5	1	5	5	4	3	3,9
PT	F	OLDER	MID	HIGH	5	4,5	3	1	4	5	5	3,9
SLO	F	YOUNG	HIGH	MID	4,5	4	2	-	-	4	4	3,7
SLO	M	OLDER	MID	MID	5	4	4	-	-	4	4,3	4,3
SLO	F	OLDER	MID	MID	5	4,5	2,5	-	-	4	4	4
SLO	M	OLDER	HIGH	LOW	4	3	3	-	-	3	3	3,2
SLO	M	OLDER	LOW	HIGH	3,5	2	3	-	-	3	2,3	2,8
			Average		4,1	4,1	3,2	2,6	3,5	4,2	3,8	3,7
55			Standard deviation		0,5	0,6	0,7	1,4	1,0	0,5	0,5	0,4

T – Tomappo, A – Agrumino, O – OPEN, I – IntegrAAL Social Engine, M – Maria, D. – Dashboard, In – Integrated solutions, Ov – Overall.

5.2 Results

The predictor (explanatory) nominal variables age, gender, country, completion time and component score were used to generate attribute rankings. The seven satisfaction indices were used as class labels (without *Overall*).

The ranked attributes (shown in Table 3) specify predictor variables' information content for the selected class variable, in the order of importance. An attribute with a higher value means that it has more influence over how the given component/item is perceived than the other ones.

For example, *country: 0.95* as the highest value in the *ISE* satisfaction list means that the *country* attribute of users (where they live) had the most influence on user satisfaction concerning *ISE*, and it had about thrice the influence as the *Age* attribute with the weight (information content) 0.26.

Task-level statistics show the first session as the most demanding one, with the longest completion times and highest assist counts. It was also found that components used were considered satisfactory regarding usability, except for *OPEN*. The exact task-wise values computed are provided in Appendix C3, the categorized answers and their respective questions in Appendix C4.

Table 3. Satisfaction index-wise ranked attributes values [14].

Ranked attribute	Individual component					D	In	Ov
	T	A	O	I	M			
Age	0.21	0.24	0.11	0.26	0.12	0.20	0.07	0.10
Country	0.37	0.59	0.63	0.95	0.62	0.46	0.31	0.73
Gender	0.05	0.28	0.23	0.17	0.55	0.23	0.21	0.23
Score	0.25	0.28	0.38	0.28	0.35	0.21	0.25	0.24
Completion time	0.26	0.17	0.52	0.82	0.62	0.06	0.16	0.25

T – Tomappo, A – Agrumino, O – OPEN, I – IntegrAAL Social Engine, M – Maria, D. – Dashboard, In – Integrated solutions, Ov – Overall.

In order to identify hidden relationships among the variables, the Apriori association rule mining algorithm was run on the data set, and 76 important rules were found (rules are like IF-THEN structures in the form of *rule head → rule body*, describing what the "pre-requisites" are for a statement to be "true"). A rule was considered "important" if it had a lift value above 4 and a conviction value above 3. The lift was computed as the ratio of the rule's measured and expected confidence (the expected value being the product of the rule body's support values and the rule head divided by the support of the rule body). The measured confidence is the percentage that shows how frequently the rule head occurs among all the groups containing the rule body. Similarly, a greater value of conviction shows that incorrect predictions (head -> body) occur less often than if these two were independent.

The important rules can be classified into the following two groups:

- Country-based rules. The country, especially Belgium is a variable that strongly influenced the satisfaction indices. For example, the Country = Belgium AND Age = YOUNGER pattern was associated with Score Integ = LOW AND Satisfaction Overall #2 = LOW. The fact that Country = Belgium appeared in numerous important association rules (ca. 50% of all) while the other three premises did not at all makes it apparent that either the system's acceptance or the testing method was quite different in Belgium from the rest.
- Related scores and satisfaction indices. In many of the rules, the scores, especially the low scores were associated with (low) satisfaction, for example, Score Integ = LOW -> Age = YOUNGER AND Score Dash = LOW AND Satisfaction Overall #2 = LOW. This phenomenon may be due to the fact that users with low scores found little

success and therefore little satisfaction in the features, and also that various kinds of low scores often occur together, as a symptom of limited computer literacy.

The following conclusions were formed based on the received free-text answers:

1. Turntable's overall acceptance was highly positive. Most users would gladly use the solution once available (this is confirmed by the high average scores of the post-session answers).
2. Users experienced no problems with the mobile technology presented (as working prototypes and mock-up applications), with only a few exceptions.
3. Most users prefer using a single integrated solution and would avoid using individual components. The *Dashboard* app should be integrated with the other component apps.
4. A significant number of the participants have no social media profiles and would prefer not to create such. This means that social functionality must be implemented in the solution to provide related features.
5. Even if Turntable is primarily aimed at healthy users (as it offers no condition-specific recommendations or features), many users missed having a health profile and related functions.
6. *OPEN* should be coupled more tightly to *Tomappo* and *Lifely*, as users had more interest in those.
7. Users considered the behavior assessment and profiling features of ISE intrusive and unwarranted. *ISE* must be better positioned and explained.

The user interface of *OPEN* should be redesigned, and some minor changes might also be beneficial for other components to improve usability. The vast majority of users preferred using checkboxes rather than toggle switches as they find the latter perplexing. Text and button sizes were adequate, but means for personalizing them should be provided. Tooltips or similar support features would greatly help those with lower technological proficiency.

6   Discussion

The initial assumption of the Turntable project was confirmed as users reported the gardening oriented approach to be quite interesting and that using information technology solutions is not problematic. Thus, Turntable has the potential to effectively assist ageing people in (re)adopting and maintaining healthy habits.

The number of 20 participating users (5 from each country) is a relatively low sample count, insufficient for providing statistically significant conclusions. Still, it still serves as a good starting point as observations made only on the trend level can be helpful [27].

The calculated satisfaction indices verified that users were contented with most of the components tested. The mock-ups of *Tomappo, Lifely*, the *Dashboard* and the *Integrated features* were liked the most and received the best remarks. Less interest was shown in *OPEN*, which might be caused by its lacking user interface design rather than its concept (this is detailed later in this paragraph). The remarks made in free-text answers concur with the low satisfaction indices calculated for *ISE*, which means most users consider its functionality too intrusive. However, it must be noted that *ISE* received highly positive remarks in Portugal, where it is developed, which might be related to its presentation or social factors. Still, this component must be better matched with users' needs and requires better positioning and introduction. Better transparency about its purposes and how it works is vital. Achieving this is important as the profiling features are solely there to aid users, without financial purposes (e.g., targeted marketing). Some discrepancies appeared between the indices calculated and other answers given for *MARIA*. Most users reported finding voice control to be more advantageous than using touch screens. However, when asked about using specific component features by voice command, and how useful that is, low(er) ratings were given. Moreover, no meaningful answers were received when asked what kind of questions they would ask the voice assistant, how would they use it. A possible reason is that these questions were formulated improperly or that the functionality was not explained well enough.

Results show the country attribute as the most important factor in users' perception of a component and which ones they prefer. This could be interpreted as a country- or culture-specific difference; however, results might be affected by subtle differences in sessions' execution or by translation. Analysis accuracy was also reduced as inaccurate or missing answers could not be substituted in some cases. If the country attribute is disregarded, the most notable factor for user satisfaction is completion time. That is, those requiring more time to complete tasks tend to dislike them more, confirming the generally accepted notion of users disliking grueling chores.

Usability and user experience had a significant impact on how users perceived components, as anticipated. *OPEN* was the least desirable service with a graphical user interface (GUI) and received the most criticism. This can be attributed to its GUI's lack of widespread and generally accepted design principles such as Material Design or Flat Design (2.0). It was no surprise that even self-declared low proficiency users required less effort to completed tasks when components' interfaces adhered to such design principles. So providing good user experience is crucial for the solution to be effective.

An intriguing observation regarding GUIs was that most participants (17 out of 20) had problems using toggle switches and preferred checkboxes instead. It is surprising as more and more software use these elements in general, and many applications that use toggle switches were among those that users admitted to use. A possible explanation is that such UI elements appear mainly in the settings menu of applications (but they are used extensively there) – a feature many users seem to ignore. But this tendency should not be accepted, both for legal and ethical reasons, especially when users' personal data is involved. Application developers should consider this during the design of user interfaces and should develop them to be accessible indeed.

7 Conclusion and Future Work

The participants of the co-creation session found the Turntable Solution's initial version, its concepts and purpose interesting and potentially beneficial. The existing features can be further improved, and future functionalities can be appropriately implemented thanks to the insights gained from their remarks and expectations.

A more complex testing procedure is being planned for Turntable to validate if beneficial effects on quality of life are measurable for users who engage with the solution for an extended period. A total of 150–180 participants are anticipated in order to obtain statistically significant results. If the data received confirms this hypothesis, the solution was developed properly to support older adults in achieving healthy living and successful ageing.

Acknowledgements. The authors thank all involved project partners and the participants for contributing to the co-creation sessions and the Turntable Solution.

Project no. 2019–2.1.2-NEMZ-2019–00003 has been implemented with support from the National Research, Development and Innovation Fund of Hungary, financed under the AAL-2018–5-163-CP funding scheme.

Appendix

Additional material is available at http://rebrand.ly/submisAppndx_ACT4AWE2021.

References

1. Amarya, S., Singh, K., Sabharwal, M.: Changes during aging and their association with malnutrition. J. Clin. Gerontol. Geriatr. **6**, 78–84 (2015)
2. McReynolds, J.L., Rossen, E.K.: Importance of physical activity, nutrition, and social support for optimal aging. Clin. Nurse Spec. **18**, 200–206 (2004)
3. Shinkai, S., Yoshida, H., Taniguchi, Y., Murayama, H., Nishi, M., Amano, H., et al.: Public health approach to preventing frailty in the community and its effect on healthy aging in Japan. Geriatr. Gerontol. Int. **16**, 87–97 (2016)
4. WHO. World Report on Aging and Health. World Heal Organ (2015)
5. Urtamo, A., Jyväkorpi, S.K., Strandberg, T.E.: Definitions of successful ageing: a brief review of a multidimensional concept. Acta Biomed. **90**, 359 (2019)
6. Howarth, Michelle, Brettle, Alison, Hardman, Michael, Maden, Michelle: What is the evidence for the impact of gardens and gardening on health and well-being: a scoping review and evidence-based logic model to guide healthcare strategy decision making on the use of gardening approaches as a social prescription. BMJ Open **10**(7), e036923 (2020). https://doi.org/10.1136/bmjopen-2020-036923
7. Soga, M., Gaston, K.J., Yamaura, Y.: Gardening is beneficial for health: a meta-analysis. Prev. Med. Reports. **5**, 92–99 (2017)
8. Gagliardi, Cristina, Piccinini, Flavia: The use of nature – based activities for the well-being of older people: an integrative literature review. Arch. Gerontol. Geriatrics **83**, 315–327 (2019). https://doi.org/10.1016/j.archger.2019.05.012
9. Spano, G., D'este, M., Giannico, V., Carrus, G., Elia, M., Lafortezza, R., et al.: Are community gardening and horticultural interventions beneficial for psychosocial well-being? a meta-analysis. Int. J. Environ. Res. Public Health. **17**, 3584 (2020)
10. Scott, T.L., Masser, B.M., Pachana, N.A.: Positive aging benefits of home and community gardening activities: older adults report enhanced self-esteem, productive endeavours, social engagement and exercise. SAGE Open Med. (2020)
11. Wannamethee, S.G., Shaper, A.G., Walker, M.: Physical activity and mortality in older men with diagnosed coronary heart disease. Circulation. **102**, 1358–1363 (2000)
12. Leng, C.H., Der, Wang J.: Daily home gardening improved survival for older people with mobility limitations: an 11-year follow-up study in Taiwan. Clin. Interv. Aging. **11**, 947–959 (2016)

13. European Commission. Digital Single Market: Digital Skills and Jobs [Internet]. Eur. Semester Themat. Fiche (2016). https://ec.europa.eu/esf/transnationality/filedepot_dow nload/1072/1048
14. Szakonyi, B., Vassányi, I., Mantur-Vierendeel, A., Loi, D., Correia, G., Blažica, B.: Co-creating digital services to promote active lifestyle among older adults: the turntable project. In: Proceedings of 7th International Conference on Information Communication Technology Ageing Well e-Health - ICT4AWE, pp. 213–220. SciTePress (2021)
15. Wang, D., MacMillan, T.: The benefits of gardening for older adults: a systematic review of the literature. Act Adapt Aging. **37**, 153–181 (2013)
16. Cheng, E., Hui, P., Pegg, S.: "If I'm not gardening, I'm not at my happiest": exploring the positive subjective experiences derived from serious leisure gardening by older adults. World Leis J. **58**, 285–297 (2016)
17. Sia, A., Tam, W.W.S., Fogel, A., Kua, E.H., Khoo, K., Ho, R.C.M.: Nature-based activities improve the well-being of older adults. Sci. Rep. **10**, 1–8 (2020). https://doi.org/10.1038/s41 598-020-74828-w
18. Akbar, M.F., Ramadhani, N.A., Putri, R.A.: Assistive and wearable technology for elderly. Bull. Soc. Inf. Theory Appl. **2**, 8–14 (2018)
19. Álvarez-Lombardía, I., Migueles, M., Aritzeta, A., Acedo-GIl, K.: Effectiveness of the "Kwido-Mementia" computerized cognitive stimulation programme in older adults. Int. J. Aging Res. **1**, 1004 (2018)
20. Honor Technology Inc. Honor Family app (2020). https://www.joinhonor.com/
21. Lekjaroen, K., Ponganantayotin, R., Charoenrat, A., Funilkul, S., Supasitthimethee, U., Triyason, T.: IoT Planting: watering system using mobile application for the elderly. In: 20th International Computer Science Engineering Conference Smart Ubiquitos Computer Knowledge, ICSEC 2016 (2017)
22. Maddali, H.T., Lazar, A.: Sociality and skill sharing in the garden. In: Conference on Human Factors Computer System – Proceedings, pp. 1–13 (2020)
23. Wherton, J., Sugarhood, P., Procter, R., Hinder, S., Greenhalgh, T.: Co-production in practice: how people with assisted living needs can help design and evolve technologies and services. Implement Sci. **10**, 1–10 (2015)
24. Harrington, C.N., Wilcox, L., Connelly, K., Rogers, W., Sanford, J.: Designing health and fitness apps with older adults: Examining the value of experience-based co-design. In: ACM International Conference Proceeding Series, pp. 15–24 (2018)
25. Wang, S., Bolling, K., Mao, W., Reichstadt, J., Jeste, D., Kim, H.-C., et al.: Technology to support aging in place: older adults' perspectives. Healthcare. **7**, 60 (2019)
26. Easton, K., Potter, S., Bec, R., Bennion, M., Christensen, H., Grindell, C., et al.: A virtual agent to support individuals living with physical and mental comorbidities: co-design and acceptability testing. J. Med. Internet Res. **21**, 12996 (2019)
27. Nielsen, J.: Why You Only Need to Test with 5 Users. Jakob Nielsens Alertbox (2000)

Extracting Color Name Features Utilized for Skin Disease Characterization and Comparing It to Other Representations Describing the ABCD Dermatological Criteria for Melanoma Inspection

Jinen Daghrir[1,2(✉)] 📷, Lotfi Tlig[2], Moez Bouchouicha[3], Eric Moreau[3],
Noureddine Litaiem[4], Faten Zeglaoui[4], and Mounir Sayadi[2]

[1] ISITCom, Université de Sousse, 4011 Hammam Sousse, Tunisia
jinen.daghrir@isitc.u-sousse.tn
[2] ENSIT, Laboratory SIME, Université de Tunis, Tunis, Tunisia
[3] Aix Marseille Univ, Université de Toulon, CNRS, LIS, Toulon, France
[4] Faculty of Medicine of Tunis, Department of Dermatology, Charles Nicolle Hospital,
University of Tunis El-Manar, Tunis, Tunisia
http://www.isitcom.rnu.tn/

Abstract. Recent development in image resolution has led to the excessive use of medical images in creating automated systems for inspecting and early detection of deadly diseases. Some computer vision diagnosis systems has focused on the inspection and analysis of skin cancers, such as melanoma. It is considered as one of the most fatal skin condition if it is caught at an advanced stage. Thus, it is important to regularly check every skin lesion for an early detection of melanoma. Many systems have been introduced in the last years. They mainly rely on visual features describing the color, border and texture to inspect the malignancy of skin lesions. The performance of such systems is impressive but still lacks the integration of many other different clues invented by dermatologist. Studying the color variegation can shed the light on some criteria already adopted by doctors of malignant lesions. Thus, extracting the different colors skin lesion contain is of high relevance. This paper presents a novel method for extracting and quantifying the different colors in a skin lesion in a supervised way that will ensure high specificity and sensitivity in classifying different skin conditions simultaneously. This paper aims to prove the effectiveness of our proposed method by making a comparative analysis of different state-of-the-art methods held on the ISIC 2017 and SD 198 datasets. Moreover, we employ a collected dataset to explore the performance of our proposed method. The application of our hand-crafted color features results in better classification performance of different skin illnesses.

Keywords: Melanoma diagnosis · Computer aided diagnosis · Skin lesions · Skin conditions classification · Color feature extraction · Machine learning · Hand-crafted features

L. A. Maciaszek et al. (Eds.): ICT4AWE 2021/2022, CCIS 1856, pp. 17–34, 2023.
https://doi.org/10.1007/978-3-031-37496-8_2

1 Introduction

With the advancement in the image technologies and machine learning techniques, Computer Aided Diagnosis (CAD) field has become an active area of research. Thereupon, many of its applications have already been proposed in the literature. These can help doctors improve and accelerate the inspection of dreadful diseases [6]. Skin cancer has been given a great interest during the last years with the increase in its death cases [4]. Skin cancer starts by a weird change in already existing moles or by the appearance of new lesions. Skin cancers range from frequent and benign conditions such as Basal and Squamous cell carcinoma to uncommon and fatal melanoma [22]. Melanomas, are less common, but they are the most fatal cancer since they can quickly spread to other parts of the body [14].

The global skin condition studies estimate about 60,000 skin cancer deaths in 2018 [22]. it represents 0.7% of all cancer deaths which is particularly worrying regarding a completely curable cancer. In this matter, receiving the appropriate professional diagnosis is of paramount importance as it can save people's lives [14]. Statistics show that the five-year survival rate of people who have been diagnosed with melanoma at an early stage is about 98% of the total number of cases. However, only 22% of people who had melanoma at an advanced stage have be alive after five years. In this regard, diagnosing melanoma at an early stage is very essential as it can increase the life expectancy [19].

The inspection of skin diseases is a delicate process since they come in different appearances and shapes. In addition, they are not straightforwardly recognized by only observing them. Sometimes, a skin lesion biopsy is needed where a small portion of skin is removed to be examined. In this case, an intelligent system can be helpful to accurately and quickly diagnose skin conditions. Moreover, doctors and dermatologists can be subjective and biased in making decisions about visual classifying a specific skin disease [13]. This is due to the complex nature of skin lesions [30]. As a result of this, a particular interest in creating automated intelligent systems for skin condition inspection has been the challenge of the healthcare management community, more specifically in inspecting melanomas [22]. Using supportive imaging techniques will serve dermatologists in detecting melanomas at an early stage when curing them is very easy, thereby reducing mortality [5].

CAD has been widely designed to improve and facilitate a diagnostic process. They are comprised of a variety of steps processing low-level pixels of skin lesion images. Generally, the whole pipeline process of recognizing melanomas is of a classical pattern recognition system, where the main design steps are: image processing, lesion segmentation, feature extraction, and classification of lesions in question [3] as shown in Fig. 1. After improving the quality of inspected skin lesion images carried out by using preprocessing techniques, a lesion segmentation process is required. It concerns the isolation of pathological skin lesions from the surrounding healthy skin to finally extract some visual cues characterizing them. The feature extraction techniques is done based on strategies invented by physicians. Conventionally, the ABCDE sign is the most used in inspecting melanomas [35]. This popular rule based on multivariate analysis of four criteria was invented by Stolz et al. and expanded to ABCDE in 2004. It represents an analytical method for differentiating malignant and benign lesions based on the manifestation of five characteristics [1], namely asymmetry (A), border irregularity (B),

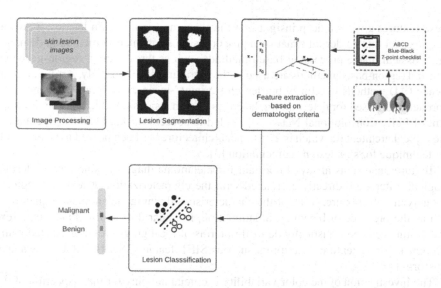

Fig. 1. The layout architecture of computer-aided diagnosis based on dermatological criteria.

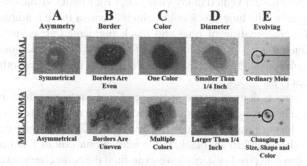

Fig. 2. ABCDEs of detecting melanoma: aspects and differences between benign and malignant skin lesions [14].

color variability (C), diameter greater than 6 mm or it can be refereed to the presence of some differential structures(D), and evolution (E) or change in the color or size (see Fig. 2). These proposed cues which are used for skin lesions characterization are examined in a way to extract relevant and discriminate primitives. These features must ensure non-redundancy, relevance, discrimination and robustness to noise [14]. Over the years many automated methods have adopted the ABCD rule in the detection and diagnosing melanomas. Other features can be employed such as the seven-point checklist [9] which contains three major aspects (change in size, shape and color), and four minor aspects (diameter, inflammation, crusting or bleeding and sensory change). All the aforementioned criteria investigate mainly the change in texture, color and border.

These features should be of high sensitivity for diagnosing melanomas. Thus, it is more important to increase the true positives and decrease the false negatives. The most used features for border characterization are asymmetry, the greatest diameter, area of skin lesions, border irregularity, circularity index, smoothness of lesion edges, etc [25].

These features give us a deep insight into the shape and area of skin lesions. To accurately extract this border information a proper lesion segmentation method is demanding. Classical image processing-based methods such as thresholding, region growing, edge and region-based methods are used in the literature [16,31]. Lately, Artificial Intelligence (AI) methods like fuzzy border, clustering C-means, and Deep Learning (DL) approaches are used for determining the edges of skin lesions [29,32,37]. The development of Fully Convolutional Networks has led to success in skin lesion segmentation. One typical architecture which is The U-net architecture has been proved to be an excellent technique for skin lesion segmentation [3].

Texture analysis is always important for melanoma diagnosis since many dermatological criteria are directly correlated with the characterization of textured regions. By analyzing the texture, some of the characteristics defining melanoma are quantified such as the presence of bleeding, inflammation, irregular dots and globules, etc. Textural features can be statistically defined in terms of local gray-level or extracted using different kinds of texture descriptors such as SIFT features, SURF, HOG or wavelet transform [13].

The investigation of the color variability is crucial not only for the inspection of the color in the ABCD criteria but also for another essential cue which is the Blue-Black rule. Dermatologists have invented many visual cues for a better visual diagnosis of skin lesions over the years. The blue-black color which is one of these features is defined by the presence of a combination of blue and black pigmented areas involving at least 10% of the lesion surface [7]. The presence of these two colors demonstrates 78.2% sensitivity for melanomas. Nonetheless, it can also help in detecting other pigmented skin malignancies [7].

Color irregularity is defined as the presence of non-uniform colors in skin lesions. Since most benign lesions mainly contain one color, often a single shade of brown, having a variety of colors is a warning signal as given by Fig. 2. Thus, malignant lesions can contain different shades of brown, black, red, white, or blue colors. Conventionally, dermatologists and computerized systems have examined the color characteristics by defining the different color shades in skin lesions. They have been using a restricted number of colors including light brown, dark brown, black, red, white, and slate blue [25]. However, this limited number of colors still faces challenges in inspecting many kinds of skin conditions. Skin lesion images can be affected by reflections, light rays, and camera resolutions, or the lesions themselves can be amelanotic in some cases. Thus, for an automated system, it is not straightforward to quantify the presence of only six colors. Even dermatologists, who are experts in inspecting skin diseases, will not be able to estimate them by the naked eye [38].

Besides, the human perception of color is very ineffectual, and men and women can differently describe a color [19]. However, women's color perception seems to be better, they are able to distinguish even the tiniest differences between two colors, contrary to men despite having normal color vision [19]. In this regard, in a study conducted in the department of Physiology, SGRRIM&HS, Dehradun, 60 young and healthy men and women 17–22 yrs of age with normal visual acuity were requested to match some test colors with a shade chart. This study concluded that females are adept to see more range of colors as compared to males [21]. Along these lines, we interviewed dermatologists on whether to use only the six basic colors to characterize skin lesions or 12 colors extracted automatically by computer from a range of skin lesions (see Fig. 3). We found that female dermatologists are statistically better than male dermatologists in observing the different colors found in skin lesions. However, it is worth mentioning that many male dermatologists showed a lot of interest in using the automatically extracted colors in inspecting melanomas.

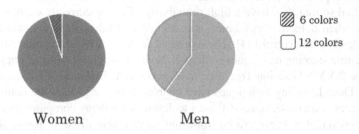

Fig. 3. Gender variation for color presence in skin lesions.

Since it is difficult to determine the various color shades, that differentiate malignant and benign lesions, our key contribution was to develop a machine learning-based method to extract the most pertinent colors characterizing melanoma. Subsequently, the classification of skin lesions will be done using these colors. Thus, our goal was to create a low-dimensional representation that is capable of accurately identifying the different colors that might be present in a skin lesion. Particularly the black and blue colors, which are reliable indicators of melanoma. This method has been already introduced and published by the international conference on information and communication technologies for aging well and e-health 2022 (ICT4AWE).

This method showed a great performance in characterizing the colors of skin lesions regarding other descriptors with high dimensionality. It was mainly designed for inspecting the colors of melanoma skin lesions. However, it showed a limitation when using a dataset containing hundreds of real-world skin disease images. In fact, we were concerned to classify only five skin conditions that may have common characteristics with melanomas. This can prove the effectiveness of our method which is not only restricted to dermoscopic images but also ordinary photographic images to diagnose melanomas. Moreover, we have used it to characterize the colors of a novel collected dataset for further skin disease classification. Additionally, extensive experimental results on the ISIC2017 dataset were conducted to show that using other handcrafted features describing the color, border, and texture can outperform a Convolutional Neural Network (CNN) model.

In the following sections, a comprehensive analysis of the most common color variability features for melanoma inspection is reported. After that, we introduce our proposed method of extracting the color names using machine learning and use them to validate the usefulness of our method by carrying out a classification process. Then, we conducted an extensive experimental analysis showing the power of hand-crafted features in classifying melanomas comparing to deep neural features. We end up with a conclusions and further work in the last section.

2 Background of Melanoma Characterization

The recent development of machine learning techniques in computer-aided diagnosis has led to great research attention over the years. Recognition and detection of melanomas have been widely carried out by a set of pattern recognition processes [23]. After accurately identifying the skin lesion over the surrounding skin in an image with a segmentation process, some visual cues are extracted [8]. These cues are described and quantified so that they have a high probability of being correctly classified. More essentially, when detecting melanoma, the decrease in false negatives (misclassified malignant lesions) is critical [14]. The extracted features are fed to some of state-of-the-art machine learning techniques such as K-Nearest Neighbor (KNN), Support Vector Machine (SVM), Decision Tree, etc., to inspect the malignancy of a lesion.

Lately, Deep Learning techniques have enabled robust and accurate feature learning, which makes them the state-of-the-art techniques for many computer vision applications. However, it is proved to be irrelevant for the skin disease classification and hand-crafted features have more advantages over them [36]. Besides, their performance is highly influenced by the large datasets used for training. Also, training them is very expensive in terms of time and memory.

Examining the shape, color and texture has been the consideration of many researchers for decades. For border characterization, many features have been used by research such as the greatest diameter, the area, the border irregularity ratio, the circularity index, asymmetry, and the smoothness of edges [25].

The clinical parameter of the differential structure was evaluated by texture analysis, which is represented based on different color channels. Textural features can be statistically defined in terms of local gray-level statistics or extracted using different kinds of texture descriptors, such as SIFT features, SURF, HOG, and wavelet [13].

Color features are also extracted to represent the uniformness of skin lesion colors. If the variance is low, then the colors are more likely to belong to a benign lesion. Color variability is an important factor for melanoma inspection. This is due to the fact that, in addition to the inspection of the C criterion of the well-known ABCD, the blue-black rule has also shown to be a good practice in the diagnosis process [7]. Color features inside skin lesions are examined and colors are determined and quantified. The spherical coordinate LAB average and variance responses for pixels, Red, Green, Blue (RGB), Hue, Saturation, and Value (HSV) representation channels, are used to study the color features. The minimum, maximum, average, and standard deviations from these channels are extracted to quantify the color consistency [25].

Color texture can also be used to determine the nature of a skin lesion, by measuring the lacunarity in the distribution of colors [26] or by using the color SIFT [2]. An interesting and simple method was proposed in [39], which examines the color variegation in a lesion by calculating the variance of the local average color. A physics-based model of healthy tissue coloration is proposed by Claridge et al. [10]. It quantifies the uniformness of the tumor color by determining the conformity of the constructed model with a lesion and the abnormal skin colors. Furthermore, in [28] a group of features connected with the color parameter is extracted which describes: the maximum change in the colors, size of the area with dominating color red, blue, or green, maximum change of brightness. Skin lesions may include six basic colors light, dark brown, black, red, white, and slate blue. Many researchers have proposed several methods to quantify the presence of these colors in a skin lesion. For instance, in [38], Yang *et al.* introduce the color by two representations: first to define the different color names and then to indicate for each pixel the probability of belonging to a color name.

3 Proposed Method

The recent development of machine learning techniques in the last decades has led to a great improvement in computer-aided diagnosis and early inspection of deadly skin cancer, more specifically melanoma. In fact, melanoma has a high mortality rate, but it can be cured if it is caught at an early stage. Many traditional systems inspecting melanoma have been proposed in the literature. Most of them use the basic approaches of pattern recognition systems, which are carried through a set of low pixel processing methods [3] image pre-processing, lesion segmentation, feature extraction, and detection of the lesion malignancy. These methods have proved their efficiency in melanoma inspection [24, 27].

Regarding the evolution of CNN, CAD has become more and more oriented toward the implementation of semantic techniques such as the Deep Learning (DL) [17, 34]. DL approaches transform the skin lesion images into low-level representations by learning the nature of skin lesions. This representation has shown limitations in some cases [36] since their performance highly depends on the training set. These kinds of models require a huge number of skin lesion images to correctly be trained, which is not straightforward for the medical imaging field. Also, it is proved that when diagnosing skin disease, other proper resources such as expert dermatologists are more accurate than fully automated systems [38].

For that, the traditionally based classification is the state-of-the-art method for the process of melanoma detection. After an accurate lesion segmentation, a feature extraction technique is applied to extract quantified characteristics for identifying the specific type of skin disease.

The popular ABCD approach has been used by dermatologists, where three main characteristics are described: the color, the border, and the texture [15]. Dermatologists also tend to use other criteria for diagnosing melanomas such as the blue-black rule [7], the seven-point checklist, and the ugly duckling [18]. The parameter color is considered to be a crucial criterion in inspecting melanomas to study the color variability and the presence of blue and black pigmented areas in skin lesions. One way to examine the color of skin lesions, some researchers defines the Color Name (CN) features which are linguistic color labels. As discussed above, the color is with a high sensitivity in the whole melanoma detection. In this regard, we introduced a new color feature extraction method that includes two phases. First, we determine the different color names from a set of skin lesion images. As a second step, we extract the most pertinent and discriminative color names that ensure an accurate melanoma detection based on a feature selection algorithm. The overall implementation of the extraction process is given in (see Fig. 4). To demonstrate the effectiveness of our proposed method, we test the selected features on a set of skin lesion images (see Fig. 5).

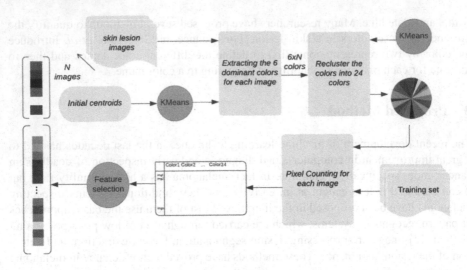

Fig. 4. Layout architecture of method of extracting color-names [14].

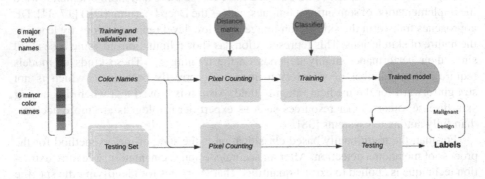

Fig. 5. Layout architecture of evaluating extracted color names [14]. (Color figure online)

3.1 Supervised Color Name Extraction

The healthy skin color and the skin disease type as well as its stage are factors that determine the colors contained in the skin lesion. Thus, it is important to choose which colors are more likely to be present in a skin lesion.

Melanomas usually include six colors with different degrees. For an effective color name representation, we extract the dominant six colors from a set of images using the K-means algorithm. Centroids for the algorithm initially depend on the six considered colors: light brown, dark brown, black, red, white, and slate blue. K-means iteratively minimizes the intra-class and maximizes the inter-class distances to create a final partition of image pixels into six groups. Each input pixel is characterized by three intensities in the RGB color space. When convergence is reached, six centroids will be assigned for each color. For more details about K-means clustering, the reader is referred to [27]. Gathering all the extracted colors will serve then to do clustering one more time to finally extract the 24 major colors, which are displayed in the pie chart shown in Fig. 6. We assume that for each color four instances are adopted.

After identifying the major 24 colors associated with skin lesions, the next step is to only preserve the colors that guarantee an effective representation of lesion color names. This is done using feature selection, which is the trend in a lot of machine learning systems. We use the infinite Feature Selection (inf-FS) [33] which is a feature selection method that performs a ranking step in an unsupervised way, followed by a cross-validation strategy to select only the most representative features. Ranking individually the relevancy of features is done utilizing class labels: malignant or benign. On the other hand, using a distance matrix, we define how the 24 various color values frequently occur in the lesion (see Fig. 5). Note that in the processed image, every pixel value is assigned to the nearest color name regarding the distance of its intensity. Finally, by counting the pixels of each color name and applying the inf-FS procedure, the suggested process generates a ranked features that refer to their characterization relevance. The six major colors found after applying the feature selection further confirm the efficiency of the black-blue clue proposed by physicians in inspecting the malignancy of skin lesions. The slight blue and black colors are highly ranked (see Fig. 5).

3.2 Classifying Skin Lesion Using Color Name Features

Once we extract the most relevant color names, We are interested to investigate the performance of these color names in recognizing clinical skin disease images. We employ a skin lesion classification based on the best-ranked color names using machine learning algorithms and training images. It seems reasonable that using them will be more accurate in the classification process. Though, when computing the distance matrix corresponding to pairwise distances between the color names and pixels' intensities will create an unfair distribution. In view of the fact that some pixels will have different yet distant colors regarding the best color names. These pixels will be assigned with the nearest color name, so it is crucial to disturb the pixels partitioning by using the six worst color names [14]. For the classification task, we used the K-Nearest Neighbor (KNN) algorithm [12]. This method demonstrates a high classification accuracy, especially when using a low-dimensional representation and imbalanced dataset.

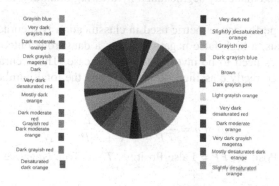

Fig. 6. The most dominant 24 colors extracted from a set of images [14]. (Color figure online)

4 Experiments and Results

In order to validate our proposed method, we conducted a lot of experiments. We employed the extracted color names as well as state-of-the-art handcrafted features describing the color and border to recognize skin diseases from different datasets. First, we used the ISIC2017(International Skin Imaging Collaboration) dataset [11] to extract the different color names. This dataset involves three unique diagnoses of skin lesions: melanoma, nevus, and seborrheic keratosis. We were interested in inspecting the malignancy of the skin lesions. Thus, the dataset is split into three sets: the training set which is used for extracting the color names using our proposed method and for training the KNN, as well as the validation and testing set which are used to evaluate the performance of our method.

We have also used the SD-198 [36], which contains 198 different skin diseases represented by 6,584 images. We have used the fifty-split strategy provided by the authors, which contains 3,292 training and 3,292 testing images. The advantage of using this dataset is that it contains different images under many illumination and point of view conditions. This is a real-world problem since the dataset contains ordinary photographic skin lesion images. In [38], extensive experiments on the SD-198 dataset were introduced to demonstrate the effectiveness of their proposed diagnosis system. They compared their representation with several standard low-level features from the three visual components: texture, color, and border. They also compared it with a deep representation derived from CNN models. For that, we compared our extracted color names with the other color features used in the literature.

In this paper, we have tested our proposed method on a new clinical skin disease dataset, which contains both clinical and dermoscopic images. Collecting medical images is not always a straightforward process due to the privacy-preserving of medical images. Besides, annotating these images require dermatologists' expertise. Our collected dataset contains four different diseases: three benign and one malignant skin disease (seborrhoeic keratosis, basal cell carcinoma, nevus, and melanoma). There are 515 skin lesion images in total.

To carry on the color name extraction process on these datasets: skin lesions are segmented using the segmentation mask provided in the ISIC2017 challenge for the ISIC2017 dataset and manually segmented by drawing bounding boxes for the other datasets.

Generally, the performance metric used in classification is accuracy. Therefore, in melanoma diagnosis, a high false negative rate is a dangerous outcome. Thus, other performance metrics need to be investigated in this case. The accuracy is quantified by the fraction of correctly classified skin lesions and the total number of skin lesion images.

$$Accuracy = \frac{TP + TN}{TP + TN + FP + FN} \tag{1}$$

where TP = True Positive, FP = False Positive, TN = True Negative and FN = False Negative.

When evaluating a binary classification, accuracy does not really indicate the relevancy of the system with imbalanced classes. Often, when inspecting rare diseases such as melanoma which appears more often than the other skin disease. Thus, balanced accuracy generally is used to overcome class imbalance, which is based on two more commonly used metrics: sensitivity known also as recall (True positive rate), and specificity(True negative rate). The sensitivity metric measures the proportion of actual positives that are correctly identified. Nevertheless, the specificity measures the negative cases correctly classified.

$$Sensitivity = \frac{TP}{TP+FN} \tag{2}$$

$$Specificity = \frac{TN}{TN+FP} \tag{3}$$

Balanced accuracy is simply the arithmetic mean of the two.This metric will properly introduce the performance of melanoma diagnosis.

$$Balanced\ accuracy = \frac{sensitivity + specificity}{2} \tag{4}$$

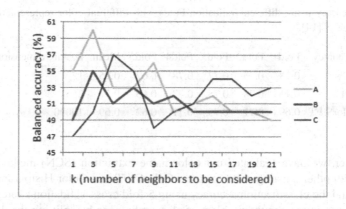

Fig. 7. Balanced accuracy using different scenarios with various values of K on validation set [14].

Table 1. Diagnosis performance of different scenarios applied on testing set [14].

	Scenario A	Scenario B	Scenario C
Accuracy(%)	**77.7**	77	62.7
Sensitivity(%)	17.4	11.6	**26.7**
Specificity(%)	87.7	**88.1**	68.8
Balanced accuracy(%)	**52.6**	49.8	47.7

To evaluate the performance of our method on the ISIC2017 dataset, we conducted experiments for two aspects. comparing the influence of the different combinations of the 24 extracted color names and evaluating the classification performance of some of the state-of-the-art color features.

Thus as a first step, we identified the most promising 24 color names that better suit the melanoma diagnosis process. Then, using the testing set, we proposed three scenarios to show how well the extracted color names function. Our proposed representation is referred as Scenario A, which combines the six best and six worst color names. The use of only the best color names is referred to as Scenario B. On the other hand, for scenario C, we employ all the 24 extracted color names. We gradually changed the hyperparameter K of the KNN algorithm to find the proper K using the different scenarios. In binary classification, K should be an even value. Figure 7 shows the performance evaluation using the balanced accuracy with many K values. Skin lesion classification is better when using a small number of K with a small number of color names. This is obvious since the KNN algorithm operates better with an unbalanced dataset characterized by a small number of features. We have also tested the performance of our proposed method using the three scenarios with K=3, the results are summarized in Table 1. The experiments show that when using the proposed color name combination(scenario A) the balanced accuracy is higher than in the other scenarios. However, when using all the 24 color names, the sensitivity gets its highest value.

Table 2. Accuracy using different validation Folds with different color representations on the ISIC2017 dataset [14].

Accuracy	Fold1	Fold2	Fold3	Fold4	Fold5	Mean	Feature dimension
SCN	0.78	0.76	0.77	0.78	0.67	0.75	12
CH	0.71	0.78	0.75	0.77	0.63	0.72	255
colorSIFT	0.69	0.71	0.75	0.71	0.62	0.69	10000

Moreover, we have evaluated our color name extraction (SCN) method by comparing it with other existing color features. ColorSIFT and Color Histogram (CH) are extracted, and the classification accuracy using 5-fold cross-validation strategy is measured. This can overcome the problem of class imbalance by splitting the dataset into different folds having different combinations of data points. Thus, 5 KNNs are evaluated with K = 3 and the performance of our proposed color names is calculated as the mean of all the accuracies (see Table 2). Obviously, our extracted color names represented by 12-dimensional features succeeded in classifying the skin diseases with a 75% accuracy unlike the others that are represented with high-dimensional features.

Our proposed method introduced precise results and potentially succeeded in diagnosing melanoma among other skin diseases. Although, diagnosing dreadful diseases should be totally accurate. For that we have also used other features describing the color and the border, so we can rigorously inspect the ABCD parameters. We suggested using the most popular border features which are: circularity index, normalized area of the lesion, its greatest diameter, asymmetry, convexity, smoothness of the border, and border irregularity which is quantified using three methods. A naive assumption of what an irregularity is, is to study how an object is circle-like. So, we calculated the intersection-over-union of a convex image and lesion image to compare the similarity between the convex hull image enclosing the skin lesion and the skin lesion mask itself.

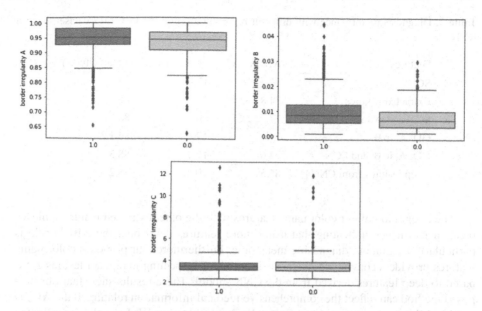

Fig. 8. Border irregularity variation in benign(0) and malignant(1) lesions.

Border irregularities B, and C are introduced as the division of the lesion perimeter over the lesion area, and the perimeter over the lesion's greatest diameter respectively [20]. We have also examined the color variability by measuring the means and the standard deviations of the color intensities in the RGB and HSV color channels. The box plots in Fig. 8 are univariate analyses of the influence of features on the malignancy of skin lesions, we can notice that many outliers badly affect the classification process. Also, when comparing the distribution of the three features for malignant and benign diagnosis, we deduce that the border irregularity B is the best in diagnosing melanoma, since the box-plots are less overlapped comparing to the others.

This is proved when we have used a feature selection procedure [33] to visualize the best features. We then verify the performance of different combinations of features for comprehensive combinations. The best ranked features with high degrees of importance are the greatest diameter(GD), the normalized area of lesion(A), and the border irregularity B(irrB). In this context, we report the diagnosis performance of different representations and their combinations in Table 3. The intuition behind having a low true positive rate is that datasets with imbalanced classes are more challenging to models. This is why we choose to work with the KNN algorithm. Convolutional Neural Networks (CNNs) have been widely used in the literature to automatically characterize skin lesions, for their notable performance [14]. We used a CNN followed by a fully-connected layer with a softmax activation function to classify malignant and benign lesions of the ISIC2017 dataset [15].

Table 3. Diagnosis performance with different representation on the ISIC2017 dataset using a KNN.

Features	Accuracy(%)	Sensitivity(%)	Specificity(%)
SCN	77.7	17.4	87.7
Extracted features	74.8	17	88.8
SCN and extracted features	77	20	88
GD, A, irrB	74.1	17.6	86.1
GD, A, irrB, and SCN	74.6	17.1	88.3
Deep features from CNN [15]	85.5	10.4	98.2

The integration of our color name features with the other extracted feature achieves better performance indicating that using more features describing the ABCD rule is particularly accurate in diagnosing melanoma. Furthermore, our proposed color name features provide a convincing diagnosis in terms of inspecting malignant lesions compared to deep features derived from the CNN model. These results show that our proposed method can reflect the comprehensive medical information relating to the ABCD and black-blue rules invented and proved by dermatologists. We have also investigated the performance of our suggested color name extraction method on the SD-198 [38] aiming to classify several skin diseases. as well. Thus, 198 skin disorders were used to test the entire procedure. The already extracted 12 color names are quantified and the skin diseases were classified using a KNN and a Support Vector Machine. We report the accuracy of using the proposed color name features, as well as the color-based features used in [38] (see Table 4). Clearly, our method is irrelevant since it only achieves 5.58% accuracy. The diversity and specificity of various skin diseases limit the process of correctly identifying them.

Table 4. Accuracy using different representations and classifiers on the SD-198 dataset [14].

Features	Dimension	K-Nearest Neighbor	Support Vector Machine
CH	256	12.33	4.19
CN	21000	20.03	20.23
colorSIFT	21000	21.29	22.51
CN-L	21000	42.50	38.91
CCV-L	21000	42.80	40.13
SCN	12	5.58	4.73
SCN	24	5.99	5.51

The authors also evaluated the classification performance of the deep features derived from tuned CNNs in [38]. In fact, a CNN classifies the 198 skin disorders with an accuracy of 53.35%.

It is observed that there is a slight increase(5.99% accuracy) in the performance of the skin disease classification when using more than 12 color names (all the 24 extracted color names). This can somehow prove the efficiency of our proposed method in precisely identifying melanoma since it manifests the presence of a very limited number of colors (generally 6 colors) [14].

Thus, the huge number of skin diseases in a dataset, limits the performance of our method, as it is shown in Table 4. In general, the overall classification can be improved when fewer skin diseases are used, which is verified in Table 5. We have also visualized the diagnosis results of our proposed representation using a subset of the SD-198 dataset (see Table 5). It contains only 5 common skin diseases that may appear similar to melanoma. As shown in Table 5, using our proposed representation, the diagnosis performance is improved when using a limited number of skin diseases.

Table 5. Accuracy using the different scenarios and classifiers on a subset of SD-198 dataset.

Features	K-Nearest Neighbor	Support Vector Machine
Scenario A	0.38	0.36
Scenario B	0.3	0.313
Scenario C	0.2	0.233

Also, the extracted color names are used to diagnose the malignancy of three types of skin diseases: melanoma, nevus, and seborrheic keratosis. The classification performance is reported in Table 6. as usual, the proposed representation achieves the best accuracies. We introduced the performance of the extracted color names in recognizing the four skin conditions of the collected data (see Table 7). The skin lesion images in the SD-198 and collected images are ordinary photographic images taken under different conditions. Considering these challenges, our proposed representation shows promising results in both clinical and dermoscopic images.

Table 6. Results of classifying lesions into malignant and benign lesions from the SD-198 dataset using a KNN (K = 3).

Representation	Accuracy	Sensitivity	Specificity
Scenario A	0.72	0.13	0.91
Scenario B	0.67	0.23	0.82
Scenario C	0.67	0.16	0.84

Table 7. Accuracy using the different scenarios and classifiers on the collected data.

Representation	K-Nearest Neighbor	Support Vector Machine
Scenario A	0.48	0.55
Scenario B	0.42	0.47
Scenario C	0.49	0.52

5 Conclusion

This paper presents a novel supervised method of color name extraction using feature selection to rank the extracted color names. A classifier with three different partitions was used to prove the extraction of color names. These color names are mainly extracted to classify skin lesions for more accurate inspection of melanomas, which are considered as the most fatal skin cancer. It is worth mentioning that we proved the already known fact, which is that females perception of colors is superior to that of males. The proposed method has shown a notable performance for diagnosing melanomas on different benchmark datasets. A comparison of different handcrafted features is presented as well, which proves the efficiency of our color name features against the state-of-the-art color representations. Accordingly, using only our proposed color-based features shows a promising result compared to automatically extracted features using deep learning. Also, we reported the melanoma diagnosis performance using further hand-crafted features. However, our proposed representation method shows limitations when using a benchmark dataset that contains several skin conditions and imbalanced datasets. Thus, data augmentation can be used to overcome the drawbacks of our proposed methods in recognizing minor classes. The use of fuzzy color based on parametric membership might be proposed further to semantically describe the colors as a dermatologist do.

Acknowledgement. We would like to acknowledge all the dermatologists who accepted to answer our questionnaire. Also, we would like to deeply thank all members of the dermatology department of Charles Nicolle Hospital, Tunis, for their help and support during the collect of data.

References

1. Abbasi, N.R., et al.: Early diagnosis of cutaneous melanoma: revisiting the ABCD criteria. JAMA **292**(22), 2771–2776 (2004)
2. Abdel-Hakim, A.E., Farag, A.A.: CSIFT: A SIFT descriptor with color invariant characteristics. In: 2006 IEEE Computer Society Conference on Computer Vision and Pattern Recognition (CVPR 2006), vol. 2, pp. 1978–1983. IEEE (2006)
3. Adegun, A., Viriri, S.: Deep learning techniques for skin lesion analysis and melanoma cancer detection: a survey of state-of-the-art. Artif. Intell. Rev. **54**(2), 811–841 (2021)
4. Adeyinka, A.A., Viriri, S.: Skin lesion images segmentation: a survey of the state-of-the-art. In: Groza, A., Prasath, R. (eds.) MIKE 2018. LNCS (LNAI), vol. 11308, pp. 321–330. Springer, Cham (2018). https://doi.org/10.1007/978-3-030-05918-7_29
5. Al-Masni, M.A., Al-Antari, M.A., Choi, M.T., Han, S.M., Kim, T.S.: Skin lesion segmentation in dermoscopy images via deep full resolution convolutional networks. Comput. Meth. Programs Biomed. **162**, 221–231 (2018)
6. Almaraz-Damian, J.A., Ponomaryov, V., Sadovnychiy, S., Castillejos-Fernandez, H.: Melanoma and nevus skin lesion classification using handcraft and deep learning feature fusion via mutual information measures. Entropy **22**(4), 484 (2020)
7. Argenziano, G., et al.: Blue-black rule: a simple dermoscopic clue to recognize pigmented nodular melanoma. Br. J. Dermatol. **165**(6), 1251–1255 (2011)
8. Barata, C., Celebi, M.E., Marques, J.S.: A survey of feature extraction in dermoscopy image analysis of skin cancer. IEEE J. Biomed. Health Inform. **23**(3), 1096–1109 (2018)

9. Betta, G., Di Leo, G., Fabbrocini, G., Paolillo, A., Scalvenzi, M.: Automated application of the "7-point checklist" diagnosis method for skin lesions: estimation of chromatic and shape parameters. In: 2005 IEEE Instrumentation and Measurement Technology Conference Proceedings, vol. 3, pp. 1818–1822. IEEE (2005)
10. Claridge, E., Cotton, S., Hall, P., Moncrieff, M.: From colour to tissue histology: physics-based interpretation of images of pigmented skin lesions. Med. Image Anal. **7**(4), 489–502 (2003)
11. Codella, N.C., et al.: Skin lesion analysis toward melanoma detection: a challenge at the 2017 international symposium on biomedical imaging (ISBI), hosted by the international skin imaging collaboration (ISIC). In: 2018 IEEE 15th International Symposium on Biomedical Imaging (ISBI 2018), pp. 168–172. IEEE (2018)
12. Coomans, D., Massart, D.L.: Alternative k-nearest neighbour rules in supervised pattern recognition: Part 1. k-nearest neighbour classification by using alternative voting rules. Anal. Chim. Acta **136**, 15–27 (1982)
13. Daghrir, J., Tlig, L., Bouchouicha, M., Litaiem, N., Zeglaoui, F., Sayadi, M.: Selection of statistic textural features for skin disease characterization toward melanoma detection. In: 2022 8th International Conference on Control, Decision and Information Technologies (CoDIT), vol. 1, pp. 261–267. IEEE (2022)
14. Daghrir, J., Tlig, L., Bouchouicha, M., Litaiem, N., Zeglaoui, F., Sayadi, M.: A supervised quantification of the color names characterizing the visual component color in the ABCD dermatological criteria for a further melanoma inspection. In: ICT4AWE, pp. 147–154 (2022)
15. Daghrir, J., Tlig, L., Bouchouicha, M., Sayadi, M.: Melanoma skin cancer detection using deep learning and classical machine learning techniques: a hybrid approach. In: 2020 5th International Conference on Advanced Technologies for Signal and Image Processing (ATSIP), pp. 1–5. IEEE (2020)
16. Emre Celebi, M., Wen, Q., Hwang, S., Iyatomi, H., Schaefer, G.: Lesion border detection in dermoscopy images using ensembles of thresholding methods. Skin Res. Technol. **19**(1), e252–e258 (2013)
17. Gonzalez-Diaz, I.: DermakNet: incorporating the knowledge of dermatologists to convolutional neural networks for skin lesion diagnosis. IEEE J. Biomed. Health Inform. **23**(2), 547–559 (2018)
18. Grob, J., Bonerandi, J.: The 'ugly duckling' sign: identification of the common characteristics of nevi in an individual as a basis for melanoma screening. Arch. Dermatol. **134**(1), 103–104 (1998)
19. Heinzerling, L., Eigentler, T.K.: Skin cancer in childhood and adolescents: treatment and implications for the long-term follow-up. In: Beck, J.D., Bokemeyer, C., Langer, T. (eds.) Late Treatment Effects and Cancer Survivor Care in the Young, pp. 349–355. Springer, Cham (2021). https://doi.org/10.1007/978-3-030-49140-6_34
20. Jain, S., Pise, N., et al.: Computer aided melanoma skin cancer detection using image processing. Procedia Comput. Sci. **48**, 735–740 (2015)
21. Jaint, N., Verma, P., Mittal, S., Mittal, S., Singh, A.K., Munjal, S.: Gender based alteration in color perception. Indian J. Physiol. Pharmacol. **54**(4), 366–70 (2010)
22. Khazaei, Z., Ghorat, F., Jarrahi, A., Adineh, H., Sohrabivafa, M., Goodarzi, E.: Global incidence and mortality of skin cancer by histological subtype and its relationship with the human development index (HDI); an ecology study in 2018. World Cancer Res. J. **6**(2), e13 (2019)
23. Koundal, D., Sharma, B.: Advanced neutrosophic set-based ultrasound image analysis. In: Neutrosophic Set in Medical Image Analysis, pp. 51–73. Elsevier (2019)

24. Magalhaes, C., Tavares, J.M.R., Mendes, J., Vardasca, R.: Comparison of machine learning strategies for infrared thermography of skin cancer. Biomed. Signal Process. Control **69**, 102872 (2021)
25. Maglogiannis, I., Doukas, C.N.: Overview of advanced computer vision systems for skin lesions characterization. IEEE Trans. Inf. Technol. Biomed. **13**(5), 721–733 (2009)
26. Manousaki, A.G., Manios, A.G., Tsompanaki, E.I., Tosca, A.D.: Use of color texture in determining the nature of melanocytic skin lesions-a qualitative and quantitative approach. Comput. Biol. Med. **36**(4), 419–427 (2006)
27. Melbin, K., Raj, Y.J.V.: Integration of modified ABCD features and support vector machine for skin lesion types classification. Multimed. Tools Appl. **80**(6), 8909–8929 (2021)
28. Mikolajczyk, A., Grochowski, M., Kwasigroch, A.: Optimal selection of input features and an acompanying neural network structure for the classification purposes-skin lesions case study. In: 2018 23rd International Conference on Methods & Models in Automation & Robotics (MMAR), pp. 899–904. IEEE (2018)
29. Mohamed, A.A.I., Ali, M.M., Nusrat, K., Rahebi, J., Sayiner, A., Kandemirli, F.: Melanoma skin cancer segmentation with image region growing based on fuzzy clustering mean. Int. J. Eng. Innov. Res. **6**(2), 91C95 (2017)
30. Naji, S., Jalab, H.A., Kareem, S.A.: A survey on skin detection in colored images. Artif. Intell. Rev. **52**(2), 1041–1087 (2019)
31. Peruch, F., Bogo, F., Bonazza, M., Cappelleri, V.M., Peserico, E.: Simpler, faster, more accurate melanocytic lesion segmentation through meds. IEEE Trans. Biomed. Eng. **61**(2), 557–565 (2013)
32. Pollastri, F., Bolelli, F., Paredes, R., Grana, C.: Augmenting data with GANs to segment melanoma skin lesions. Multimed. Tools Appli. **79**(21), 15575–15592 (2020)
33. Roffo, G., Melzi, S., Cristani, M.: Infinite feature selection. In: Proceedings of the IEEE International Conference on Computer Vision, pp. 4202–4210 (2015)
34. Saeed, J., Zeebaree, S.: Skin lesion classification based on deep convolutional neural networks architectures. J. Appl. Sci. Technol. Trends **2**(01), 41–51 (2021)
35. Stolz, W., et al.: Multivariate analysis of criteria given by dermatoscopy for the recognition of melanocytic lesions. In: Book of Abstracts, Fiftieth Meeting of the American Academy of Dermatology, Dallas, Tex: Dec, pp. 7–12 (1991)
36. Sun, X., Yang, J., Sun, M., Wang, K.: A benchmark for automatic visual classification of clinical skin disease images. In: Leibe, B., Matas, J., Sebe, N., Welling, M. (eds.) ECCV 2016. LNCS, vol. 9910, pp. 206–222. Springer, Cham (2016). https://doi.org/10.1007/978-3-319-46466-4_13
37. Vesal, S., Ravikumar, N., Maier, A.: SkinNet: a deep learning framework for skin lesion segmentation. In: 2018 IEEE Nuclear Science Symposium and Medical Imaging Conference Proceedings (NSS/MIC), pp. 1–3. IEEE (2018)
38. Yang, J., Sun, X., Liang, J., Rosin, P.L.: Clinical skin lesion diagnosis using representations inspired by dermatologist criteria. In: Proceedings of the IEEE Conference on Computer Vision and Pattern Recognition, pp. 1258–1266 (2018)
39. Zhang, Z., Moss, R.H., Stoecker, W.V.: Neural networks skin tumor diagnostic system. In: International Conference on Neural Networks and Signal Processing, 2003. Proceedings of the 2003, vol. 1, pp. 191–192. IEEE (2003)

Evaluating the Depression Level Based on Facial Image Analyzing and Patient Voice

Alexander Ramos-Cuadros, Luis Palomino Santillan, and Willy Ugarte[✉]

Universidad Peruana de Ciencias Aplicadas, Lima, Peru
{u201520019,u201512610}@upc.edu.pe, willy.ugarte@upc.edu.pe

Abstract. Depression is regarded as a widespread mental condition that affects people of all ages. It has a negative impact on a variety of aspects of life, including mood, vigor, and interests in enjoying activities. In the most severe cases, depression can also result in suicide. creating the chance for collaboration between mental health professionals and the use of technical tools to enhance the assessment of the severity of depression to offer the patient with an ideal clinical diagnosis and an appropriate referral to begin treatment. The COVID-19 epidemic in Peru has decreased face-to-face interaction and quick access to medical professionals, making it more difficult for patients' mental health to be identified or treated effectively, which results in the disease becoming chronic, psychological suffering, and high costs associated with specialized care. The implementation of a technology model that assesses degrees of recurrent depression by examining facial photos and voice to identify the chronicity of depressive symptoms in young Peruvians is thus one of the research's problems. Our findings demonstrate that, based on the functions of the mobile application, adolescent patients were predisposed to complete a self-administered depression questionnaire in a simulated setting with an optimal feeling of satisfaction and usefulness.

Keywords: Depression · Facial detection · Audio analysis

1 Introduction

According to the World Health Organization (WHO)[1], it was estimated that depression was one of the most common mental disorders that affected around 264 million people of all ages, being one of the main causes of disability in the world. Depression is characterized by affecting the mood of the sufferer, which is why it is also known as a mood disorder or affective disorder which causes suffering and disability in family, work and social environments, and this can be classified between the levels: mild, moderate and severe, depending on the amount and severity of symptoms presented[2,3]. For the most serious cases of depression, this disease can lead to suicide, and it is estimated that about 800 thousand people conclude this act, considering it the fourth leading cause of death in people aged 15 to 29 years Likewise, it is considered that not addressing cases of depression during the patient's adolescence stage may lead to the impact of the

---

[1] "Adolescent mental health" - WHO.
[2] Depression - National Ministry of Health (in Spanish).
[3] "Depression" - WHO.

© The Author(s), under exclusive license to Springer Nature Switzerland AG 2023
L. A. Maciaszek et al. (Eds.): ICT4AWE 2021/2022, CCIS 1856, pp. 35–55, 2023.
https://doi.org/10.1007/978-3-031-37496-8_3

mental disorder extending into adulthood, causing the opportunities for a full life to be limited.

Currently, it is estimated that in Peru, 80% of suicides are related to severe depression, and the Peruvian entities in charge of treating mental health are not sufficiently of people who suffer from the disorder[4]. Either, due to the limited number of mental health specialists available to attention to these cases or technological deficiencies to provide efficient health services, which have been important barriers to accessing mental health services during the COVID-19 pandemic, which has led to a deterioration in mental health and the vital functions of people who already suffered from a mental disorder previously deteriorate due to the multiple factors experienced during the state of health emergency[5]. The percentage of cases that received some treatment per year from 2014 to 2018 is approximately 14%, the remaining 86% do not usually receive some type of treatment for depression symptoms [14]. According to the National Institute of Mental Health (INSM)[6], it is reported that among the population with this disability, young people between the ages of 17 and 25 in Peru suffer the most from this disorder, seeing a considerable increase in mental health problems in Peru's children and adolescents, so it became a priority to address these cases in specialized centers in order to provide the corresponding mental health services. However, the care gaps continued to be high, considering that not only the prescription for a medical drug was enough but also the support of mental health professionals for comprehensive recovery and reintegration into society.

Artificial intelligence (AI) and cloud services are progressively focused on supporting the health sector, which are used to make better decisions based on the large amount of data that they analyze. For example, in [3] point out that AI generates benefits in terms of the detection and diagnosis of mental disorders due to its algorithms and the ability to extract information from a data source, which provide a better understanding of the prevalence of these disorders in the population allowing health professionals to focus mainly on the human aspects of medicine and doctor-patient treatment while AI would focus on cases of self-administered smart health treatments that improve the limited time of patient care. Likewise, the potential of AI is focused on complementing existing treatments, providing value in optimizing their availability and effectiveness, because health technology solutions that incorporate AI, such as chatbots, and diagnostic tools, such as questionnaires self-administered depression, they can meet the needs of large groups of populations unlike the effort that a mental health specialist can provide [8]. The mental health sector can obtain various benefits from this technology, as well as how it benefited in the digitization process to improve patient care, now AI must be used to make a more efficient, accurate and personalized diagnosis or treatment selection in less time for the well-being of patients.

The analysis of emotions is very important in these cases, since many people do not receive adequate attention because they believe that the symptoms, they present do not need medical attention, when in fact these first symptoms are essential to identify depression in time. On the one hand, facial perception is one of the key indicators of

---

[4] "Severe depression is the principal cause of death by suicide" - MINSA (2019).

[5] "COVID-19 and the need of act in relation with mental health" - UN (2020).

[6] Ending stigma towards people with mental health problems, the challenge of psychiatry.

social interactions allowing to determine clues about thoughts and emotions through the facial expressions of an individual, likewise, mental disorders can be determined through negative facial expressions, without However, it is a challenge to be able to differentiate between the facial recognition of a person suffering from a mental disorder and someone with optimal health controls [13]. On the other hand, speech has the potential to provide characteristics that help detect a mental disorder, since the vocal anatomy is a unique structure that provides the ability to vocalize various acoustic signals in a coordinated and meaningful way, making it a marker suitable for detecting health conditions [1]. This research will focus on the evaluation of the level of depression considering the implementation of a technological model whose components can detect the chronicity of depressive symptoms and address them with the help of technological tools and experts in mental health. The main contributions of the proposed model are the following:

- We propose a technological model to support the treating mental health professional to optimize the diagnosis and level of depression by analyzing facial images and voice, signals that will help detect the chronicity of depressive symptoms.
- Our technological solution benefits from the facial recognition characteristics that will be obtained through the camera of a mobile device, and these will be evaluated with algorithms in the Azure Cognitive Services cloud.
- Our technological solution benefits from the voice recognition features that will be obtained through the microphone of a mobile device and these will be transcribed from audio to text with the IBM Watson Speech to Text service and then analyzed with IBM Watson Tone Analyzer.
- We propose to obtain a better diagnosis through the support of mental health specialists so that the patient begins with the corresponding treatment, which will be presented in our experiments.

This paper is organized as follows. In Sect. 2, we will address the key concepts for the development of our solution; then, in Sect. 3, we will address the core of our approach in the evaluation of depression level with facial and voice analysis and the aggregated value of the our work according to the evaluation of the level of depression. In Sect. 4, we will describe the differences and comparisons with other works about the evaluation of the level of depression; subsequently, in Sect. 5 we will present the validation of the technological model functionalities in a simulated scenario that includes young patients and mental health specialists. Finally, in Sect. 6 we will specify our main conclusions and results of the finished application.

2 Background

In this section, the main concepts involved in our research will be developed. We propose that, for each concept, there is a definition and a respective example based on a review of the literature on depressive disorder and facial and voice recognition.

Facial Recognition

Definition 1 (Facial recognition [6]**).** *When compared to other bio-metric character-istics such as fingerprints, palms, etc., it has several advantages in obtaining these characteristics, since they can be extracted through the images of the cameras in a non-intrusive way.*

Example 1 (Face Detection). Given the Fig. 1, the procedure for obtaining multiple face detection is displayed. Figure 1a shows the detected face-like regions, Fig. 1b shows the rough face detection result, Fig. 1c shows the spatial distribution of facial features, and Fig. 1d shows the refined result.

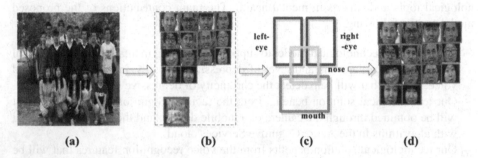

(a)   (b)   (c)   (d)

Fig. 1. Face recognition [6]. The proposed multi-face dectection procedure. (a) Detected face-like regions. (b) Rough face detection result. (c) Spatial distribution of facial features. (d) Refined result.

Definition 2 (Facial expression [17]**).** *This is one of the key social indicators which allows us to determine clues about thoughts and emotions from the movements and positions of the facial muscles under the skin of the face. These movements are a form of non-verbal communication and transmit the emotional state to an observer.*

Example 2 (Detection of facial expressions). Given the Fig. 2, the features to obtain the emotional expressions of are: i)The distance between the two eyes is identified, ii) The width of the nose is estimated, iii) The vertical distance between the eyes and the center of the mouth is calculated and iv) The distance between the eyes and the eyebrows is measured.

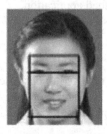

Fig. 2. Facial expressions detection [17].

Voice Recognition

Definition 3 (Voice recognition [1]**).** *Speech has the potential to provide character-istics that help detect a mental disorder, since the vocal anatomy is a unique structure that provides the ability to vocalize various acoustic signals in a coordinated and mean-ingful way, making it a suitable marker to detect health conditions.*

Example 3 (Detection of facial expressions). Given the Fig. 3, the muscles and struc-tures that produce the voice signal are shown, which supports being an identifier of different health conditions.

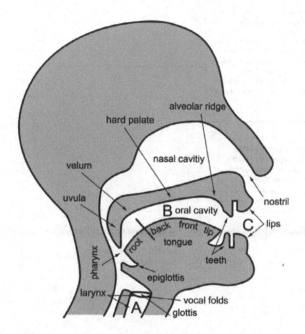

Fig. 3. Muscular key groups to produce an speech [12].

Depression

Definition 4 (Depression). *Depression is a common mental disorder considered one of the main causes of disability worldwide that can lead to suicide, where the individual who suffers from it experiences a depressed mood, losing enjoyment and interest in developing activities. Likewise, depressive episodes can be categorized by levels: mild, moderate, or severe, depending on the severity of the symptoms and the impact on the person's functionality (WHO, 2021).*

Example 4. Some typologies of mood disorder indicated by the WHO are: i) Single episode depressive disorder, ii) Recurrent depressive disorder and iii) Bipolar disorder.

According to the National Ministry of Health (MINSA) , depressive disorder is considered a disease that mainly affects the mood of an individual, which is why it is

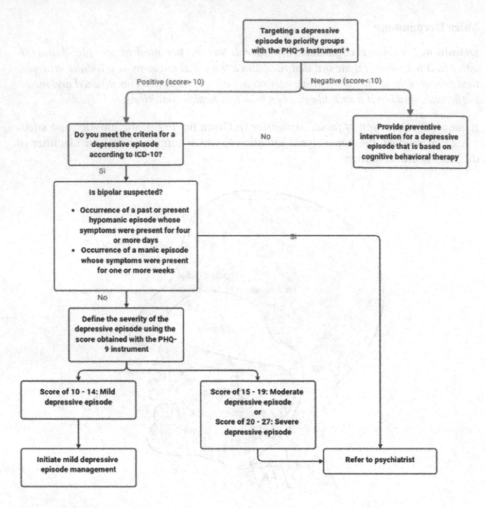

Fig. 4. Screening and diagnosis flowchart for mild depressive episode [9].

known as a mood disorder or affective disorder. In addition, individuals who experience the disorder often experience deep feelings of sadness, which can hinder their family relationships and work responsibilities, due to the loss of desire to perform activities. MINSA indicates that the most common types of depression are:

- Severe depression
- Dysthymia
- Bipolar disorder

In [9], the authors point out that the clinical practice and screening guide for the management of mild depressive episode in the first level of care of the Social Security of Peru in the entity Essalud addresses the screening, diagnosis, management and prevention of patients through six questions: which allow:

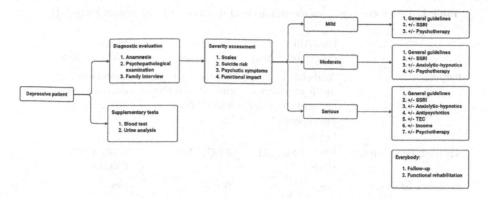

Fig. 5. Diagnostic and therapeutic protocol for depression [10].

Table 1. Analysis of key characteristics in self-administered medical questionnaires [12].

	PHQ-9	CES-D	BDI-II	Zung SDS	MDI
Estimated time (minutes)	5 to 10	5	5 to 10	10	5 to 10
Target Audience	General Public	Older than 12 years	Older than 13 years	General Public	General Public
Number of items (questions)	10	20	21	20	12
Sensitivity	.88	.98	.88	.79	.86
Specificity	.88	.57	.98	.72	.82

- Search for interventions to prevent depressive episodes
- Conduct screening test using the Patient Health Questionnaire (PHQ-9) instrument to measure the severity of depression and refer a mental health specialist.
- Diagnose the cases and determine whether to carry out psychotherapy or pharmacological therapy
- Question what psychotherapy to use
- Question what drug therapy will be used
- Define the usefulness of physical exercise

In this way, it is ensured that patients who reach the first level of medical care can minimize their partial or total exposure to developing a mild depressive episode.

In Fig. 4, the depressive episode screening flow is shown, using the PHQ-9 instrument. Where it depends on the score obtained and the medical criteria evaluated, the patient can start a treatment of the depressive episode level or in cases of moderate or severe episodes be referred to a psychiatrist (Fig. 5).

3 Depression Detection with Images and Voice

In this section, we will present the design of a model to assess the level of depression by analyzing facial images and a patient's voice. To explain the design process, it will be

Table 2. Analysis of key characteristics in cloud services for facial images analysis [12].

	Face API (Microsoft Azure)	Amazon Rekognition (AWS)	Vision AI (Google Cloud)
Purpose	Artificial intelligence service that analyzes faces in imagesand videos	Automate image and video analysis with machine learning	Detect emotions, interpret text and images
Supported image format	JPEG, PNG, GIF, BMP	JPEG, PNG	JPEG, PNG8, PNG24
Real-time analysis	Yes	Yes	Yes
Service availability	.99	.99	.99
Face attributes that it detects	Emotions, age, blur, exposure, gender, head position, hair, noise, occlusion, smile	Gender, smile, emotions, face landmarks, posture, beard, glasses	Emotions, age, nose, ears, mouth, face position, blur

divided into three sections: component analysis and benchmarking, technology model design, and solution architecture.

3.1 Benchmarking and Analysis of Components

First, looking for components in the technological model to assess the level of depression using facial and voice analysis with three layers: The technique used to segment the components was to consider three layers:

- Front Office Layer: It will make it possible to identify the way in which customers will go to acquire the product and service[7].
- Middle Office Layer: It will be related to the intermediate section of the business architecture focused on the execution of external and / or internal rules that satisfy the needs of the business logic[8].
- Back Office layer: It will be related to the software in charge of managing the core functions of the solution[9].

According to the National Institute of Statistics (INEI)[10], in the first quarter of 2020, 93.3% of households have at least one member who has a mobile phone, and of the total number of people who have internet access, 87.9% do so through this device.

Likewise, regarding Tablets, the devices that were delivered by the Peruvian government during 2020 are considered, since these were provided to primary and secondary

---

[7] "Front Office scanning: from the back room to the counter" - IBM.
[8] "Data office as part of enterprise architecture".
[9] "Back office software" - FinancialForce.
[10] Statistics of information and communication technologies in households (in Spanish).

Table 3. Analysis of key characteristics in cloud services for voice recognition [12].

	Watson Speech to Text (IBM Cloud)	Amazon Transcribe Medical (AWS)	Speech to Text (Google Cloud)
Purpose	Use speech recognition to convert a language to text	Add speech-to-text functionality for the medical field	Convert speech to text with precision using AI technology
Supported audio size	≤ 100 MB	≤ 2 GB	≤ 10 MB
Detect voice in real time	Yes	Yes	Yes
Complementary services to analyze the text	Tone Analyzer (IBM Cloud)	Twinword API	Natural Language API
Service availability	.99	.99	.99
Classification of feelings	By type of feeling	By type of feeling	Positive, negative, neutral

school students in rural areas, as well as to teachers[11]. Due to these facilities provided by the mobile device, in addition to its components such as the integrated camera and microphone, it is for this reason that various scientific investigations on depression rely on to carry out the evaluation of depressive symptoms or the level of depression that occur in people.

For example, there is a bachelor thesis[12] that developed a mobile application which allowed to obtain video recording and audio recording from a mobile device, whose characteristics of the device had to record a 640×480 video with a frequency of 30 FPS and the audio frequency was between 0.3 Hz and 35 Hz, to obtain the parameters related to the variability of respiration and heart rate to monitor patients with depression during the development of the stress test. Likewise, the essential tools used to carry out the depressive disorder detection procedure in patients were a minimum recording camera of 30 FPS and a microphone with a frequency of 16 kHZ [16]. In the Middle Office layer, the analysis and benchmarking of self-administered medical questionnaires (Screening Test) to evaluate the level of depression, facial image analysis cloud services and voice analysis cloud services were considered. Regarding the Screening Tests to assess the level of depression, five medical tools were considered:

- Patient Health Questionnarie (PHQ-9)
- Center for Epidemiologic Studies-Depression scale (CES-D)
- Beck Depression Inventory (BDI-II)
- Zung Self-Rating Depression Scale (Zung SDS)
- Major Depression Inventory (MDI)

---

[11] "In October, the distribution of tablets to students and teachers will begin" - shorturl.at/ahuP6.
[12] "App development to monitor depressed patients during the performance of stress tests" - shorturl.at/rJMSU.

Table 4. Analysis of key characteristics in NoSQL databases [12].

	Mongo DB	Cassandra	Redis	Couchbase
Data storage	Documents (BSON, XML, etc.)	Oriented to flexible columns	Data structures such as lists, strings, ordered sets, bitmaps	Documents (JSON, XML, etc.)
Use cases	Real-time analysis, mobile applications	E-commerce, fraud detection, IoT	Chat or messaging, real-time analysis, cache storage	Mobile apps
Open Source	Yes	Yes	Yes	Yes
DBaaS	ScaleGrid, MongoDB	-	Redis Enterprise, Cloud	-
Provider	AWS, GCP, Microsoft Azure	AWS, GCP, Microsoft Azure	AWS, GCP, Microsoft Azure	AWS, GCP, Microsoft Azure

Table 1 shows the analysis of key characteristics about the self-administered medical questionnaires mentioned to measure the level of depression. As a result of the benchmarking estimation, the Screening Test with the best fit for our proposal was the Zung Self-Rating Depression Scale (Zung SDS), since it covers a General Public, and it has a good trade-off between sensitivity and specificity. This was considered as the component that will support the evaluation of the level of depression. Regarding the facial image analysis cloud services that contributed to the detection of depressive symptoms, three cloud services were considered: i) Face API (Microsoft Azure), ii) Amazon Rekognition (AWS) and iii) Vision AI (Google Cloud).

Table 2 shows the evaluated criteria according to cloud services of analysis of facial images. As a result of the benchmarking estimate, the facial image recognition and analysis cloud service with the highest score was Face from Microsoft Azure. This service will be considered as part of the solution due to its functionalities. It should be noted that the educational institution has an agreement with Microsoft Azure, which benefits the project team in terms of the acquisition and management of the tool for the student credit that is granted. Regarding voice recognition cloud services that contributed to the detection of depressive symptoms, three cloud services were considered: i) Watson Speech to Text (IBM Cloud), ii) Amazon Transcribe Medical (AWS) and iii) Speech to text (Google Cloud).

Table 3 shows the evaluated criteria of the voice recognition cloud services. As a result of the benchmarking estimate, the speech recognition and text analysis cloud services with the highest scores were the Speech to Text and Tone Analyzer services. These services were considered as part of the solution due to their functionalities.

NoSQL databases store data in documents rather than relational tables. NoSQL database technology stores information in JSON documents instead of columns and rows used by relational databases. To be clear, NoSQL stands for "not only SQL" rather than "no SQL" at all In the Back Office layer, the analysis and benchmarking of NoSQL databases was considered, since these are designed specifically for specific data models and you have flexible schema to create applications, compared to a relational SQL database that is a collection of Predefined data elements among them, being organized as a set of tables with columns and rows [5]. Regarding NoSQL databases, non-relational databases were considered table: i) Mongo DB, ii) Cassandra, iii) Redis and iv) Couchbase.

Table 4 shows the evaluated criteria of the NoSQL databases. As a result, we have that the databases that satisfy the most these criteria were MongoDB and Redis, this is because both present facilities for the migration of the database to a cloud environment. However, a higher score was obtained by MongoDB since the data storage is document oriented and this will be essential for better data collection.

3.2 Design of the Technological Model

Second, we carry out the design of the technological model, incorporating the components of the first section of component analysis and benchmarking. In Fig. 6. the proposed model is shown.

To explain the attributes of the technological model in greater detail, we will indicate the model input, phases of the model and the model output.

Model Input. It begins when a young patient seeks institutions or mental health professionals due to the recurrent presence of depressive symptoms that hinder their daily activities. We consider the age between 18 and 29 years, considered as the stage of youth[13]. The initial inputs would be, on the one hand, the demographic data of the young patient, and on the other hand, the self-administered Screening Test that will allow knowing presumptively the level of depression suffered by the patient. Both the demographic data and those of the Screening Test are planned to be hosted on a Backend of a mobile application deployed in the Microsoft Azure cloud environment with its Service App service.

Phases of the Model

Devices. The model contemplates the use of mobile devices, both smartphones and tablets, which will allow the young patient to access a mental health counseling application. Likewise, the patient will be able to perform the self-administered Screening Test to assess the level of depression, and the device's camera and integrated microphones will be used to capture emotions in the face and voice to reinforce the results obtained during filling.

Internet Connection. An important aspect for accessing the mental health counseling application is having an internet connection, for this reason it is estimated that patients can contact it, through their WI-FI network or through their mobile data from net. This to be able to access the services within the application, such as facial and voice analysis, data storage or information listing in real time, which will be deployed in the Microsoft Azure Service App cloud environment.

---

[13] "Health Situation of Adolescents and Young People in Peru" (in Spanish) - MINSA.

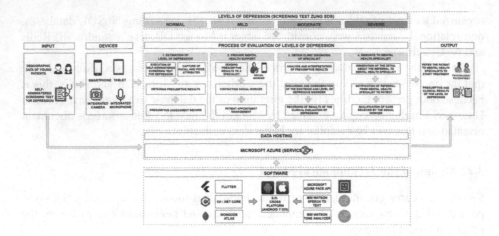

Fig. 6. Our proposal [12].

Depression Level Assessment Process. To begin with the process of evaluating the level of depression, it is necessary to indicate that the levels of depression that will be considered in this project are those that are granted by the Screening Test of the Zung Self Depression Scale (SDS), which based on the score obtained by the patient depression is classified into levels: normal, mild, moderate, and severe. Regarding data hosting, this will be done in the Backend deployed in the Microsoft Azure cloud environment with its Service App service, which is planned to be designed so that the mental health advisory application can be run on cross-platform mobile devices (Android and iOS). In addition, regarding the software, the tools that will allow the construction of the Backend would be C# and the .NET CORE framework for the construction of code and business logic, integrating through libraries the cognitive cloud services of facial analysis (Face-Microsoft Azure) and speech analysis (Speech to Text and Tone Analyzer-IBM Watson), and the Mongo DB Atlas which will allow the storage of non-relational data; Regarding the Frontend construction tools, they would correspond to the Flutter framework for the user interface.

Estimation of the Level of Depression. The first step to assess the level of depression has been the estimation of the level of depression, where only the young patient intervenes, who will perform the Zung SDS self-administered Screening Test, which consists of 20 questions and 4 alternatives, to obtain a result presumptive level of depression. It is planned that the young patient can carry out this activity within the proposed mobile application, where the capture of facial and voice attributes will also be executed at the same time, to reinforce the results obtained from the Screening Test.

In this way, a presumptive result would be obtained indicating the level of depression that is being experienced, in addition to considering the emotions collected during the capture of facial and voice attributes, aspects that are mostly involuntary on the part of the patient and can reach be a signal to determine symptoms related to depression. After that, it is planned that the data obtained from the presumptive evaluation can be registered within the platform, so that a history of evaluations carried out and the option of being able to contact See a mental health specialist of your choice to receive mental health support.

Provide Mental Health Support. The second step to assess the level of depression takes place when the young patient sends the presumptive results to a mental health specialist, who will provide the necessary support based on their knowledge and the battery of psychological or medical evaluations. that you consider necessary to carry out. For this scenario, it is planned that the young patient will have the possibility of contacting a social worker who will help as a first filter in the evaluation of the level of depression.

The social worker will manage the appointment with the patient once the presumptive results and data have been obtained. It is proposed that the management of the appointment can be carried out within the mental health counseling application where the details of the meeting are indicated so that both the patient and the specialist can follow up.

Obtain a Clinical Diagnosis from a Specialist. The third step to assess the level of depression relies mainly on the analysis and interpretation of presumptive results by the social worker in the meetings that have been held together with the patient. In this way, the mental health specialist will have the possibility to rule out symptoms and corroborate the existence of the depressive disorder. Since the mental health of the patient is a very delicate subject, the best option he chose for the research is that the social worker as the first mental health filter can determine if the result of the level of depression obtained from the Screening Test is related with the true level of depression experienced by the patient. Likewise, it is planned that the social worker consolidates a clinical diagnosis for the patient which can allow them to access help by referring them to mental health professionals who can provide optimal treatment, where said clinical diagnosis has the possibility of being registered and consulted. within the mobile application.

Refer to a Mental Health Specialist. The fourth step to assess the level of depression has been the referral to mental health specialists, where the social worker will generate a detail that involves the presumptive results and clinical diagnosis of the patient, in addition to incorporating the corresponding referral to the mental health specialist so that a treatment can be executed. With the referral detail, the social worker will notify the patient through the mobile application which specialist will be recommended. For these cases, in [9] where the authors point out that patients suffering from mild depression should be referred to a psychologist, while cases of moderate or severe depression are linked to referral to a psychiatrist. In addition, it is planned that once the patient receives the details of the referral notification, they will have the option of being able to rate the care received by the specialist from the first mental health filter.

Model Output. To finalize the flow of the proposed model, the outputs generated would be to refer the patient to a mental health specialist to initiate optimal treatment, thus depending on the level of depression identified by the social worker as the first mental health filter, the referral will allow timely attention from psychologists or psychiatrists according to the level of depression experienced. Likewise, another of the outputs would be the presumptive results and clinical diagnosis of the level of depression, carried out first by the young patient and second by the social worker within the process of evaluating the level of depression.

Solution Architecture. Once the technological model was mentioned, the proposed integrated architecture sketch of the mobile solution that would be built was carried out to validate the functionalities of the model.

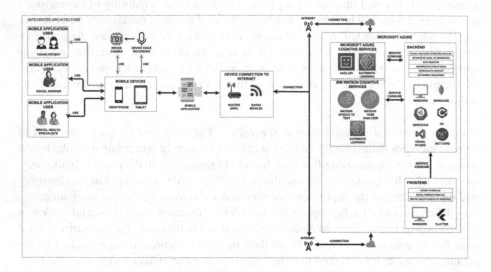

Fig. 7. Integrated architecture of the solution.

From Fig. 7. we can point out that we consider as actors the young patient, social worker, and mental health specialists (psychologist or psychiatrist), where they will use mobile devices such as Smartphones or Tablets to access the mental health counseling application. It is considered that the mobile application requires internet connectivity which can be done through Wi-Fi or mobile data to interact with the services of the mobile application. Within these services, it is shown that they will be deployed in the Microsoft Azure Service App service where the Frontend, Backend and cognitive services that correspond to the mobile application are contemplated.

In the Frontend, the tools to be used are mainly based on Flutter which is a tool provided by Google to design the user interface of mobile, web or desktop applications. The reason for the use of this tool can be seen reflected in [2], where they used the Flutter cross-platform framework to create a voice recognition mobile application. They also pointed out that this tool is mostly used today due to its simplicity of development using the Dart programming language.

In the Backend, Microsoft's open-source framework, .NET Core, was incorporated, which will allow the creation of cross-platform applications in Android and iOS environments, using the C# programming language to perform the business logic of a mobile application[14]. Also, to achieve the development of the validation solution, the Integrated Development Environment (IDE) with which it would work would be Visual Studio or Visual Studio Code. Likewise, the IDE allows incorporating the services of the connection to the MongoDB non-relational database with which the data will be managed in the application, as well as the cognitive services for facial and voice analysis.

Regarding the possibility of integrating the Microsoft Azure facial analysis service, Face, there is the possibility of coupling it with .NET Core, since the framework accepts the integration of Microsoft Azure cognitive services through the consumption of programming libraries. Likewise, the voice and text analysis service by IBM Cloud Watson can be integrated thanks to the Nuggets (packet consumption tool) provided by the .NET framework. Also considering that these services have the possibility of machine learning to train the services if it deserves it.

Once the integrated architecture has been defined, we carry out the development of the mobile application to start with the validation of functionalities of the technological model, which will be detailed in Sect. 5.

4 Related Works

In this section, the main works that have been of important relevance and influence in the development of our work will be discussed.

In [7], the authors describe that the problem related to the persistence of anxiety and depression in the population due to the COVID-19 pandemic was addressed. They present a technique related to the analysis of potential risk factors in different types of population associated with the symptoms of the mental disorders mentioned above, where self-administered medical instruments were used to measure levels of depression (Zung SDS) and anxiety (Zung SAS) to measure the severity of symptoms. In contrast to this research, we contemplate the use of the Zung SDS test, also used in public health entities in Peru, to identify the level of depression based on the symptoms evidenced in the patient considering the quality that allows it to perform the test without the mandatory need for the accompaniment of a mental health professional.

In [4], addressed the risk of suffering from health problems in older adults, and the limitations to implement technological solutions for routine surveillance. Therefore, they developed an intelligent model that detects emotions in real time using facial images using the Microsoft Azure Face API cognitive service. We extend this work with the idea of analyzing facial emotions with the help of the Face API cognitive service to obtain the main emotions that are related to depressive disorder and provide a greater number of characteristics to specialists.

In [11], the authors addressed the need to provide a better user experience and a better understanding of complex behaviors in different conditions through the integration of emotional capabilities in Chatbots. They provide a comparison of different Chatbot APIs where interactivity with these could support different languages and analyze the tone of voice and mood of the user with services from IBM, Amazon, and Google. Unlike his work, we adapted the IBM Watson Tone Analyzer technology tool

---

[14] "Introduction to .NET" - Microsoft.

to detect emotions in texts, but we complemented it with the IBM Watson Speech-To-Text speech-to-text transcription tool to be able to perform the analysis of the patient's voice.

In [15], the authors addressed the limitations of capacity for clinical office visits by patients by automatically estimating depression from facial and voice analysis. The technique used by the authors is to develop an algorithm that estimates articulatory coordination of speech from audio and video signals and uses these coordination characteristics to allow you to learn the prediction model and track the severity of depression using the scale of Hamilton (HAM-D). Unlike the authors, our approach is aimed at obtaining a presumptive result of the level of depression in the first instance where facial and voice analysis are used during the execution of a medical questionnaire (Zung SDS), in this way we couple the facial and speech analysis tools from cognitive services to reinforce Zung SDS test results.

5   Experiments

In this section, the procedure and the necessary tools will be shown to carry out the deployment of the prototype of the technological model of the research that will support the evaluation of the level of depression of a patient and the corresponding referral.

5.1   Experimental Protocol

For this study, a prototype was developed that served as support to validate the technological model, which is a mobile application that has the following services.

Table 5. Services used in the development.

Service	Provider
App Service	Microsoft Azure
Service Cognitive Face API	Microsoft Azure
Non-Relational Database	Mongo DB
Service Cognitive Speech-To-Text	IBM Watson
Service Cognitive Tone Analyzer	IBM Watson

First, an account was created in the MongoDB Atlas database and the "Free & Hobby" cloud database implementation plan was chosen. After that, the connection to the cluster was made where the connection to the IP address and the creation of the database user were selected, also the selected driver is C# .Net, since our backend is created with that technology and version 2.13 or later (Table 5).

Second, the Backend was deployed, that is, the cognitive services of Microsoft Azure and IBM Watson. To do this, a Microsoft Azure App Services is created in the .NET Core 3.1 LTS environment and Windows Operating System where they gave us a Basic B1 plan with a total size of 1.75 GB of memory.

Finally, to generate the APK of the mobile application called "Help +" a key.properties file is created, the signature is configured in gradle, the application is changed to relread mode and finally the command to finish flutter build apk is executed to generate the file APK to be installed on a mobile device. The APK to install is in the following path: https://github.com/LuisPA-ui/AYUDA-.

5.2 Results

Participants. The research focused on supporting young Peruvians between 17 and 25 years old, for that reason we were able to contact 60 young people between the age ranges to participate and interact with the prototype made. These were selected randomly by sending invitations by mail to faculty students. Besides, mental health specialists were contacted, a psychiatrist and a social worker that were contacted by mail, they gave us their support to validate the technological model by confirming whether the technological model presents the benefits that we wish to obtain for young Peruvians.

Validation. For validating of the prototype, we aim to prove these strategies: desirability, feasibility, usability, and satisfaction, which will be explained below.

Desirability. To satisfactorily develop the desirability of the technological model and Identifying if a problem worth solving is being solved, surveys were conducted for young people and specialists, and a Show & Tell was held with both stakeholders. Regarding the survey designed in Google Forms to validate the functionalities of the Technological Model aimed at the role of:

– Patient: which was carried out by 57 young Peruvians:
  - 75.4% would be willing to look for a mobile App to be able to address depressive disorder.
  - 63.2% intend to contact a specialist to deal with depression.
  - 80.7% would be willing to run a medical questionnaire (Zung SDS Test) with the functionalities of facial and voice analysis.
  - 89.5% would like to receive the clinical diagnosis from the specialist in the same App
– Specialist: which was carried out by 18 mental health professionals:
  - 44.4% indicate that the largest number of cases are related to adolescents and young people.
  - 50% indicate that the moderate level of depression is mostly evident in the Peruvian population.
  - 75% agree that a worker or social worker is a first filter to diagnose symptoms and refer the patient to the specialist.
  - Zung SDS, BDI-II and PHQ-9 are some depression diagnostic questionnaires that specialists consider to be most effective.

Regarding the show & tell for:

– Participants: the meeting was held with 20 users, between 18 to 29 years old, through videoconference rooms, where:

- The research project was explained
- The depressive disorder context was explained.
- A demo of a mobile app based on the technological model function was presented from the patient's perspective (Video format).
– Specialists: the meeting was held with two mental health professionals, through videoconference rooms, where:
  - The research project objective was explained.
  - The prototype of a mobile app based on technological model functions was presented.
  - The main benefits of the technological model presented were identified.

Feasibility. For the defined solution to be feasible, the necessary components were identified so that it is possible to implement both at a technical and operational level as shown in Fig. 8.

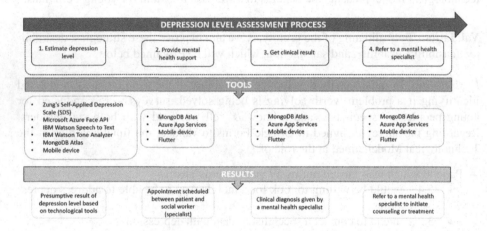

Fig. 8. Implementation of the technological model.

Usability. Unit Tests were performed on the young patients who used the prototype during the previously mentioned interviews, where they were given the APK of the mobile application so that they could perform the respective tests. After, they gave their opinions regarding its functionalities and usability, where it was obtained as a result that 70% of users identified that it is easy to use, as shown in Fig. 9.

Satisfaction. The level of satisfaction was also carried out during the interviews with the young patients and at the end of the tests 85% of the users indicated that they were satisfied with the results and the ease of contacting a mental health specialist to support the depression, as shown in Fig. 10.

Regarding the precision of effectiveness of the cognitive services of Microsoft Azure and IBM Watson of facial and voice recognition used respectively in the research project, the following is presented (Table 6):

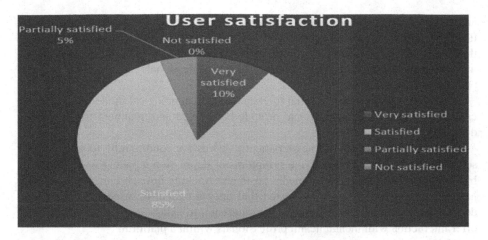

Fig. 9. Usability of the prototype.

Table 6. Precision of the cognitive services [12].

Service	Accuracy
Microsoft Azure Face API	90%–95%
Watson Tone Analyzer	41%–68%

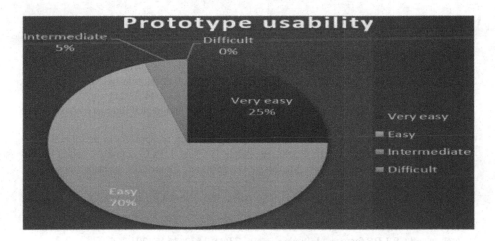

Fig. 10. User satisfaction [12].

6   Conclusions and Perspectives

We were able to learn about the current state of this process and the shortcomings it exhibits thanks to the research we did on the methodologies currently employed to assess a patient's level of depression. The areas for improvement are not only the use of technological tools to gauge the severity of depression, but also the inclusion of quicker and more efficient contact with a specialist. Due to the validation strategy's foundation in desirability, feasibility, usability, and satisfaction, we were able to determine that young Peruvians are willing to use technological tools in order to be supported in improving their mental health, and mental health professionals recognize a significant opportunity to advance in this field.

Additionally, there are potential to enhance the technological model that has been created to enhance patient flow and provide better care and treatment for depressive disorders.

A technology method to track a patient's depressive condition by looking at their social media postings can track the symptoms of depression a patient is experiencing by looking at their daily social media posts and tracking how chronic the symptoms have become over time. It is suggested that once a patient is suspected of having a depressive condition, applications can be suggested to assess and treat the disorder or offer interaction with mental health professionals within a platform.

Using strategies that encourage healthy coping in people with the aid of virtual assistants, a preventive model to deal with suicidal depressive episodes aims to stop suicidal thoughts brought on by severe episodes of depression. Since it is believed that a depressive episode can happen at any time in a person's life, it is planned to create a virtual assistant that can accompany and offer mental health support during severe episodes of depression, allowing for the recommendation or direct contact of a mental health professional once the level of depression has subsided.

References

1. Cummins, N., Baird, A., Schuller, B.W.: Speech analysis for health: current state-of-the-art and the increasing impact of deep learning. Methods **151**, 41–54 (2018)
2. Faisol, M., Ramlan, S.A., Hafizah, A., Mozi, A., Zakaria, F.F.: Mobile-based speech recognition for early reading assistant. J. Phys. Conf. Ser. **1962**, 012044 (2021)
3. Graham, S., et al.: Artificial intelligence for mental health and mental illnesses: an overview. Curr. Psychiatry Rep. **21**, 1–18 (2019)
4. Khanal, S., Reis, A., Barroso, J., Filipe, V.: Using emotion recognition in intelligent interface design for elderly care. In: Rocha, Á., Adeli, H., Reis, L.P., Costanzo, S. (eds.) World-CIST'18 2018. AISC, vol. 746, pp. 240–247. Springer, Cham (2018). https://doi.org/10.1007/978-3-319-77712-2_23
5. Khasawneh, T.N., AL-Sahlee, M.H., Safia, A.A.: SQL, NewSQL, and NOSQL databases: a comparative survey. In: ICICS (2020)
6. Li, C., Wei, W., Li, J., Song, W.: A cloud-based monitoring system via face recognition using Gabor and CS-LBP features. J. Supercomput. **73**(4), 1532–1546 (2017)
7. Li, X., et al.: Depression and anxiety among quarantined people, community workers, medical staff, and general population in the early stage of COVID-19 epidemic. Front. Psychol. **12**, 638985 (2021)
8. Lovejoy, C.A.: Technology and mental health: the role of artificial intelligence. Eur. Psychiatry **55**, 1–3 (2019)
9. Macciotta-Felices, B., et al.: Clinical practice guideline for the screening and management of the mild depressive episode at the first level of care for the Peruvian Social Security (EsSalud). Acta Medica Peruana **37**(4) (2020)

10. Pereira-Sánchez, V., Molero-Santos, P.: Protocolo diagnóstico y terapéutico de la depresión. Medicine - Programa de Formación Médica Continuada Acreditado **12**(86) (2019). enfermedades psiquiátricas (III) Psicosis. Trastornos del humor

11. Ralston, K., Chen, Y., Isah, H., Zulkernine, F.H.: A voice interactive multilingual student support system using IBM Watson. In: IEEE ICMLA (2019)

12. Ramos-Cuadros, A., Palomino-Santillan, L., Ugarte, W.: Model to assess the level of depression by analyzing facial images and voice of patients. In: ICT4AWE, pp. 26–36 (2022)

13. Simcock, G., et al.: Associations between facial emotion recognition and mental health in early adolescence. Int. J. Environ. Res. Public Health **17**, 330 (2020)

14. Villarreal-Zegarra, D., Cabrera-Alva, M., Carrillo-Larco, R.M., Bernabe-Ortiz, A.: Trends in the prevalence and treatment of depressive symptoms in Peru: a population-based study. BMJ Open **10**(7), e036777 (2020)

15. Williamson, J.R., Young, D., Nierenberg, A.A., Niemi, J., Helfer, B.S., Quatieri, T.F.: Tracking depression severity from audio and video based on speech articulatory coordination. Comput. Speech Lang. **55**, 40–56 (2019)

16. Zeghari, R., et al.: Correlations between facial expressivity and apathy in elderly people with neurocognitive disorders: exploratory study. JMIR Form. Res. **5**(3), e24727 (2021)

17. Zhang, Y., et al.: Facial emotion recognition based on biorthogonal wavelet entropy, fuzzy support vector machine, and stratified cross validation. IEEE Access **4**, 8375–8385 (2016)

Advantages of Oversampling Techniques: A Case Study in Risk Factors for Fall Prediction

Gulshan Sihag[1(✉)], Pankaj Yadav[2], Vivek Vijay[2], Veronique Delcroix[1], Xavier Siebert[3], Sandeep Kumar Yadav[2], and François Puisieux[4]

[1] Univ. Polytechnique Hauts-de-France, CNRS, UMR 8201 - LAMIH, 59313 Valenciennes, France
{Gulshan.Sihag,Veronique.Delcroix}@uphf.fr
[2] Department of Mathematics, Indian Institute of Technology, Jodhpur, Jodhpur, India
{yadav.20,vivek,sy}@iitj.ac.in
[3] Faculté polytechnique Département de Mathématique et Recherche Opérationnelle, Univ. de Mons, Mons, Belgium
xavier.siebert@umons.ac.be
[4] Dépt. de Gérontologie, Hôpital Universitaire de Lille, 59037 Lille Cedex, France
francois.puisieux@chru-lille.fr

Abstract. The evaluation of risk factors for falls (RFF) is a key point in fall prevention for the elderly. Since the information of the main actionable RFF can not always be regularly re-evaluated by medical factors, their automatic prediction would allow providing useful recommendations to reduce the risk of falls. This article explores the advantages of three oversampling methods to improve the quality of the prediction of 12 target RFF on the basis of a real imbalanced data set. We first present the data set, together with the selection of 45 variables and 12 target variables and other pre-processing steps. Second, we present the three oversampling methods, SMOTE, SMOTE-SVM, and ADASYN, the classifiers (Logistic Regression, Random Forest, Bayesian Network, Artificial Neural Network, and Naive Bayes), and the quality measures that we use in this study (balanced accuracy, area under ROC curve, area under Precision-Recall curve, F1 and F2 score). Each target is successively evaluated from all other variables. Results are presented by the classifier (averaging over targets) and by target (averaging over classifiers), for each oversampling method and quality measure. Finally, statistical tests validate the interest of using oversampling methods. The three methods demonstrate a clear advantage in comparison with the imbalanced data set, and SVM-SMOTE provides the best increment.

Keywords: Classification · Oversampling · Risk factors for falls · Imbalanced data

1 Introduction

Preventing falls in the elderly is a major public health issue [16]. The regular evaluation of risk factors for fall (RFF) is a key point in fall prevention [22]. Indeed, giving the right recommendations at the right time reduces the number of risk factors for a given

L. A. Maciaszek et al. (Eds.): ICT4AWE 2021/2022, CCIS 1856, pp. 56–78, 2023.
https://doi.org/10.1007/978-3-031-37496-8_4

person and thus reduces his risk of falling. However, information of the main actionable RFF can not be regularly re-evaluated by medical actors, and their automatic prediction is very interesting. In real life, when a RFF is not identified for a person, it prevents her from receiving the appropriate advice that could help reduce that risk. This case corresponds to a false negative in the context of RFF prediction, showing the importance of reducing false negative. On the other hand, false positive also have to be reduced; indeed, when a RFF is wrongly identified, it may lead to useless cost (for example useless further investigation) and other recommendations may not be followed.

This study was conducted based on a real, imbalanced data set involving 1810 patients from the fall prevention service at Lille's Hospital in France. These patients are placed in that service due to the potential for a significant fall risk. We concentrate on 12 target variables, each of which is a modifiable risk factor for falling, out of the 45 selected variables. We tackle a binary classification problem for every one of them. The presence of the risk factor, which is what the positive value signifies, is what we're trying to find. The 12 risk factors for falling that were chosen are modifiable, which means that there are suggestions and steps that can be taken to lessen each of these risks and the likelihood of falling. The ultimate goal is to create a fall prevention application that offers a limited number of well-suited recommendations for a specific person based on the prediction of fall risk factors. Such a program aims to take part in active aging as well. The positive value in the first group of these 12 targets corresponds to the majority class, whereas the positive value in the second group corresponds to the minority class.

Imbalanced data set occurs when there is an unequal representation of classes. Severe imbalance in data set may raise a problem in machine learning algorithm. These algorithms are more likely to classify a new observation in the majority class since the probability of belonging to the majority class is higher and the algorithm tries to minimize errors [11].

One of the oversampling techniques to address the imbalance issue is SMOTE (synthetic minority oversampling technique) [5]. By increasing minority class examples at random and duplicating them, it seeks to balance the distribution of classes. SMOTE creates new minority instances by combining minority instances that already exist. For the minority class, it creates virtual training records using linear interpolation. For each example in the minority class, one or more of the k-nearest neighbors are randomly chosen to serve as these synthetic training records.

SVM-SMOTE [27] is an additional oversampling technique. After training SVMs on the initial learning set, SVM-SMOTE uses support vectors to roughly estimate the borderline area. Each minority class support vector will be connected at random to a few of its closest neighbors by lines of synthetic data.

Another SMOTE variant that doesn't concentrate on neighbors or borders is adaptive synthetic sampling (ADASYN) [10]. Instead, it emphasizes data density and generates fictitious data in line with that.

We encounter the imbalanced classification problem when our training data's class distribution has a significant skew. Even though the skew may not always be extreme (it can vary), we still consider imbalanced classification to be a problem because it can affect how well our machine learning algorithms perform. One way of handling imbalanced data is oversampling. Oversampling is the duplicating of samples using the minority class. Another way is undersampling which includes deleting samples from majority class. We can also handle the imbalanced data using the hybrid methods which include both oversampling and undersampling.

Medical data classification examines patient medical information to identify illness risks. Data mining techniques were extensively utilised to classify medical data and identify disorders. Numerous approaches now in use make use of different classifiers and feature selection to enhance classification performance. Although the issue of data imbalance must be fixed to improve performance. In a recent study [9], Recurrent Neural Network (RNN) is utilised for classification, and Synthetic Minority Over-sampling Technique (SMOTE) is used to solve the problem of data imbalance. The SMOTE approach uses over- and under-sampling of the attributes based on the k Nearest Neighbor (kNN) algorithm. For categorization, the RNN processes the instance without reference to the prior instance [9].

In the real world, classifying imbalanced data is a difficult task for many data sets. In another study [4], SMOTE, Borderline-SMOTE, and ADASYN are put to the test to see how well they handle data set imbalance and what effect it has on classification accuracy . In this study, a classifier based on gradient boosting is deployed across seven datasets, and F1-Score, AUC, accuracy, recall, and precision are used to gauge classifier performance. Studies for the data sets Mammography, Liver Disorders, Diabetes (Pima Indian), Indian Liver, Habberman, and Immunotherapy indicated that oversampling technique increased accuracy from 2% to 11% . When compared to other oversampling techniques, borderline-SMOTE boosts accuracy more significantly. Surprisingly, Breast Cancer Wisconsin consistently achieves accuracy, whether oversampling is used or not [4].

In this article, we explore the advantages of three oversampling methods to improve the quality of the prediction of 12 target RFF on the basis of a real imbalanced data set. This article is an extended version of [23]. In the current article, we consider three variants of the SMOTE oversampling method, SMOTE, SVM-SMOTE and ADASYN, instead of a single one (SMOTE) in the first article. We use two more classifiers: Support vector machine and Naive Bayes, in addition with the previous four classifiers. Third, we evaluate the classifiers using five metrics instead of four previously (using now the area under the Precision Recall curve in addition). Finally, we present the results by target (averaging over classifiers) and by classifiers (averaging over targets). In the first article, only the results averaged by classifiers were presented. We perform new additional statistical tests to evaluate all these new results.

We first present the data set, together with the selection of 45 variables and 12 target variables and other pre-processing steps. In the second section, we present the methodology that we follow, the three oversampling methods, SMOTE, SMOTE-SVM and ADASYN, the classifiers (Logistic Regression, Random Forest, Bayesian Network, Artificial Neural Network and Naive Bayes), and the quality measures that we use in this study (balanced accuracy, area under ROC curve, area under Precision-Recall curve, F1 and F2 score). The third section includes results and analysis. Results are presented by classifier (averaging over targets) and by target (averaging over classifiers), for each oversampling method and quality measure. In both case, we achieve statistical tests to evaluate the interest of using oversampling methods. The conclusion summarizes the approach and the key points of our analysis.

2 Real Data Set and It's Characteristics

In this section we first illustrate, the process of collecting data and different steps of cleaning this row data. Furthermore, we describe the selected and target variables used in this study.

2.1 Data Source

The study included the 1810 patients who visited the service of fall prevention in University Hospital of Lille, France between January 2005 and December 2018, of which 28% of them are male and 72% are female. The age of patients ranges from 51 years old to 100 years old, with an average age of 81 years old. The patients are admitted to the service for a full day, during which they interact with various medical professionals who each look into a variety of factors, including past falls, diet, physical activity, and medical tests like a balance test. The patient's information is recorded at each step. The patient's case file is then discussed among a group of experts in the subject of elderly falls, and they discuss the best course of action based on the patient's known risk factors. At the end of the day, the patient receives a few suitable recommendations. The patient is invited to return to the hospital six months later for a brief consultation so that the recommendations and the number of falls over the previous six months can be evaluated. This data has been added to the file that was given to us for analysis.

2.2 Preprocessing of Data

Due to the possibility of incorrect outputs from unreliable samples, data pre-processing has a significant impact on the performance of machine learning models [1]. Before the data is pre-processed, the domain should either be thoroughly researched or the domain expert should be included in the data analysis [15]. For a better understanding of the data in this study, we used expert knowledge. The best subset of pertinent data is additionally selected using conventional pre-processing techniques like data set creation, data cleaning, variable sampling, and variable selection. Below, we go into more detail about these steps.

Cleaning. The data may contain a great deal of irrelevant and incomplete variables as well as missing data. To extract information that can be understood from this type of data, cleaning is necessary [7]. We removed variables with unusable content in the first step (free text, very heterogeneous type of values). Then, variables with missing values of more than 30% are eliminated. This cutoff was chosen in order to preserve the quality of the data and keep the important information accessible.

Reducing the Number of Variables. The dimension of data has been a key issue in data analysis. Thus, reducing the size plays an important role in analysing the data [1]. Following an incremental methodology, we start with a small model size, go through the entire process, and then create a second loop where the model and each step can be improved. Here are some general guidelines we have established to cut down on the number of variables:

- In case of two variables X, nbX with X a binary variable and nbX the number of X, we keep only the binary variable (for example, presence of environmental factors);
- in case of two variables X, Y where X is a specific case of Y, meaning that Y is more general, we keep Y (for example, fracture, hip fracture)
- in case of two variables X, Y within the same category but in different sub classes, create a new var $V = X$ or Y (for example, variable $newTrOst$ that regroups biphosphonate and other treatment against osteoporosis)

Moreover, some continuous variables and discrete variables with large domain were transformed into discretized variables with small domain (mainly binary or tertiary).

Missing Values Imputation. Real-world data sets frequently have issues with missing data. Any number of things, such as incomplete variables, missing files, incomplete information, data entry errors, etc., can result in missing data. Missing values should be treated differently depending on the type, generally classified as missing completely at random (MCAR), missing at random (MAR), and "missing not at random (MNAR)", and the cause of the missing values. Various types of techniques, including mean imputation, k nearest neighbors (knn), EM algorithms, Maximum Likelihood Estimation, and Multiple Imputation, have been proposed in numerous studies to impute missing values [19]. Each of these approaches has advantages and disadvantages of its own; we favor knn Imputation since (1) it is very straightforward and user-friendly compared to other methods, and (2) it can be applied regardless of the type of data, whether MCAR, MAR, or MNAR [26] (which is the same situation we have with our data). The number of neighbors are set to five after weighing the different options.

2.3 Description of the Selected Variables

We now go over the list of 45 variables that the aforementioned steps led to (see Table 1). Age, sex, body mass index, and number of falls in the previous six months are direct characteristics of the person and the following 24 variables directly represent the major fall risk factors identified in the ontology about fall prevention [8], which was developed previously with the same service of fall prevention of Lille's Hospital. The remaining 17 variables, which relate to additional fall risk factors and related variables, are as follows: diabete (*diabete*), unipedal stance test more than 5 s (*apUniGt5*), cardiac arrhythmia (*arythm*), cardiopathy (*cardiop*), drives her car (*conduit*), difficulty using the toilets (*difWC*), diuretic (*diuretiq*), avoids going out by fear of falling (*evitSort*), get up and go test greater than 20 s (*GUGOgt20*), high blood pressure (*HTA*), lives in a retirement home (*maisRet*), podiatric problem (*pbPodo*), pneumopathy (*pneumo*), urologic pathology (*pathUro*), goes out of his/her house (*sort*), environmental factors (*factEnv*), tobacco (*tabac*). All the variables are binary (yes: 1, no: 0), except the variables *nbMed3* and *BMI4* (discretized in 3 or 4 intervals).

Table 1. List of variables regrouped by categories.

Variable description	short name	Variable description	short name
personal characteristics		predisposing factors	
age greater than 80	$agegt80$	balance impairment	$trEq$
sex	sex	gait impairment	$trMar$
body mass index	$BMI4$	sarcopenia	$dfOuFaiM$
$\geq$ falls in last 6 months	$nbChu2$	activities of daily living <5	$ADLinf5$
precipitating factors		depression	dep
number of drugs	$nbMed3$	stroke or TIA	$AVCAIT$
orthostatic hypotension	$newHypoT$	parkinson disease (PD) or	$parkOuSP$
at least 1 psychotropic drug	$gt1psych$	parkinsonian syndrome	
severity factors		hearing disorder	$trAudit$
fracture during a fall or	$fracturA$	arthritis or rheumatoid	$arthPoly$
vertebral collapse		dementia	$demence$
confirmed osteoporosis	$osteoConf$	vision disorder	$trVision$
anti osteoporosis treatment	$newTrOst$	neurological disorder other	$auTrNeur$
lives alone	$vitSeul$	than stroke, TIA, PD or	
		dementia	
remained on the ground for	$gt1hSol$	behavioral factors	
more than one hour		walking aids	$utiATM$
was able to get up off	$aSuSeRel$	alcohol consumption	alc
floor on his own		fear of falling	$peurTom$

2.4 Variables Selected as Target

Twelve target variables have been chosen for prediction from the list of variables in Table 1 because it is important to assess their value. Indeed, outside of specialized fall prevention services, information about these risk factors is frequently unavailable. It's interesting for a number of reasons to assess how likely it is that these factors will exist in the present or the future:

1. All of these factors go into determining fall risk, and since they are all modifiable, it is possible to take certain steps to lower that risk.
2. Since depression, dementia, orthostatic hypotension, Parkinson disease, and other neurological disorders are not always diagnosed, assessing the likelihood of their occurrence enables one to alert a doctor to the need for additional testing.
3. In order to prevent osteoporosis and loss of autonomy, it's interesting to evaluate their likelihood of developing positively in the future even if they don't already exist.

Table 2 provides the list of target variables and their prevalence. We distinguish two groups among these target variables:

– Group *M0* - the risk factors with majority class 0
– Group *M1* - the risk factors with majority class 1.

The target variables are listed by decreasing order of their prevalence.

Table 2. Target Risk Factors for Fall and their group.

Group	Target variable	prevalence of the RFF	Group	Target variable	prevalence of the RFF
M1	trMar	83.3%	M0	demence	42.2%
M1	peurTom	77.2%	M0	newHypoT	32.5%
M1	trEq	74.5%	M0	dep	28.4%
M1	auTrNeur	70.1%	M0	ADLinf5	25.5%
M1	dFouFaiM	66%	M0	osteoConf	19.2%
M1	nbChu2	58.4%	M0	parkOuSP	16.5%

3   Methodology

In this article, we compare the outcomes of classifiers that evaluate 12 different target risk factors using imbalanced data and data that has been balanced using an oversampling method. A general overview of the methodology is shown in Fig. 1.

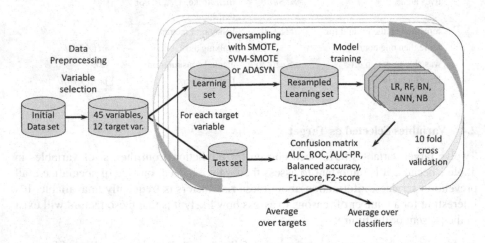

Fig. 1. Methodology.

We employ 10-fold cross validation, where 90% of the data is used as the training set and 10% as the test set for each fold. The balancing method is only applied to the training set when using oversampling techniques. While balancing the test set may artificially enhance the results, the situation would change if the classifier were used in actual situations.

The various classifiers and measurements used in our study are presented below, along with a description of the balancing methods.

3.1   Oversampling Techniques

Resampling methods consist in adding or removing samples from the training dataset. We use oversampling methods, that duplicate or create new synthetic samples in the minority class in order to increase the number of cases of the minority class and change the class distribution. We present below the three methods that we use in this work.

SMOTE. By using an interpolation method, SMOTE [5] generates fresh observations from the minority class. Instead of extracting data at random, the minority class is over-sampled by creating synthetic examples. SMOTE stops data from being duplicated. The new observations produced using the minority class will differ from the original observations in some ways. In order to subtract one of the k samples from the original minority instances, the algorithm first determines the k nearest samples for each minority instance. Then it creates a new instance by multiplying the difference by alpha, where alpha is a random number between (0,1), and adds that instance to the data matrix.

SMOTE-SVM. The supervised classifier support vector machine (SVM) algorithm is frequently used to address classification and regression issues. SVM was first introduced as an upgrade to the maximum - margin classifier, which is limited to working with the data that is simply linearly separable [18]. Since data points from different classes are infrequently clearly distinguished from one another, linear classification can result in significant misclassification. SVM can handle these frequently encountered situations because it maps the feature set into a greater dimensional space where non-linear data samples are converted into points that can be separated along a linear path. Consequently, the boundaries between data points belonging to various classes are more distinct [2]. The high-dimensional space is created by non-linearly expanding the original space using the kernel function. In addition to linear kernels, polynomial kernels and radial basis function kernels are other varieties of kernel functions. Equations 1, 2, and 3 describe them, respectively, where k() stands for the kernel function and the result is represented by the product of two sample vectors z_i and z_i'. We have used linear kernel function because generally it is used in the literature. The reinvented feature space is denoted by the symbol and the product of the two vectors is written as $\phi z_i \phi z_i'$ [17].

$$k\left(z_i, z_i'\right) = \sum_{j=1}^{p} z_{ij} z_{ij}' \tag{1}$$

$$k\left(z_i, z_i'\right) = \left(1 + \sum_{j=1}^{p} z_{ij} z_{ij}'\right)^d \tag{2}$$

$$k\left(z_i, z_i'\right) = \exp\left(-\gamma \sum_{j=1}^{p} (z_{ij} - z_{ij}')^2\right) \tag{3}$$

SVM-SMOTE is a variant of SMOTE in which SVM approach is used to determine the classification errors rather than K-nearest neighbors. After training SVMs on the initial training set, SVM-SMOTE uses support vectors to roughly estimate the borderline area. Every minority class support vector will be connected at random to a few of its closest neighbors by lines of synthetic data. More data are synthesized away from the area of class overlap in SVM-SMOTE especially in comparison to the SMOTE, which is unique. It concentrates more on how the data is divided [27].

ADASYN. Another SMOTE variant that doesn't concentrate on neighbors or borders is adaptive synthetic sampling (ADASYN). Instead, it emphasizes data density and generates fictitious data in line with that. The density of the minority class is inversely related to the generation of synthetic data. This means that where minority class density is low within feature space, more synthetic data are generated, whereas where minority class density is high, few (or no) such data are generated. In other words, the frequency of the creation of synthetic data is higher in the feature space where the minority class is less dense; otherwise, no synthetic data are produced [10].

Let n_{min} and n_{maj} represent the number of minority class samples and the number of majority class samples, respectively. Beginning with an assessment of the degree of class imbalance, which is defined as $d = \frac{n_{min}}{n_{maj}}$.

The number of synthetic datapoints that must be generated is determined if d is less than the actual maximum acceptable threshold for imbalanced class degree. It is stated by $G = (n_{min} - n_{maj}) * \gamma$, where the expected balance level following resampling is indicated by the $\gamma \epsilon [0, 1]$. In a subsequent step, the density distribution $r_i = \frac{\delta_i}{k}$ is calculated for each observation x_i belonging to the minority class.

The nearest neighbors to sample x_i of the minority and majority classes are determined by the k and δ_i parameters, respectively. The Euclidean distance metric is used to determine which samples are the most similar. The normalized form of the density distribution, $r_i^{'} = \frac{r_i}{\sum_{i=1}^{n_{min}} r_i}$, can also be used to express it.

Calculating how many synthetic data samples g_i are necessary to create for observation x_i is the last step. This is defined by $g_i = G * r_i^{'}$.

Then, each synthetic sample s_i for observation x_i is created using $s_i = (x_{yi} - x_i) * random(0, 1)$, where $(x_{yi} - x_i)$ denotes the difference vector between sample x_i and a sample drawn at random from the k-nearest neighbors.

3.2   Classifiers

The six different classifiers used for the analysis are presented below.

Logistic Regression (LR). The technique of logistic regression has grown in significance in the field of machine learning. It enables to categorize incoming information based on previous data by examining the correlation between one or more already present independent variables and forecasts a dependent data variable. Furthermore, it reduces complicated probability calculations to simple arithmetic problems. Although the calculation itself is admittedly somewhat complicated, most of the tedious work is automated by modern statistical software. This helps to significantly reduce the impact of confounding factors and dramatically clarifies analyzing the impact of various variables. The algorithms become more accurate at making predictions classifications within data sets as new pertinent data is added [12].

Random Forest (RF). The wisdom of crowds is the basic idea behind random forest, which is a straightforward but effective idea. A random forest is made up of numerous individual decision trees that work together as an ensemble. The key is the low correlation between models. Uncorrelated models have the ability to generate ensemble predictions that are more accurate than any of the individual predictions, much like investments with low correlations (like stocks and bonds) combine to form a portfolio that is greater than the sum of its parts. As long as they don't consistently all err in the same direction, the trees shield each other from their individual errors, which accounts for this wonderful effect. Many trees will be right while some may be wrong, allowing the group of trees to move in the right direction. More precisely, every single tree in the random forest spits out a class prediction, and the classification that receives the most votes becomes the prediction made by our model [3].

Support Vector Machine (SVM). uses supervised learning to classify or predict the behavior of groups of data. The algorithms create hyperplanes (lines) to divide the groups into various configurations. It works to maximize the boundary around the hyperplane and maintain equality between the two sides in order to achieve the best data separation. An SVM needs labeled training data, just like other supervised machine learning algorithms. The training materials are organized into distinct groups and classified separately at various locations in space. SVMs can also be used to perform unsupervised learning after processing a large number of training examples. Also, SVMs are referred to as non-probabilistic, binary linear classifiers based on these functions. It has the ability to employ techniques like Platt Scaling in probabilistic classification settings [13].

Artificial Neural Networks (ANN). In some ways, neural networks resemble how the human brain learns. Neurons are the building blocks of an artificial neural network, and they in turn create layers. Each layer has a unique nonlinear activation function that aids in the learning process and the layer's output. The output of each layer is transferred to the following layer. Each epoch updates the weights connected to the neurons and in charge of the overall predictions. Several optimisers are used to optimize the learning rate. Every Neural Network has a cost function, which is minimized as learning progresses. Then, the weights that produce the best results according to the cost function are used. The relationship between the neuron's input and output can be described as follows:

$$y = f(\sum_{i=1}^{n} w_i x_i + b),$$

where x_i denotes the input signal, w_i denotes the weight, y denotes the output, b denotes the threshold, and f denotes the activation function. These neurons are linked together to form ANN.

The ANN prediction algorithm has the advantage of not requiring an exact mathematical relationship between input and output parameters. Incorporation of spatial information, for example, does not necessitate its explicit parameterization. Another advantage of the ANN prediction algorithm is that as more data sets become available, the training sample sizes can easily be increased. The computational time of the ANN prediction algorithm rapidly increases as the number of parameters (layers) increases [21,25].

Naive Bayes (NB). The supervised machine learning algorithms that are primarily employed for classification also include Naive Bayes. It is referred to as "naive" because of the presumption that the input features used to build the model are independent. Therefore, altering one input feature will have no impact on the others. It is therefore naive in the sense that it is highly unlikely that this assumption is accurate. Furthermore, it is based on Bayes theorem and are often suitable for very high-dimensional data sets. Bayes theorem can be described as follows:

$$P(A|B) = \frac{P(B|A) * P(A)}{P(B)}$$

where, $P(A|B)$ is called posterior which represents probability of hypothesis A on the observed event B, and $P(B|A)$ is called likelihood which means probability of the evidence given that the probability of a hypothesis is true, and $P(A)$ is called prior which represents the probability of hypothesis before observing the evidence, and $P(B)$ is marginal that represents probability of evidence [20]. We have used multinomial naive bayes (MNB) for our analysis because our data is in nominal form.

Bayesian Networks (BN). A particular kind of probabilistic graphical model called Bayesian networks (BNs) [6, 14] is an effective tool for capturing uncertainty and evaluating risk. The Bayes theorem and conditional probability theory are used to structure BNs. By computing the posterior probability of input data given new data input in a specific state, Bayes' theorem allows us to reason in a logical, rational, and consistent manner. More formally, a Bayesian network is a graphical representation of a set of variables U = $\{X_1, X_2, \ldots, X_n\}$ with a joint probability that can be factorized as follows:

$$P(X_1, X_2, ..., X_n) = \prod_{i=1}^{n} P(X_i | Parent(X_i))$$

where $Parent(X_i)$ is the set of variables that correspond to direct predecessors of X_i in the graph. It consists of a directed acyclic graph graph where each node represents a distinct random variable and each edge represents a conditional dependency. It also contains a set of the local probability distributions for each node/variable.

Baseline Classifier. In order to evaluate a classifier, we compare it to a baseline classifier which always predicts the majority class. For the target variables in group M0, the baseline always predict 0, whereas it always predict 1 for targets of group M1.

3.3 Evaluation Metrics

A number of techniques can be used to assess machine learning models. Analytical research is anticipated to expand with the use of a variety of evaluation tools. Our data are imbalanced, so we use the F1-score, F2-score, area under ROC curve (AUC-ROC), area under precision recall curve (AUC-PR) and balanced accuracy to evaluate the performance of a given classifier. Reducing false negatives is the first goal in fall prevention because they correspond to positive cases where the risk factor is not found (no recommendation is given to patient at risk). Since the majority class and the minority class are given the same importance, we do not use accuracy because it is typically inappropriate for data that are unbalanced.

A classification model's (or "classifier's") performance on a set of test data for which the true values are known is described by a confusion matrix. Shown in Table 3, where TN (TP) is number of negative (positive) samples correctly classified, and FP (FN) is number of negative (positive) samples incorrectly classified as positive (negative) [24].

Table 3. A confusion matrix.

	Predict Positive	Predict Negative
Actual Positive	TP	FN
Actual Negative	FP	TN

Balanced Accuracy. Both binary and multi-class classification use balanced accuracy. It is widely used when working with imbalanced data, or when one of the target classes shows up much more frequently than the other. It is the arithmetic mean of sensitivity and specificity.

$$Balanced\ Accuracy = \frac{1}{2}(\frac{TP}{TP+FN} + \frac{TN}{TN+FP})$$

Area Under ROC Curve (AUC-ROC). Area Under the Receiver Operator Characteristic Curve provides a summary of the trade-offs between true positive rates and false-positive rates for the given predictive model. When the observations are evenly distributed among the classes, ROC produces good results.

Area Under PR Curve (AUC-PR). A simple graph with precision values on the y-axis and recall values on the x-axis is what makes up a PR curve.

$$precision = \frac{TP}{TP+FP}; \ recall = \frac{TP}{TP+FN}$$

Remember that precision is also known as the Positive Predictive Value (PPV).

Remark that for a target variable in group M0, the precision of the baseline classifier is undefined and recall is null.

The F-score uses precision and recall to assess a test's accuracy in binary classification analysis.

F1 Score. F1-score maintains a balance between recall and precision. F1 score (also known as F-measure, or balanced F-score) is an error metric which measures model performance by calculating the harmonic mean of precision and recall for the minority positive class.

$$F1 - score = \frac{2 * precision * recall}{recall + precision}$$

For variables in group M0, F1 and F2-score of the baseline classifier equals 0. Usually, the majority class is referred to as the negative outcome, which is the case in group M0, and F-scores are frequently used in those case. We have to be careful about their interpretation when the majority class is the positive outcome.

F2 Score. The F2 score is based on the premise that recall should be given more weight than precision. As a result, the F2 score is more appropriate.

$$F2 - score = \frac{5 * precision * recall}{4 * recall + precision}$$

4   Analysis of Results Using Oversampling Techniques

We have compared the outcomes for six different classifiers namely Logistic Regression (LR), Random Forest (RF), Artificial Neural Networks (ANN), Support Vector Machine (SVM), Naive Bayes (NB), and Bayesian Networks (BN), in order to see the differences between utilizing imbalanced data for classifications and using the data after balancing with various balancing approaches, with the aim of predicting separately 12 target variables. In this section, first, we show the results for each classifiers when averaging over all targets. Second, we present the results for each target when averaging over each classifiers. In each case, we demonstrate the statistical t-test to summarize our finding.

4.1   Results by Classifier, Averaging over Targets

Figs. 2, 3, 4, 5 and 6 present the results when averaging over all targets for each classifier regarding (1) AUC-ROC, (2) AUC-PR, (3) Balanced accuracy, (4) F1-score, (5) F2-score, using imbalanced and balanced data (with the above balancing methods). Horizontal axis represents the different classifiers used. Vertical axis represents the percentage of increment or decrement from the baseline results.

Regarding the results of all measures except F2-score (Figs. 2, 3, 4 and 5), it can be seen that when using unbalanced data, the average improvement regarding the baseline classifier is variable depending on the classifier. For example, regarding AUC-ROC (Fig. 2), ANN improves the baseline by about 6 points on average while the Bayesian network improves it by about 16 points when using the unbalanced data. On the other hand, the use of an oversampling method makes the improvement of all classifier very similar with differences of only a few points.

A second remark is that using an oversampling technique provides improvement for all classifier except Bayesian network that performs generally better when using unbalanced data, and for all measures, except F2-score.

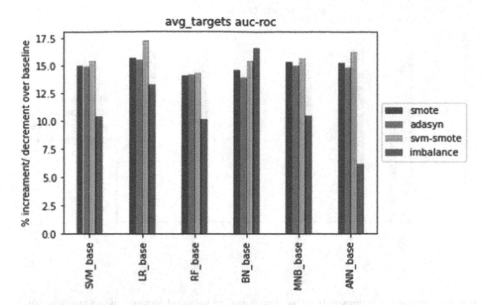

Fig. 2. Percentage of increment from baseline regarding AUC-ROC, when averaging over all targets for each classifier, using imbalanced and balanced data with SMOTE, ADASYN and SVM-SMOTE respectively.

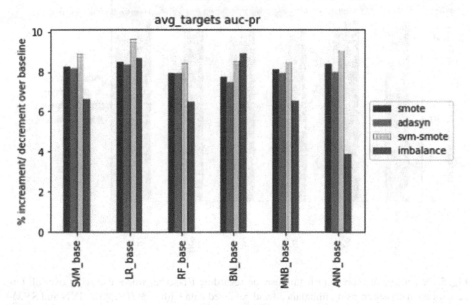

Fig. 3. Percentage of increment from baseline regarding AUC-PR, when averaging over all targets for each classifier, using imbalanced and balanced data with SMOTE, ADASYN and SVM-SMOTE respectively.

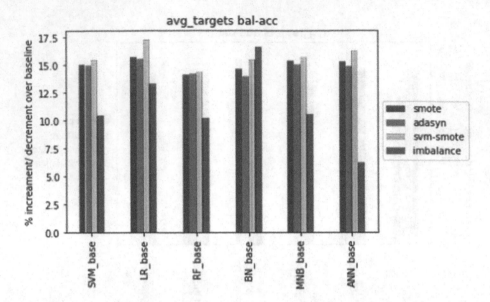

Fig. 4. Percentage of increment from baseline regarding balanced accuracy, when averaging over all targets for each classifier, using imbalanced and balanced data with SMOTE, ADASYN and SVM-SMOTE respectively.

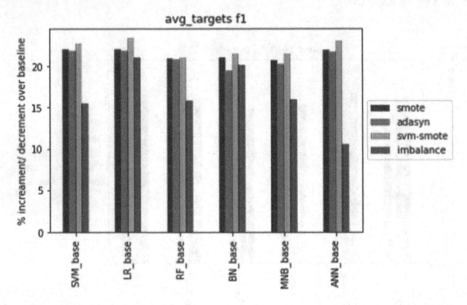

Fig. 5. Percentage of increment from baseline regarding F1-score, when averaging over all targets for each classifier, using imbalanced and balanced data with SMOTE, ADASYN and SVM-SMOTE respectively.

A third point to be noted is that SVM-SMOTE always lead to a slightly better improvement than SMOTE and ADASYN.

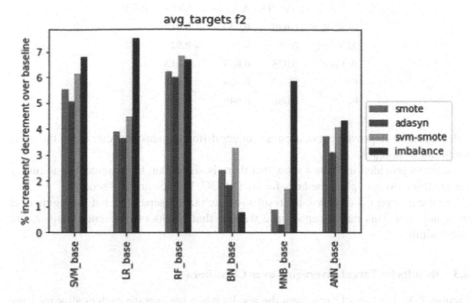

Fig. 6. Percentage of increment from baseline regarding F2-score, when averaging over all targets for each classifier, using imbalanced and balanced data with SMOTE, ADASYN and SVM-SMOTE respectively.

Regarding F2-score, no oversampling method can improve the results, whatever the classifier, except for Bayesian network.

A first conclusion is that results of different classifiers are rather similar for all the considered measures, except Bayesian network whose results using unbalanced data are comparable with results of other classifiers when using balanced data.

In order to evaluate the significance of the improvement after using oversampling techniques, we present the p-values below.

4.2 Statistical Tests When Averaging over Targets

We now use t-test to check the significance of improvement in the accuracy after using the oversampling techniques. We use classification techniques, SVM, LR, RF, BN, MNB and ANN, to classify the averaged target variable for the original (imbalance) dataset and obtain the corresponding values of accuracy measures; AUC-ROC, AUC-PR, Bal-acc, F1 and F2 scores. Similarly, we obtain the values of each of these accuracy measures after using the oversampling techniques; SMOTE, ADASYN and SVM-SMOTE, corresponding to each classifier. We then use one tailed t-test to test the null hypothesis which states that there is no improvement in the accuracy by using oversampling techniques. If the p-value is smaller than 0.05 then we reject the null hypothesis and conclude that the improvement is significant. Table 4 presents the p-values of one

Table 4. Average over targets.

	p-values		
	SMOTE	ADASYN	SVM-SMOTE
AUC-ROC	**0.025**	**0.033**	**0.013**
AUC-PR	0.08	0.1	**0.022**
Bal-acc	**0.025**	**0.033**	**0.013**
F1	**0.013**	**0.024**	**0.008**
F2	0.086	**0.046**	0.199

tailed t-test for improvement of accuracy under different measures after using the over-sampling techniques.

Results provided in Table 4 show that there is significant improvement in accuracy for the three oversampling methods for AUC-ROC, Bal-acc and F1- score.

In the next part, we analyse the results for each target separately but averaging over the classifiers. This makes sense since we saw that results of different classifiers are rather similar.

4.3   Results by Target, Averaging over Classifiers

Figures 7, 8, 9, 10 and 11 represent the results when we average each quality measure over the five classifiers for each target, using imbalanced and balanced data (with different balancing methods) respectively. Horizontal axis represents the different targets predicted. Vertical axis represents the percentage of increment or decrement from the baseline results.

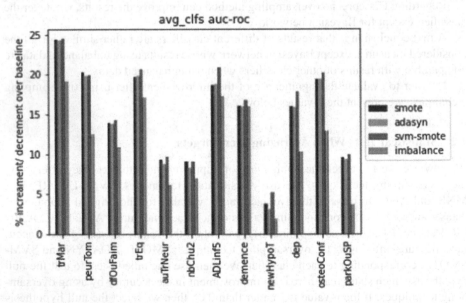

Fig. 7. Percentage of increment or decrement from the baseline results regarding AUC-ROC when averaging over classifiers for each target.

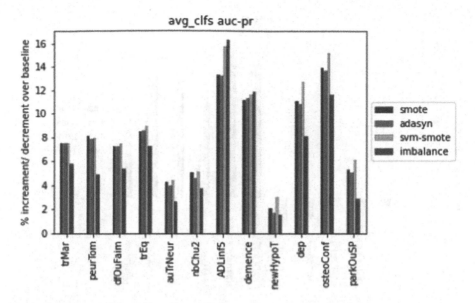

Fig. 8. Percentage of increment or decrement from the baseline results regarding AUC-PR when averaging over classifiers for each target.

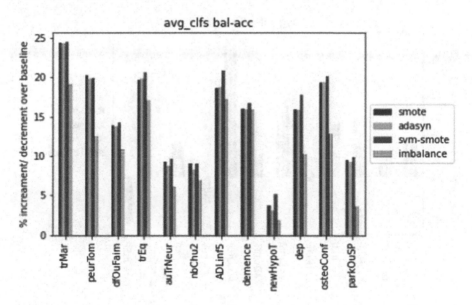

Fig. 9. Percentage of increment or decrement from the baseline results regarding balanced accuracy when averaging over classifiers for each target.

Regarding AUC-ROC, AUC-PR and balanced accuracy (Figs. 7, 8 and 9), using balanced data provide better results than imbalanced data for 10 targets out of 12 whatever the balancing method (the prediction of the variables *demence* and *ADLinf5* is not, or

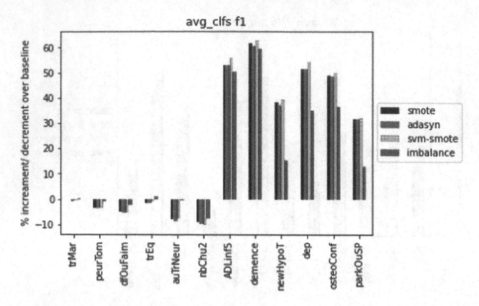

Fig. 10. Percentage of increment or decrement from the baseline results regarding F1-score when averaging over classifiers for each target.

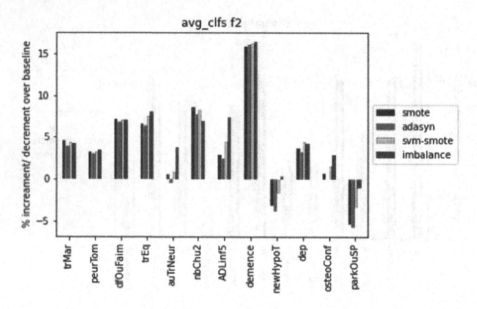

Fig. 11. Percentage of increment or decrement from the baseline results regarding F2-score when averaging over classifiers for each target.

very slightly, improved for those measures). Let's also remark that the prediction of the variable *newHypoT* is hardly better than the baseline, whatever the data set. Looking more in detail, this result also not depends on the classifier; thanks to a discussion with an expert, it appears that some important variables that could help to predict hypotension are not part of the 45 selected variables. For these three measures (AUC-ROC, AUC-PR and balanced accuracy), the balancing using SVM-SMOTE most often provides slightly better improvement than SMOTE and ADASYN.

Regarding F1-score, Fig. 10 clearly shows the difference between targets of group M1 (on the left) whose majority class is 1, and those of group M0, on the right. As mentioned above, F1-score is usually used for targets with majority class 0. When majority class is 0, since the F1-score of the baseline equals zero, the difference of the F1-score of any other classifier and the baseline is always positive. For the targets in group M0, the use of oversampling method clearly improves the F1-score, except for the two variables mentioned above (*demence* and *newHypoT*).

4.4   Statistical Tests When Averaging over Classifiers

We use t-test to check the significance of improvement in the results for each of the 12 target variables after using the oversampling techniques, averaging over all the classifiers. We use classification techniques, SVM, LR, RF, BN, MNB and ANN, to classify target variables for the original (imbalance) dataset and obtain the values of evaluation measures; AUC-ROC, AUC-PR, Bal-acc, F1 and F2-scores for each target variable. Similarly, we obtain the values of each of these evaluation measures after using the oversampling techniques, SMOTE, ADASYN and SVM-SMOTE, for each of the target variables. After averaging the values of the evaluation measures of different classifiers, we use one tailed t-test to test the null hypothesis which states that there is no improvement in the results by using oversampling techniques. If the p-value is smaller than 0.05 then we reject the null hypothesis and conclude that the improvement is significant. Table 5 presents p-values for each of the oversampling techniques using all evaluation measures except f1 score.

Table 5. Average over classifiers.

	p-values		
	SMOTE	ADASYN	SVM-SMOTE
AUC-ROC	0	0	0
AUC-PR	0.011	0.018	0
Bal-acc	0	0	0
F2	*0.011*	*0.003*	*0.022*

It is clear from table 5 that there is significant improvement in all evaluation measures presented for all the target variables. Moreover, Fig. 11 clearly shows that f2 score is better when using imbalanced data. This difference is significant as confirmed by the t-test (see italic values). Below in Table 6 we show the p-values for group M0 using f1 score when averaging over classifiers. As can be seen in Fig. 5, F1-scores for targets in group M1 (whose majority value is 1) are most often negative, compared with the

F1-score for baseline which is always 0). So, we only perform the t-test using F1-score for target variables in group M0. The results of t-test shows that there is significant improvement in F1-score when using oversampling techniques.

Table 6. p-values for group M0 using f1 score when averaging over classifiers.

	SMOTE	ADASYN	SVM-SMOTE
F1	0.007	0.009	0.004

5   Conclusion

In this study, we have discussed the problem of classification with imbalanced data and analysed the impact of three oversampling methods SMOTE, SMOTE-SVM and ADASYN. A real data set from Lille's Hospital in France, corresponding to 1810 patients from the service of fall prevention is used, which is highly imbalanced. In order to see the difference when using imbalanced data versus the data after balancing with given oversampling methods, we have compared the results using several classifiers namely Logistic Regression, Random Forest, Artificial Neural Networks, Naive Bayes, and Bayesian Networks. To evaluate the performance of different classifiers, we use several measures: Balanced Accuracy, F1-score, F2-score, area under the Precision-Recall curve, and area under the Receiver Operating Characteristic curve. We have presented the results summarised by classifier (averaging over targets) and by target (averaging over classifiers).

As observed, results of different classifiers used on Lille's data set when averaging over all targets are rather similar for all the considered measures, except Bayesian network whose results using imbalanced data are comparable with results of other classifiers when using balanced data. Similarly, results of different targets when averaging over all classifiers shows the improvement in each type of measure used when using the balanced data with oversampling methods versus using imbalanced data. In addition, we also see that SVM-SMOTE gives slightly better results as compared to other oversampling techniques.

Furthermore, the one-tailed t-test confirms our findings that when averaging over targets there is significant improvements in AUC-ROC, AUC-PR, F1-score, and balanced accuracy for all classifiers when using oversampling methods. Also from one-tailed t-test when averaging over classifiers we can conclude that there is significant improvements in AUC-ROC, AUC-PR, and balanced accuracy when using oversampling methods. For F1-score the results are dominated by target variables in group M0.

Also, recall that fall prevention requires to provide a small number of recommendations depending on the risk factors present for a person. Thus the evaluation of risk factors is the basis of fall prevention. Also, in real life imbalanced data sets are very common. So based on the results and discussion presented we propose the use of balancing techniques specifically SVM-SMOTE as a possible solution to the problem of data imbalance.

References

1. Alasadi, S.A., Bhaya, W.S.: Review of data preprocessing techniques in data mining. J. Eng. Appl. Sci. **12**(16), 4102–4107 (2017)
2. Apsemidis, A., Psarakis, S.: Support vector machines: a review and applications in statistical process monitoring. Data Anal. Appl. 3: Comput. Classif. Financ. Stat. Stochastic Methods **5**, 123–144 (2020)
3. Azar, A.T., Elshazly, H.I., Hassanien, A.E., Elkorany, A.M.: A random forest classifier for lymph diseases. Comput. Methods Programs Biomed. **113**(2), 465–473 (2014)
4. Cahyana, N., Khomsah, S., Aribowo, A.S.: Improving imbalanced dataset classification using oversampling and gradient boosting. In: 2019 5th International Conference on Science in Information Technology (ICSITech), pp. 217–222. IEEE (2019)
5. Chawla, N.V., Bowyer, K.W., Hall, L.O., Kegelmeyer, W.P.: SMOTE: synthetic minority over-sampling technique. J. Artif. Intell. Res. **16**, 321–357 (2002)
6. Cheng, J., Greiner, R.: Comparing Bayesian network classifiers. arXiv preprint arXiv:1301.6684 (2013)
7. Chu, X., Ilyas, I.F., Krishnan, S., Wang, J.: Data cleaning: overview and emerging challenges. In: Proceedings of the 2016 International Conference on Management of Data, pp. 2201–2206 (2016)
8. Delcroix, V., Essghaier, F., Oliveira, K., Pudlo, P., Gaxatte, C., Puisieux, F.: Towards a fall prevention system design by using ontology. En lien avec les Journées francophones d'Ingénierie des Connaissances, Plate-Forme PFIA (2019)
9. Francis, S., Prasad, P., Zahoor-Ul-Huq, s.: Medical data classification based on smote and recurrent neural network. Int. J. Eng. Adv. Technol. **9** (2020). https://doi.org/10.35940/ijeat.C5444.029320
10. He, H., Bai, Y., Garcia, E.A., Li, S.: ADASYN: adaptive synthetic sampling approach for imbalanced learning. In: 2008 IEEE International Joint Conference on Neural Networks (IEEE World Congress on Computational Intelligence), pp. 1322–1328. IEEE (2008)
11. He, H., Garcia, E.A.: Learning from imbalanced data. IEEE Trans. Knowl. Data Eng. **21**(9), 1263–1284 (2009)
12. Hosmer, D.W., Jr., Lemeshow, S., Sturdivant, R.X.: Applied Logistic Regression, vol. 398. Wiley, Hoboken (2013)
13. Huang, X., Shi, L., Suykens, J.A.: Support vector machine classifier with pinball loss. IEEE Trans. Pattern Anal. Mach. Intell. **36**(5), 984–997 (2013)
14. Koller, D., Friedman, N.: Probabilistic Graphical Models: Principles and Techniques. MIT Press, Cambridge (2009)
15. Kotsiantis, S.B., Kanellopoulos, D., Pintelas, P.E.: Data preprocessing for supervised leaning. Int. J. Comput. Sci. **1**(2), 111–117 (2006)
16. Lin, J.T., Lane, J.M.: Falls in the elderly population. Phys. Med. Rehabil. Clin. **16**(1), 109–128 (2005)
17. Nalepa, J., Kawulok, M.: Selecting training sets for support vector machines: a review. Artif. Intell. Rev. **52**(2), 857–900 (2019)
18. Obiedat, R., et al.: Sentiment analysis of customers' reviews using a hybrid evolutionary SVM-based approach in an imbalanced data distribution. IEEE Access **10**, 22260–22273 (2022)
19. Rahman, M.M., Davis, D.N.: Machine learning-based missing value imputation method for clinical datasets. In: Yang, G.C., Ao, S., Gelman, L. (eds.) IAENG Transactions on Engineering Technologies. Lecture Notes in Electrical Engineering, vol. 229, pp. 245–257. Springer, Dordrecht (2013). https://doi.org/10.1007/978-94-007-6190-2_19

20. Rish, I., et al.: An empirical study of the naive bayes classifier. In: IJCAI 2001 Workshop on Empirical Methods in Artificial Intelligence, vol. 3, pp. 41–46 (2001)
21. Russell, S., Norvig, P.: Artificial intelligence: a modern approach (2002)
22. Sihag, G., et al.: Evaluation of risk factors for fall in elderly using Bayesian networks: a case study. Comput. Methods Program. Biomed. Update **1**, 100035 (2021)
23. Sihag., G., et al.: Evaluation of risk factors for fall in elderly people from imbalanced data using the oversampling technique smote. In: Proceedings of the 8th International Conference on Information and Communication Technologies for Ageing Well and e-Health - ICT4AWE, pp. 50–58. INSTICC, SciTePress (2022). https://doi.org/10.5220/0011041200003188
24. Sokolova, M., Japkowicz, N., Szpakowicz, S.: Beyond accuracy, F-score and ROC: a family of discriminant measures for performance evaluation. In: Sattar, A., Kang, B. (eds.) AI 2006. LNCS (LNAI), vol. 4304, pp. 1015–1021. Springer, Heidelberg (2006). https://doi.org/10.1007/11941439_114
25. Wu, T.K., Huang, S.C., Meng, Y.R.: Evaluation of ANN and SVM classifiers as predictors to the diagnosis of students with learning disabilities. Expert Syst. Appl. **34**(3), 1846–1856 (2008)
26. Zhang, S., Li, X., Zong, M., Zhu, X., Cheng, D.: Learning k for KNN classification. ACM Trans. Intell. Syst. Technol. (TIST) **8**(3), 1–19 (2017)
27. Zheng, X.: SMOTE variants for imbalanced binary classification: heart disease prediction. University of California, Los Angeles (2020)

Exergaming with the GAME2AWE Platform: Design, Implementation and Evaluation Insights

Christos Goumopoulos[1]([✉]) and Georgios Koumanakos[2]

[1] Information and Communication Systems Engineering Department, University of the Aegean, Samos, Greece
goumop@aegean.gr
[2] Frontida Zois, Patras, Greece
gkoumanakos@frontidazois.gr

Abstract. In this paper, the GAME2AWE platform is introduced that combines multiple technologies and intelligent software to create adaptive gaming experiences aimed at improving the physical and cognitive functioning of the elderly. The GAME2AWE platform supports the claim that game-based exercising (i.e., exergaming) provides significant health benefits for older adults. Enhancing strength and balance through exercises, in particular, is an effective action to prevent falls. Analysis of the relevant literature and the use of qualitative methods (e.g., multidisciplinary focus group) have provided guidance for the design of the exergames. Insights on the implementation of the exergaming platform are also provided. An evaluation study was conducted with twelve participants (N = 12) including end users (i.e., healthy elderly) and healthcare experts. The evaluation examined the GAME2AWE platform in terms of usability, usefulness, safety and applicability. The positive results provide evidence that the GAME2AWE platform is comfortable and fun to use, the exercises integrated in the exergames are safe to perform and overall the platform could assist the elderly to reinforce their strength and balance and consequently reduce frailties and fall risk.

Keywords: Exergames · Fall risk · Focus group · Kinect sensor · Virtual reality Smart floor · Elderly · Usability evaluation

1 Introduction

Elderly have an increased risk of falling. Almost 30% of the elderly over 65 years of age experience various injuries caused by falls and this figure increases to 50% in elderly over 80 [1]. Representative injury examples are contusions, twists, injured bones and haunch fractures, while more severe falls can be fatal. Fall sufferers experience depression, loss of independence, confusion and fear of activities [2]. This reduces potential daily activities resulting in further physical and cognitive deterioration.

Studies have shown that combining strength and balance exercises along with walking is quite powerful for fall reduction and injury prevention in the elderly [3]. Likewise, other researchers argue that physical exercise and strength training in combination with

© The Author(s), under exclusive license to Springer Nature Switzerland AG 2023
L. A. Maciaszek et al. (Eds.): ICT4AWE 2021/2022, CCIS 1856, pp. 79–102, 2023.
https://doi.org/10.1007/978-3-031-37496-8_5

activities such as Tai Chi, walking or dancing can improve balance and decrease falls in the elderly [4].

Consequently, interventions based on new technologies that can support elderly to be active are of great importance and can improve the quality of life and well-being of older people. The term exergame stems from the combination of the words "exercising" and "game" and indicates exercise through playing games. An exergame is a form of digital game that requires aerobic physical effort, which exceeds the level of sedentary activity and includes activities related to strength, balance or flexibility, by the player who determines the outcome of the game [5]. Exergames combine physical activity with entertainment and can benefit older adults physically, cognitively and socially. It's an enjoyable and fun method of meeting a set goal of physical activity or encouraging inactive people to become more active.

In this paper, the GAME2AWE platform is introduced that combines hardware and intelligent software to create adaptive gaming experiences aimed at improving the physical and cognitive functioning of the elderly. GAME2AWE supports the claim that game-based exercise provides significant health benefits for older adults. Enhancing strength and balance through exercises, in particular, is an effective action to prevent falls. In addition, cognitive improvements and mental benefits for the elderly can be achieved through physical exercising. Studies show that weekly physical activity can help prevent mild cognitive impairment or prevent it from progressing to dementia [6].

The innovation of the proposed platform is found in the combination of three technologies: the smart floor, movement and gesture recognition and virtual reality. Technologies that do not require the user to use a complex environment such as the proposed smart floor are more suitable for use by the elderly to improve their physical condition and cognitive level. Furthermore, incorporating into the game mechanics tests that have been shown to predict fall risk such as the Choice Step Reaction Time test [7] will enable the platform to be used as a diagnostic tool. Finally, by using machine learning algorithms and modern artificial intelligence technology (e.g., multi-regression models) to record the characteristics of the environment and the user, it will be possible to dynamically adapt the system to these characteristics (e.g., adjustment of difficulty of exercises). The above features make the GAME2AWE platform a novel platform for game-based exercise applications.

2   Related Work

A lot of research has been done on the development of systems that provide to elderly the ability to exercise in the form of games (exergames). In this section, we will review the relevant literature with the aim of documenting interesting findings.

Important issues to consider when developing games for the elderly have been documented in the relevant literature [8–11]. Elderly people often suffer from decreased visual acuity, impaired hearing, movement difficulties and decreased cognitive functions. Furthermore, technological barriers may exist for many seniors. Therefore, the researchers suggest that it is required to tailor the game mechanics to the specific needs of each participant. The properties of the displayed information should be adjustable and should be provided in various alternative media formats including audio and video, besides text. The size of the game elements should be adequately large whereas the speed of interaction with them should be adequately low. The entire user interface should be uncomplicated and sufficient information and guidance should be provided throughout the game relieving the player from remembering earlier information provided in the gameplay. Games should also provide positive feedback in the form of encouraging messages to the player. Moreover, the literature emphasizes the significance of social features of games and suggests the potential for multiplayer support. Finally, in order to keep players engaged in the training, it is suggested that the game content should correspond to their cultural diversity and different lifestyles.

The literature has also documented the potential of Virtual Reality (VR) technology in the creation of exergames [12]. This technology can also contribute to improving the cognitive level of the elderly [13]. VR platforms can induce natural activities in a controlled environment that can be customized in accordance with the elderly needs. Additionally, such virtual environments can divert the players from current worries. As these researches note, there is also a strong concern with the existing exergames in VR technology that they are quite complex for the group of people represented by the elderly. Consequently, it is necessary to build games explicitly for the elderly, taking into account the cognitive and physical conditions, along with the interests of the elderly.

Other studies suggest using persuasive strategies to motivate older adults to practice with games [14, 15]. It is recommended to avoid excessive information regarding the progress of the players. Such feedback should be displayed in a visual way, for instance instead of points an image (e.g., a fish) may reflect the training progress (Fig. 1). Positive feedback should be provided to the players on achieving goals. This feedback should be provided at proper instances without disturbing the player. The game should provide a simple, clear and aesthetic interface to interact with the player. The researchers consider social interaction to be significant and suggest to include this aspect in the design of the games. This is based on findings that activity engagement is more efficient when more people are involved, especially in the case of elderly who frequently experience isolation and sadness [16].

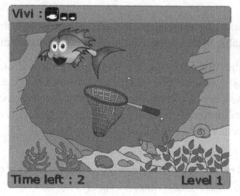

Fig. 1. Catch the Fish game [14].

Another work describes the development of an interactive exercise system for the elderly [17]. The elderly fall risk was the key incentive for this system. The work refers to studies showing that strength and balance exercises are suitable for reducing the risk of falling. The researchers reviewed studies done on treating this problem for elderly people in order to find suitable exercises to integrate in the practice system. The exercises included in the system are: "sitting walk", "sitting weight shift", "standing weight shift on both sides", "standing forward and backward weight shift", "standing on one leg" and "from sitting to chair position to standing position". The system is composed of motion tracking sensors and a computing device. The sensors are detecting movements which are displayed on a TV or computer screen. The concept of the training system is to support in a home environment personalized training assistance to the elderly. Elderly people with the help of a therapist create a user profile and then choose a practice program, an avatar and the preferred landscape. Seniors are guided during the game by a virtual trainer. Exercises must be completed with a specific sequence of moves, and completing a sequence the players will be rewarded by unlocking a new game. The therapist can supervise the practice schedule and by monitoring the training success and progress can perform appropriate game adjustments. Researchers recognize that the systems' success depends on user approval, and thus a user-friendly interface and the incorporation of inspirational features are essential.

Other studies discuss some special issues concerning the design of systems for the older population [8, 10, 18]. There is a need to create a methodology to support the software design process as close as possible to the principles of universal accessibility. Furthermore, they consider several essential characteristics of the elderly:

- As people age, the diversity in physical, sensory and cognitive functioning capabilities increases;
- Functional decline accelerates as people age;
- Cognitive problems occur, such as impaired memory and the ability to learn new things;
- Older people may have different wishes and needs;
- Usability of systems is affected by how people live, e.g., if they need a walker to walk;
- Older people are more experienced in life than younger people and thus their maturity and experience, enable them to confront problems in a different way.

A number of studies focus on the use of human-centered design as a method of developing exergames systems [9, 19–21]. Such a method focuses on the end users and in particular on their needs and abilities. It aims to develop easy-to-use applications adapted to the user's requirements/capabilities. Some suggested guidelines for designing game application screens aimed at the elderly are as follows:

- Large icons with clear meaning.
- Large fonts (14–18 pt. for web applications), use sans serif style (e.g., Arial, Verdana), avoid special styles (italics, underline, all caps).
- Simple and consistent design and arrangement of the layout, left-aligned text, fixed spaces between words and 1.5 line spacing, avoiding large sections of text.

- Clear contrast between background and foreground colors (e.g., black text on a white/yellow background or vice versa), avoiding different background colors on different pages.
- It is preferable that images do not contain text. The image will make the text more difficult to read as it draws attention. If necessary, the text should be placed in light areas of the image.
- The information should also be provided by means other than the text (e.g., sound, image, video for people with visual impairments).
- Allow enough time for users to digest the content.
- The language used for the content of the screens should be simple and understandable.
- Games should be given feedback messages. Messages should be encouraging and rewarding rather than negative criticism.

Many studies conducted on older adults and game use suggest that social interaction is important [8, 16, 22]. Social interaction can be either in the form of face-to-face multiplayer games or online games. The second case could provide an effective means to enhance sociability in elderly people who may experience mobility limitations and loneliness. Researchers did a study where the goal was to examine how elderly experience playing together under various forms of social presence [22]. A digital game was tested with forty elderly who played the game with the following modes of social presence: a) pairwise live at the same location and time, b) using a computer as an opponent, and c) pairwise online. The study outcomes revealed that in the case of online gaming the participants experienced low enjoyment, indicating that they did not like online playing. It also turned out that between playing alone with a computer and playing online they preferred the first mode. Elderly prefer to have direct physical interaction with their co-players when playing the game. Older adults experience more fun, a sense of competence, a sense of challenge, and absorption in the game when they play together in the same room than when they play with others over the Internet. The study suggests that when incorporating social interaction into games, this should be done with a cooperative character instead of a competitive one.

3 GAME2AWE Platform Design

3.1 Research Background

The GAME2AWE platform is developed in the context of the homonymous research and development project (https://game2awe.aegean.gr/) which deals with two main issues. On the one hand, the development of exergames suitable for the elderly by combining different technologies and adhering to the principles of participatory and human-centered design, and, on the other hand, the evaluation of exergames in three axes, namely motor, cognitive and technological [23].

The use of exergames in health-related applications such as exercise and rehabilitation can bring positive results. Nevertheless, prior research shows that off-the-shelf exergames are not suited for the elderly as they are not tailored for this user group [24, 25]. Based on the analysis of relevant literature, game design theory, the importance of usability, and system design knowledge, we attempt to answer the following research question:

RQ1: What issues should be considered when designing exergames to be suitable for the elderly, and what are the requirements of the GAME2AWE platform that implements these games?

Part of the answer to research question RQ1 is provided by framing the design of the platform with appropriate exergame design guidelines and pushing the GAME2AWE platform development with adequate requirements. To be able to understand the end users we look at what are the challenges in motivating older people in activities that involve physical exercise. In addition, by analyzing the relevant literature, important themes related to the development of games for the elderly emerge and are recorded as a set of design guidelines that should be followed when developing the GAME2AWE platform.

The conceptual and functional specifications of the exergames to be developed in the GAME2AWE project complement the answer to research question RQ1. An understanding of the various components involved in a digital game and considering system design issues in general are essential to the development of exergames. The importance of the participation of end users in the development process of exergames is reflected in the formation of a Focus Group which evaluates with qualitative research methods the prototypes of exergames from a design point of view and provides feedback for their improvement, as indicated in our previous work [23].

Regarding the evaluation of the GAME2AWE platform, it focuses on proving the effectiveness of exergames. The question is whether we can gather evidence to show that the GAME2AWE technology can have some significant effect, such as contributing to improving balance in the elderly. Consequently, the second research question is formulated as follows:

RQ2: Can the use of the GAME2AWE gaming platform by older adults lead to a statistically significant improvement in physical functioning parameters that are also fall predictors and secondarily to an improvement in cognitive functions?

The main method of evaluating the evidence on this topic is to conduct a randomized controlled trial. This method is chosen because it is considered suitable for determining the causal relationship between an intervention and its results.

3.2 Exergames Design Guidelines

This section outlines important design guidelines for exergames according to the literature that framed the development of the GAME2AWE platform.

Physical Condition. The physical condition of the elderly is an essential element that must be taken into account when designing games. Age-related diseases and general deterioration of health combined with limitations in mobility and the level of cognitive functions determine the ability of older people to play a game and therefore must be considered for injury prevention. In addition, it should be possible to participate in games both in a sitting and standing position due to age-based modifications in the musculoskeletal system. Also, due to balance problems and reduced endurance, rest breaks are necessary. Furthermore, games based on body tracking sensors should avoid the requirement for high-precision motion recognition, but allow a wider range of acceptance in their operation [8].

Body Movement. Games involve a range of different body kinetics to control the game or interact with the game environment. Consequently, the elderly people should be allowed to try out the necessary moves in trial sessions to familiarize themselves with the equipment and feel comfortable with it. Skillful users should be able to omit the tutorial videos however in other cases the game should provide a reminder of the moves to assist people with cognitive deficiencies [26].

Visual Condition. Age-based modifications disturb the visual system and therefore games with small-sized interfaces and quick-moving objects can cause anxiety and fear, and consequently are not appropriate for older people with visual problems [8]. Game design guidelines propose large characters and icons and emphasize on forming the requested tasks to be unambiguous and intelligible [9].

Feedback. Older people do not have the same familiarity with technology as younger people and this can automatically lead to stress. To avoid stress during the development phase of exergames, visual and auditory feedback systems should be integrated into the game. The feedback type plays a vital role as older people are inclined to blame themselves if something goes wrong or if sudden complications arise [10]. For this reason, negative feedback should be avoided and a positive approach should be preferred since older people benefit more through it in terms of their connection to the game [8].

Difficulty Adaptation. Physical and motor skills as well as cognitive abilities vary among older adults. Consequently, exergames should provide players with the ability to set the difficulty of the game and adjust it according to their level of personal condition [27]. As a result, in the long term the motivation of the players will be enhanced because the game will have the element of challenge. Still, this challenge should not frustrate the players, but on the contrary, the game objective should be achievable and fun to fulfill. An example of efficiently changing the game difficulty is to introduce components randomly to force players to act variously whenever they play it [8].

Friendly User Interfaces. Since typically the elderly have a low understanding of technology and games, it is crucial to design user-friendly interfaces that are clear, simple and easy to comprehend [28]. Ideally, older players should be able to handle the game without support from others, with the intention of making the exercise the main interest. Likewise, all excessive information should be removed from the user interface in order to minimize the risk of misunderstanding.

Game Themes. Researchers have found that older adults reject violence and disturbing content in games, and therefore it is important that game themes are chosen from topics of interest to older adults [29]. Games offering instructional or inspirational content are more likely to motivate older adults to participate in exercise. So real-world topics such as gardening or themes about animals are examples of suitable topics.

Social Interactions. Building or maintaining connections, interrelating with other people, and participating in the community become more challenging with older age [30].

Exercises allow seniors to participate in interactions with other people. Through discussions about playing and daily life, motivation to exercise is increased and social interactions are fostered among group members and between the elderly and younger family members such as their grandchildren. The development of the social health of older adults may influence cognitive health and may contribute to the reduction of anxiety and depression [31].

Flow State as a Design Goal. Exergames following the aforementioned design guidelines set all the critical elements to assist older players to arrive at a "flow state." The game flow model of player enjoyment describes the "flow state" as a state where players are fully immersed in the game, their minds are not centered on the challenging exercise, but more on enjoying the game, disconnected from all disruptions [32]. One of the major challenges a game design should face is maintaining commitment and adherence to the game's exercise program. For older people with chronic conditions, games need to provide the right incentives to enable long-term engagement in exercises for functioning progress. Motivation, enjoyment and self-confidence are important ingredients for achieving long-term commitment to continued exercise in older adults, while also emphasizing the importance of appropriate exercise.

3.3 Requirements

Based on the literature research conducted, it is clear that the elderly have characteristics that must be considered when developing technological systems aimed at them. For the development of the GAME2AWE platform, a list of requirements has been assembled as a result of literature analysis and analysis of qualitative data acquired by applying relevant research methods in the context of a multidisciplinary focus group [23]. This list is outlined in the following.

R1. The theme of a game should use environments and activities with which the participants are familiar. For example, activities from everyday life such as excursions in nature, vacation, swimming, fishing, life on a farm, gardening, sports, dancing, puzzle games, home tasks, shopping at the supermarket.

R2. The scenario of a game should be compatible with the diversity of people (gender, age, educational level, social/cultural background) and the diversity of lifestyles.

R3. The environment and characters of a game should be rendered in 3D format for enhancing the experience of using the game.

R4. A game should be enriched with appropriate music and appropriate sounds, depending on its theme and activities, in order to achieve the most effective immersion of the player.

R5. A game should integrate exercises that are safe and suitable for the elderly.

R6. A game should provide the ability to interact both when the player is sitting and standing.

R7. A game should include exercises that combine both physical movement and cognitive skills training (i.e., dual tasks).

R8. Game mechanics should avoid excessive and abrupt movements.

R9. A game should be able to adapt to the needs, interests and situation of each player.

R10. A game should not include numerous tasks but provide the potential to add more tasks after mastering the existing tasks.

R11. A game should provide different levels of difficulty so that gradual achievement of goals is possible.

R12. The players should be able to adjust the difficulty levels themselves.

R13. Games should provide opportunities for social interaction such as by supporting multiplayer and/or installing and using the games in common areas or in elderly care centers.

R14. Multiplayer support should focus more on cooperation than competition.

R15. Adequate instructions and information should be provided both before and during a game. On occasions, it may be needed to remind elderly of previous information.

R16. A game should provide information on how the player will operate the game, why the player should perform the exercise and what the benefit will be. Also, how the player will perform various activities, challenges and exercises.

R17. Constructive feedback should be provided to guide and correct exercises.

R18. Appropriate feedback should be provided to encourage and motivate to continue playing.

R19. Feedback information should be provided at the proper occasion so as to avoid players' disturbance.

R20. A game should provide the players with information about their progress and the results they have achieved. This information should not be overly extensive.

R21. A game should provide an easy menu to navigate the player to the different options of the game.

R22. The user interface should be simple and not loaded with many elements while the objects should be of adequate size.

R23. The user interface should provide information by means other than text (e.g., audio, image, video).

R24. The user interface should offer adjustable font, size and colors.

R25. Important elements should be highlighted in the user interface.

R26. A game should allow progress to be made to enhance self-efficacy and self-esteem of the players.

R27. The progress and results of the players should be able to be saved to their profiles.

4   GAME2AWE Platform Implementation

4.1   Architecture

The implementation of the games and components of the GAME2AWE platform is governed by the architecture shown in Fig. 2.

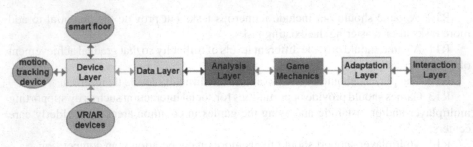

Fig. 2. GAME2AWE architecture [23].

The Device Layer is responsible for the communication of external devices with the platform. For example, the microprocessors of the tiles in the smart floor send data to this layer using the MQTT protocol. The data collected by the devices is sent to the Data Layer for preprocessing and structuring to be used by machine learning algorithms. The collected data sets are then used by the Analysis Layer to accept or reject an activity. In the case of Kinect technology, this layer evaluates input data based on recorded activities stored in training files using pattern matching algorithms to assess whether the user is performing a known movement. If accepted, the activity data is perceived by the player through Game Mechanics. The game mechanics inform the player's progress in the gameplay in order to adjust the game parameters accordingly. The Adaptation Layer provides the system intelligence to create customizable gaming experiences by adjusting the parameters and elements of each game. The Interaction Layer updates graphical elements in the user interface that provide useful/helpful information to the player.

4.2 Smart Floor

The smart floor is a technology that enables the development of a form of exergames. It is assembled from artifact tiles that have force sensors and a LED array that can display a spectrum of colors. The many colors allow for a wide range of patterns and games. To play a game on the smart floor platform a player moves to step on the tiles according to the rules of each game. The various exergames can either be played by one person or set up so that more people can cooperate or compete against each other. Interactive tiles were manufactured which are connected to each other thus allowing the creation of a smart floor whose dimensions can vary according to the needs and space of the user (Fig. 3). Each tile is connected to its neighbor while they all communicate with a central controller where all information is collected [33].

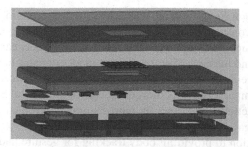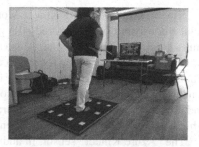

Fig. 3. Modular smart floor assembled from autonomous tiles; exergame Whack a Mole implemented on the smart floor.

An example of an exergame implemented with the smart floor technology is the game Whack a Mole (Fig. 3). The aim of the game is to repel the moles when they appear in random positions. The player stands on the two central tiles of the smart floor and observes the surrounding tiles. When one of the tiles lights up, it signals the outgoing movement of a mole and the player must quickly step on it to repel the mole and earn points. If the player delays the stepping reaction, the mole will disappear and the opportunity will be lost. The difficulty level of this game is determined by how often the intruders appear and how long the mole remains visible. This game aims to train both physical and cognitive skills.

4.3 Kinect-Based Exergames

One of the most well-known technologies used in exergames is the Microsoft Kinect motion sensor (Fig. 4), which allows the user to interact with applications through the use of gestures, movements and voice commands. The GAME2AWE platform leverages on the Xbox one version and the latest Azure version. The latter supports connection to the Microsoft Azure platform that provides machine learning technologies.

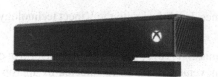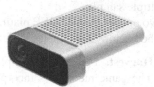

XBOX ONE KINECT MOTION SENSOR   **Azure Kinect DK**

Fig. 4. Kinect technology for exergame developing.

Kinect 2.0 (Xbox One Kinect Motion Sensor) is an interactive motion detection device consisting of an infrared (IR) projector, an IR camera, an RGB camera and a multi-dimensional microphone. It also supports voice input and recognition. Kinect can quickly scan a human body (or more) and locate a 25-joint skeletal model in real time when an elderly person is present in the field of view. Therefore, users do not need to wear sensors because interactions with the computer can be achieved through various gestures and movements. Kinect simplifies interactions and allows for more natural involvement, which makes it easier for the user to engage with the game.

The "Azure Kinect" sensor, in addition to providing body tracking for gesture and movement detection, also provides advanced functionality through the "Azure Cognitive Services" platform. The addition of cognitive services enables the detection and recognition of emotions. Specifically, using the "Face API" of this platform, 8 different emotions can be recognized ("anger", "contempt", "disgust", "fear", "happiness", "neutral", "sadness" and "surprise") during the game. Each of these emotions can be extracted, along with an accuracy value ranging from 0 to 1 that represents the confidence with which the Face API produced the prediction for a particular recognized emotion. Emotion detection is used to implement the Adaptation Layer component of the GAME2AWE architecture, as described in the corresponding section.

To recognize the games' activities, a training process was followed using a motion recording tool and the machine learning algorithms of the Kinect SDK (AdaBoost and Random Forest). To build the activity model, the Kinect Studio tool was used to observe how the sensor captures the environment. This tool also made it easy to record the movements and gestures used in game mechanics.

During the training process one issue that required attention was the fact that different elderly people have different body sizes. Thus, the system could not recognize gestures and movements effectively when it was trained on a limited number of people. Furthermore, it is expected that older people would not perform a certain movement in the same way. For example, it is expected that older people will not lean left or right in the same way. To address this problem, a focus group was organized with the participation of eight elderly people with different weight/height characteristics who were asked to perform each activity of the games to record and store the movement patterns as multiple samples.

Two of the GAME2AWE platform games developed with the Kinect technology are described below as examples (Fig. 5).

Olive Harvest. In this game, the players' mission is to collect olives from a farm of olive trees. The game mechanics incorporate movements that were selected as appropriate exercises to prevent falls while simultaneously serving a specific gameplay objective. For example, sidesteps are used to select a tree to harvest. A rowing motion is used to spread the olive collection sheet, while raising arms to harvest the crops. At more advanced difficulty levels of the game, more challenging movements are used for harvesting, such as side extension with arm lift and one leg stand with arm lift.

Fruit Harvest. The objective of this game is for the player to collect as many ripe fruits (e.g., oranges, apples) as feasible in a specified time period and place them in buckets in the field. The game mechanics incorporate a complex movement that serves the purpose of harvesting fruits. The player raises the right hand up to reach the fruit and lowers it to drop the fruit into the bucket on the left side. Alternatively, the player can raise the left hand to reach the fruit and drop it into the bucket on the right side. The avatar that appears on the screen is controlled by the players' movements.

When the fruit appears on the tree it will be colored green which means it is not ready to harvest. Ripe fruits for harvest will be colored red. On the other hand, if the ripe fruit is left too long on the tree it will rot (color is black) and fall down. Points will be awarded depending on how many fruits the player has collected and placed in the bucket. Points will be lost if green fruits are collected or if the fruits are left to rot.

The difficulty level determines the rate at which fruit will appear and ripen on the tree. As the level of difficulty increases more fruits are appearing on the tree simultaneously and at a quicker rate of ripening. An extra difficulty is to have two buckets (one at the right and one at left of the player) where the position of the fruit on the tree determines where the collected fruit will be placed. This approach provides on the one hand the possibility for cognitive training and on the other hand the possibility for a greater variety of movements and exercises.

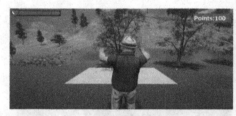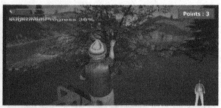

Fig. 5. Screenshots of the Kinect-based exergames Olive Harvest (on the left) and Fruit Harvest (on the right).

4.4 VR-Based Exergames

Virtual Reality (VR) technology is being used as a new way to practice in a more realistic environment. From a technical point of view, VR systems are based on three axes: immersion, interaction and imagination. Immersion is the degree to which the user feels that he is actually inside the virtual environment and is not distracted by the real one. Interactivity has to do with the computer's ability to shape the virtual world according to the user's movements. Imagination refers to whether the user perceives the virtual world and its components such as objects, behaviors and physics, as real.

Facebook's Oculus Quest 2 technology is used to develop VR games. Oculus Quest 2 is a wireless standalone virtual reality headset that creates virtual environments with the ability to navigate and interact with objects within them. A powerful Snapdragon processor for mobile devices, it runs an embedded Android-based operating system that allows running applications and games directly from the headset, without the need for a game console or PC. The device combines a light body, ease of use and high performance, features which form a satisfactory basis for developing VR applications. In the following, two example games developed with the VR technology in the GAME2AWE platform are described (Fig. 6).

Bazaar. This is mainly a cognitive exercise game in which the player is in the setting of a Fun Park and in particular in front of a stand with various objects (e.g., toys) placed on the surface. The player is asked to hand to customers who come by the stand a specific object. On the one hand, the player has to locate the correct toy indicated by the gameplay among a variety of toys, and on the other hand, the object has to be given to the customer within a certain time.

Darts. This game provides both cognitive and physical training by asking the player to virtually throw a dart repeatedly in order to break a number of balloons that are displayed in front of the player. Half of the balloons are labeled with numbers and half with letters of the alphabet. The aim of the game is the player to break all the balloons in a specific order and in the available time. In order to break a balloon it is required to raise the hand and target a balloon for a short time. To impose cognitive training, the game invites the player to hit the balloons in the following order: 1 - "A", 2 - "B", and so on.

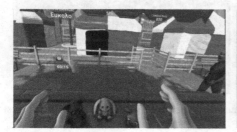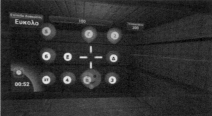

Fig. 6. Screenshots of the VR-based exergames Bazaar (on the left) and Darts (on the right).

4.5   Data Model

In the context of the game platform development, a data model is defined that describes the basic abstract concepts involved in the operation of the platform and the relationships between them. This model is illustrated in Fig. 7 in the form of a UML domain model.

During the use of the platform, the system collects and stores performance data such as the score of each game, interaction time with the game screens, frequency of game use, games completed successfully, number of errors, etc. The stored data is used by machine learning algorithms to determine the appropriate level of difficulty of the exercise individually for each user.

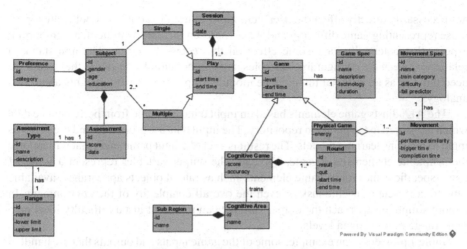

Fig. 7. GAME2AWE data model.

Based on the domain model of the GAME2AWE platform, the schema of the database is defined which will maintain the game data and user performance both for the support of the Adaptation Layer and for the support of screening procedures. In the second case, the discovery of patterns in the stored data can be exploited to detect the cognitive/physical level of the subject with the aim of supplementing and/or replacing related traditional diagnostic tools.

4.6 Adaptation Layer

The Adaptation Layer (AL) is an important component of the GAME2AWE platform architecture. AL is responsible for adjusting parameters and elements of each game. A key concern in the design of the AL is to allow customization of elements related to the difficulty of the game [34]. More specifically, transforming the main concept into measurable targets, the AL aims to improve the user's motor and cognitive functions, to increase interest in the game and prevent the user from giving up training, to improve user experience and playability and to increase the number of recorded positive emotions. These targets are measurable by a series of metrics that derive from data gathered throughout the gameplay, such as game completion time, success rate, current face expression, user's answers to game questions and other in-game data relative to measurable targets.

The game variables that are configurable by the AL can be distinguished into two main categories. The first category concerns variables related to the regulation of the game difficulty. The second category concerns variables, such as audiovisual effects and themes of in-game objects that could potentially affect the emotions of a subject. Sometimes there is a direct relation between a configurable variable and recorded metrics, for example increasing the number of tasks the user is asked to carry out affects the completion time and success ratio metrics of the game. But this kind of relation does not always apply with all variables and metrics. For example, the music theme might not necessarily directly affect the user's emotion. Thus, all variables in both categories, those representing game difficulty and those representing user sentiment, are important aspects that potentially have some effect on the recorded metrics. The non-standard relation between the configurable variables and the measurable metrics is the reason we need the AL, as an artificial intelligence module, to provide us with insights about this analogy.

The AL adjusts game elements based on input data that come from performance data which are stored in the platform repository. The input data are processed and are given as input to machine learning models. The result is a set of output parameters that will modify the adaptable elements of a game. Typically the output variables represent a series of game-specific values for in-game elements such as rate of objects appearance, available time to complete a specific task or even the overall complexity of the environment. In a more simplified approach the output variable can represent just a difficulty level on a scale range of predefined levels.

Table 1 provides as an example, some of the game inputs and outputs that are handled by the AL, grouped for three of the platform games. For the Olive Harvest game, for example, input variables may be game metrics from current and previous game sessions and output variables may be the growing speed of olives, and the required number of physical exercises to complete the game task.

Table 1. Example input and output game variables handled by the Adaptation Layer.

Game	Input	Output	
		Difficulty Adjustment Elements	Emotion Adjustment Elements
Healthy Garden	Profile characteristics such as demographics, preferences, and lifestyle.	Frequency and number of insects Insect speed Insect location Insect category	Variation of all audiovisual elements that can be adjusted such as musical theme, colors, natural sounds (air, birds, water flowing).
Olive Harvest	Game metrics from current and previous game sessions such as collected points, health bar level, completion time, failures, statistics of reaction time (average, standard deviation, quantiles), idle time percentage, etc.	Growing speed of olives Requested number of repetitions for physical exercises	
Excursion in the Nature	Recognized emotions in the current session such as fear, happiness, neutral, sadness and surprise.	Type of physical exercise Number of repetitions Difficulty of quiz questions	

To determine the game difficulty with a machine learning model, both a classifier and a more sophisticated model are involved. The choice depends on the available data and the desired output. For example, the lack of available game data in the beginning of the platform usage restricts the AL to use a simple classifier to determine a difficulty level based on the subject's demographics and other profile information such as the cognitive and physical assessments that have been performed before the intervention.

After spending some time in the game platform, the gathered data allow the AL to use advanced multi-output machine learning models that automatically determine a series of values for the configurable parameters. Furthermore, regarding the multi-output models, since they are trained with in-game gathered data, either it would require to train one model per game, or use a model of multi-regression type. The latter allows us to take into account the fact that the data model of a subject could be radically different for each game. Ideally, the AL could be set up to include a process to automatically re-train the machine learning models, either periodically or upon the gathering of a certain amount of new data.

Appropriateness of the adjustment is one of the biggest challenges for the AL, because the newly selected difficulty level determines if the game would still be within the reach of the capabilities of the subject and still make the game interesting enough for the subject to keep playing. Another challenge is to configure the AL system well enough to estimate the appropriate difficulty level for a subject before any session with a minimum amount of data, mostly based on demographic and other data apart from the actual game data. Fortunately, even in case of an ill prediction, the subject would have the difficulty automatically readjusted in the following rounds or even during the game depending on the AL configuration. Apart from directly adjusting the difficulty to improve a subjects' performance, another indirect way to achieve this is by affecting a subject's emotions. The main challenge here is the complexity of the parameters by which the emotions of a subject can be affected. Additionally, the accurate measurement of a subject's emotions at a given time is a challenge of its own, since it includes face recognition techniques.

4.7 Development Environment

Exergames were developed using the Unity 3D game development platform in combination with Microsoft Visual Studio and the C# language for programming the logic and interactivity of the games (Fig. 8). Unity engine is one of the most popular and modern options for developing a 3D (or even 2D) game world, thanks in part to its user friendliness and the large community that has been built around it, which contributes to the fast development and experimentation. A major advantage of this platform is the ability to export a developed game to multiple platforms and operating systems, running either on standard computing devices (e.g., desktop or laptop) or on mobile devices. This flexibility is particularly important, since it makes it unnecessary to learn different tools and develop code in different programming languages for deployment on different platforms.

A Unity application serves as a central point for handling GAME2AWE platform exergames, offering services such as user account creation/authentication, game selection from the main menu (Fig. 9), and in the case of the smart floor providing a visual representation of the game on a screen with the aim of improving the gaming experience. Such a case was the 'Whack a Mole' game discussed earlier (Fig. 3).

A number of demo videos of exergames developed in the GAME2AWE platform can be found in the projects' YouTube channel: Game2AWE - YouTube.

96   C. Goumopoulos and G. Koumanakos

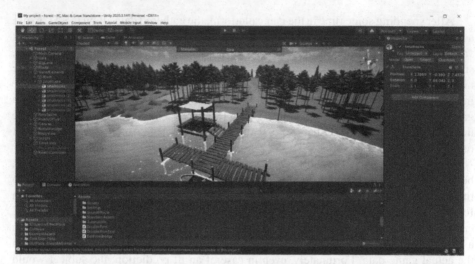

Fig. 8. Screenshot of the Unity development platform used in GAME2AWE implementation.

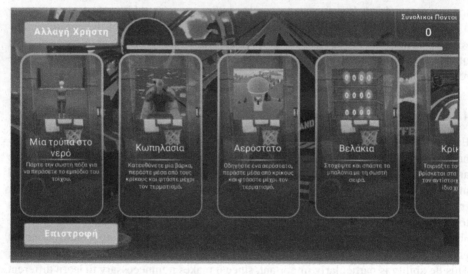

Fig. 9. Game menu in the central Unity application.

5 Evaluation

A preliminary evaluation study was conducted in the premises of an elderly care center with twelve participants (N = 12) classified as end users (i.e., healthy elderly) and healthcare experts including an orthopedic doctor, a physiotherapist, an exercise professional and a psychologist. The main characteristics of the participants are shown in Table 2. Technology familiarity, concerning the use of computing devices and services, was assessed with suitable questionnaire items in a scale of 0 to 4. The evaluation goal was to test in a pre-pilot phase the current version of the exergames in order to evaluate their usability and functionality. Informed written consent was provided by all participants prior to the beginning of the study. The evaluation examined the following aspects of the GAME2AWE platform exergames: usability, usefulness, safety and applicability. Figure 10 illustrates indicative moments from the evaluation study.

Table 2. Basic characteristics of the participants.

Characteristic	Ends Users	Experts
N	8	4
Age (mean ± stdev)	71.3 ± 4.3	38.3 ± 4.9
Gender (female/male)	6/2	2/2
Education years	9.4 ± 3.7	≥16
Technology familiarity	1.8 ± 1.0	4

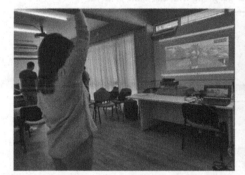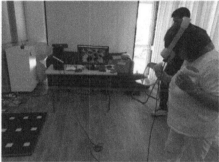

Fig. 10. Instances from the preliminary evaluation of the GAME2AWE platform.

Perceived usability and usefulness were assessed using the System Usability Scale (SUS) questionnaire [35]. The questionnaire includes ten statements with answers on a five-point scale from 1 (strongly disagree) to 5 (strongly agree). Half of the statements have a positive meaning (S1, S3, S5, S7, S9) and the other half have a negative meaning (S2, S4, S6, S8, S10). To reflect the context of the study, the word "system" in the original questionnaire items was replaced with the phrase "game platform", as shown in Table 3. The rating for each statement was transformed so that the original total scores on the 0–40 scale were converted to the 0–100 scale according to best practices [36]. An above average SUS score suggesting a good usability is a score above 68.

The SUS results for the GAME2AWE platform are shown in the form of boxplots for the different participant categories in Fig. 11. The total mean SUS score is 84.2 (SD = 10.1). The domain experts rated usability higher and with lower variability (mean SUS score 86.9 ± 3.1) than the end-users (mean SUS score 82.8 ± 12.3). Overall, the results suggest a high user acceptance by all the participants. This evaluation pointed out that the goals of the game tasks were clearly understood and were adequately engaging to be pursued.

Table 3. SUS items with alternating positive and negative statements.

ID	Statement
S1	I think that I would like to use this game platform frequently
S2	I found the game platform unnecessarily complex
S3	I thought the game platform was easy to use
S4	I think that I would need the support of a technical person to be able to use this game platform
S5	I found the various functions in this game platform were well integrated
S6	I thought there was too much inconsistency in this game platform
S7	I would imagine that most people would learn to use this game platform very quickly
S8	I found the game platform very cumbersome to use
S9	I felt very confident using the game platform
S10	I needed to learn a lot of things before I could get going with this game platform

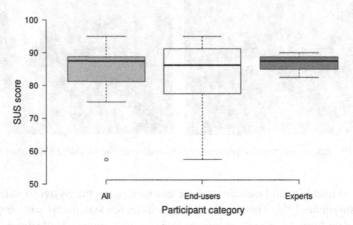

Fig. 11. Perceived usability as conveyed by SUS score for the different participant categories.

A more detailed analysis of the assessment received by the end-users is shown in Fig. 12 which outlines the distribution of the ratings for each SUS statement. The elderly have a strong view that training with the game platform is characterized by simplicity, accessibility and consistency while the learning effort is acceptable. This is indicated by the responses in S2, S6, S8 and S10 which refer to items with negative meaning and the answers laying in the lower part of the scale are more intense. On the other hand, a clear concern emerges from the answers of the end users to the statement S4 (mean value 3.5 ± 1.5). Since this item determines the participants' ability to use the system independently, it is interpreted that it may reflect the low technological familiarity that characterizes the majority of the participants and the general viewpoint that new technology may cause anxiety to older people.

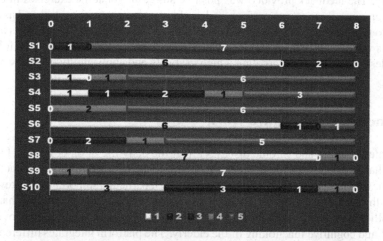

Fig. 12. SUS questionnaire item ratings by the end-users only.

To evaluate the usability and acceptance of the platform qualitative data were also collected using a semi-structured interview with the participants. The collected data revealed that there was a high motivation to exercise since all participants responded that they enjoyed and had fun with exergaming on the GAME2AWE platform, they agreed that the exergames tested can contribute to the improvement of their physical and cognitive abilities and consequently to their well-being. They unanimously expressed a wish to continue training with the platform.

The safety of the participants in the VR-based exergames was measured using the Virtual Reality Sickness Questionnaire (VRSQ) [37]. The VRSQ assesses nine different simulator sickness symptoms, including general discomfort, fatigue, headache, eye strain, etc. A 4-point Likert scale is used to rate the severity of each symptom. By adding all item scores, a total score is computed and then is converted to a percentage score. Higher severity in VR sickness is indicated by a higher score. To examine safety for the other exergames in the platform, an open-ended question was asked to the participants i.e., "Did you experience any worries or unpleasant symptoms during and after the use of the exergaming platform?", at the end of the evaluation to identify other possible ill effects.

Regarding unpleasant effects, the majority of the end users (63%) never suffered any symptoms of VR sickness. Overall, only very mild symptoms were identified (such as eye strain and fatigue) as indicated by a mean VRSQ score in the end user group (N = 8) of 2.92/100 (STDEV 4.03). Regarding other concerns for the rest of the platform, it was suggested that adding a protective extension around the edges of the smart floor would maximize its safe use in the case of tile boundary moves.

To assess the applicability of the exergames a discussion with the domain experts was conducted after testing all the exergames. The discussion focused on the applicability of the exergames for elderly training to reduce fall risk with questions on topics such as the suitability of the exercises, the effectiveness and safety of the movements, the appropriateness of the difficulty levels and how well the movements are integrated in the gameplay. The feedback provided was positive suggesting that the exercises integrated in the exergames were safe to perform and could improve postural control and assist the elderly to reinforce their strength and balance and consequently reduce frailties and fall risk. This was actually expected since a participatory design approach had been followed for the design of the games targeting a high usability and applicability of the exergames [23].

6   Conclusion and Future Work

Age-related changes and chronic diseases affect the daily life of older people. Physical activity has been shown to delay and reduce age-related symptoms and risk factors. In particular, strengthening and balance exercises are of particular importance in preventing falls. In this paper, the GAME2AWE platform was presented that combines hardware and intelligent software to create adaptive gaming experiences aimed at improving the physical and cognitive functioning of the elderly. The platform integrates different technologies (Kinect motion tracking sensor, virtual reality and smart floor) to provide the user with a greater variety of interactions and exercises to reduce fall risk.

An extensive evaluation of the developed game platform in the near future will provide more sound evidence on the usefulness of the proposed exergames in relation to fall prevention. The evaluation methodology includes a control group and an intervention group applying a randomized controlled trial. For all users, measurements of motor and cognitive functions are recorded before and after using the GAME2AWE platform. Measurable success metrics of the game platform will be to achieve improvement on indicators of motor and cognitive function. This evaluation study will provide answers to the second research question of the GAME2AWE research approach.

Acknowledgements. This research has been co-financed by the European Regional Development Fund of the European Union and Greek national funds through the Operational Program Competitiveness, Entrepreneurship and Innovation, under the call RESEARCH – CREATE – INNOVATE (project code: T2EDK-04785). The authors would like to thank the fellow researchers in the GAME2AWE project for their valuable support in the performed research and the volunteers that took part in the reported evaluation study.

References

1. Sterling, D.A., O'connor, J.A., Bonadies, J.: Geriatric falls: injury severity is high and disproportionate to mechanism. J. Trauma Acute Care Surg. **50**(1), 116–119 (2001)
2. Rivasi, G., Kenny, R.A., Ungar, A., Romero-Ortuno, R.: Predictors of incident fear of falling in community-dwelling older adults. J. Am. Med. Dir. Assoc. **21**(5), 615–620 (2020)
3. Finnegan, S., Seers, K., Bruce, J.: Long-term follow-up of exercise interventions aimed at preventing falls in older people living in the community: a systematic review and meta-analysis. Physiotherapy **105**(2), 187–199 (2019)

4. Cadore, E.L., Rodríguez-Mañas, L., Sinclair, A., Izquierdo, M.: Effects of different exercise interventions on risk of falls, gait ability, and balance in physically frail older adults: a systematic review. Rejuvenation Res. **16**(2), 105–114 (2013)
5. Oh, Y., Yang, S.: Defining exergames & exergaming. In: Proceedings of Meaningful Play, 2010, pp. 21–23 (2010)
6. Lautenschlager, N.T., Cox, K., Kurz, A.F.: Physical activity and mild cognitive impairment and Alzheimer's disease. Curr. Neurol. Neurosci. Rep. **10**(5), 352–358 (2010)
7. Lord, S.R., Fitzpatrick, R.C.: Choice stepping reaction time: a composite measure of falls risk in older people. J. Gerontol. A Biol. Sci. Med. Sci. **56**(10), M627–M632 (2001)
8. Planinc, R., Nake, I., Kampel, M.: Exergame design guidelines for enhancing elderly's physical and social activities. In: AMBIENT 2013, The Third International Conference on Ambient Computing, Applications, Services and Technologies, pp. 58–63 (2013)
9. Chartomatsidis, M., Goumopoulos, C.: A balance training game tool for seniors using Microsoft Kinect and 3D worlds. In: ICT4AWE, pp. 135–145 (2019)
10. Gerling, K.M., Schulte, F.P., Smeddinck, J., Masuch, M.: Game design for older adults: effects of age-related changes on structural elements of digital games. In: Herrlich, M., Malaka, R., Masuch, M. (eds.) ICEC 2012. LNCS, vol. 7522, pp. 235–242. Springer, Heidelberg (2012). https://doi.org/10.1007/978-3-642-33542-6_20
11. Larsen, L.H., Schou, L., Lund, H.H., Langberg, H.: The physical effect of exergames in healthy elderly—a systematic review. Games Health Res. Dev. Clin. Appl. **2**(4), 205–212 (2013)
12. De Vries, A.W., Van Dieën, J.H., Van Den Abeele, V., Verschueren, S.M.: Understanding motivations and player experiences of older adults in virtual reality training. Games Health J. **7**(6), 369–376 (2018)
13. Sayma, M., Tuijt, R., Cooper, C., Walters, K.: Are we there yet? Immersive virtual reality to improve cognitive function in dementia and mild cognitive impairment. Gerontologist **60**(7), e502–e512 (2020)
14. Kostaki, C., Goumopoulos, C.: Development and evaluation of an exergaming application for improving seniors' well-being. In: Proceedings of the 20th Pan-Hellenic Conference on Informatics, pp. 1–6 (2016)
15. Petsani, D., Kostantinidis, E.I., Diaz-Orueta, U., Hopper, L., Bamidis, P.D.: Extending exergame-based physical activity for older adults: the e-coaching approach for increased adherence. In: Bamidis, P.D., Ziefle, M., Maciaszek, L.A. (eds.) ICT4AWE 2018. CCIS, vol. 982, pp. 108–125. Springer, Cham (2019). https://doi.org/10.1007/978-3-030-15736-4_6
16. Li, J., Erdt, M., Chen, L., Cao, Y., Lee, S.Q., Theng, Y.L.: The social effects of exergames on older adults: systematic review and metric analysis. J. Med. Internet Res. **20**(6), e10486 (2018)
17. Kiselev, J., Haesner, M., Gövercin, M., Steinhagen-Thiessen, E.: Implementation of a home-based interactive training system for fall prevention: requirements and challenges. J. Gerontol. Nurs. **41**(1), 14–19 (2015)
18. Marinelli, E.C., Rogers, W.A. Identifying potential usability challenges for xbox 360 kinect exergames for older adults. In: Proceedings of the Human Factors and Ergonomics Society Annual Meeting, vol. 58, no. 1, pp. 1247–1251. SAGE Publications, Los Angeles (2014)
19. Väätänen, A., Leikas, J.: Human-centred design and exercise games. In: Kankaanranta, M., Neittaanmäki, P. (eds.) Design and Use of Serious Games, pp. 33–47. Springer, Dordrecht (2009). https://doi.org/10.1007/978-1-4020-9496-5_3
20. Sanders, E.B.N.: From user-centered to participatory design approaches. In: Design and the Social Sciences, pp. 18–25. CRC Press (2002)
21. Brox, E., Konstantinidis, S.T., Evertsen, G.: User-centered design of serious games for older adults following 3 years of experience with exergames for seniors: a study design. JMIR Serious Games **5**(1), e6254 (2017)

22. Gajadhar, B.J., Nap, H.H., De Kort, Y.A., IJsselsteijn, W.A.: Out of sight, out of mind: co-player effects on seniors' player experience. In: Proceedings of the 3rd International Conference on Fun and Games, pp. 74–83 (2010)

23. Goumopoulos, C., Chartomatsidis, M., Koumanakos, G.: Participatory design of fall prevention exergames using multiple enabling technologies. In: ICT4AWE, pp. 70–80 (2022)

24. Nyman, S.R., Victor, C.R.: Older people's participation in and engagement with falls prevention interventions in community settings: an augment to the Cochrane systematic review. Age Ageing **41**(1), 16–23 (2012)

25. Valenzuela, T., Okubo, Y., Woodbury, A., Lord, S.R., Delbaere, K.: Adherence to technology-based exercise programs in older adults: a systematic review. J. Geriatr. Phys. Therapy **41**(1), 49–61 (2018)

26. Mason, L., Gerling, K., Dickinson, P., Holopainen, J., Jacobs, L., Hicks, K.: Including the experiences of physically disabled players in mainstream guidelines for movement-based games. In: CHI Conference on Human Factors in Computing Systems, pp. 1–15 (2022)

27. Cantwell, D., Broin, D.O., Palmer, R., Doyle, G.: Motivating elderly people to exercise using a social collaborative exergame with adaptive difficulty. In: Proceedings of the 6th European Conference on Games Based Learning, Cork, Ireland, pp. 4–5 (2012)

28. Gerling, K., Mandryk, R.: Custom-designed motion-based games for older adults: a review of literature in human-computer interaction. Gerontechnology **12**(2), 68–80 (2014)

29. De Schutter, B., Brown, J.A.: Digital games as a source of enjoyment in later life. Games Cult. **11**(1–2), 28–52 (2016)

30. Bookman, A.: Innovative models of aging in place: transforming our communities for an aging population. Community Work Fam. **11**(4), 419–438 (2008)

31. Li, J., Theng, Y.L., Foo, S.: Effect of exergames on depression: a systematic review and meta-analysis. Cyberpsychol. Behav. Soc. Netw. **19**(1), 34–42 (2016)

32. Sweetser, P., Wyeth, P.: GameFlow: a model for evaluating player enjoyment in games. ACM CIE **3**(3), 1–24 (2005)

33. Goumopoulos, C., Ougkrenidis, D., Gklavakis, D., Ioannidis, I.: A smart floor device of an exergame platform for elderly fall prevention. In: Proceedings of the 25th Conference on Digital System Design, Maspalomas, Gran Canaria, Spain, pp. 1–8 (2022)

34. Danousis, M., Goumopoulos, C., Fakis, A.: Exergames in the GAME2AWE platform with dynamic difficulty adjustment. In: Proceedings of the 21st IFIP International Conference on Entertainment Computing, Bremen, Germany, pp. 585–592 (2022)

35. Brooke, J.: SUS-A quick and dirty usability scale. Usability Eval. Ind. **189**(194), 214–223 (1996)

36. Sauro, J.: A practical guide to the system usability scale: background, benchmarks & best practices. Measuring Usability LLC (2011)

37. Kim, H.K., Park, J., Choi, Y., Choe, M.: Virtual reality sickness questionnaire (VRSQ): motion sickness measurement index in a virtual reality environment. Appl. Ergon. **69**, 66–73 (2018)

Don't You Worry 'bout a Thing? Identification and Quantification of Relevant Privacy Parameters Within the Acceptance of AAL Technology

Caterina Maidhof[✉][ID], Julia Offermann[ID], and Martina Ziefle[ID]

Chair of Communication Science, Human Computer Interaction Center, RWTH Aachen University, Campus Boulevard, Aachen, Germany
{maidhof,offermann,ziefle}@comm.rwth-aachen.de

Abstract. To combat healthcare challenges Ambient Assisted Living (AAL) technologies offer the opportunity to support an independent life in older age. Although the potential and advantages of such technology are acknowledged, perceived barriers in particular referred to privacy still represent a hurdle for their acceptance. Applying a two-step empirical approach, this study aimed at the identification and quantification of relevant privacy parameters for the acceptance of visual AAL technology. First, a qualitative study investigated the participants' cognitive privacy representations in a scenario in which AAL was installed in their own home to support life in older age. 12 participants (age range: 23–81 years) shared their opinions within semi-structured interviews. Based on these findings, an online survey (N = 134) study was applied in a second step in order to quantify the identified privacy parameters. Overall, the paper presents the qualitative key findings as well as the descriptive results of the quantitative study. The results show the usefulness of both methods to a) identify and understand thought processes of potential users regarding privacy requirements as well as b) to get insights into the relevance and meaning of the identified privacy parameters. The qualitative and quantitative findings are useful to inform technical designers as well as lawmakers to consider the privacy parameters during technology or law development.

Keywords: Privacy perceptions · Qualitative insights · Quantification · Privacy parameters · AAL technology · Life in older age

1 Introduction

In the last decades, Ambient Assisted Living (AAL) technologies were developed aiming at being an integral part of the everyday life of older adults in need of care [1,2]. By improving the quality of life for older adults in need of care, supporting an independent life within the own home, and relieving formal as well as informal caregivers, AAL technologies and approaches offer the capability to address and combat healthcare challenges [3,4]. A broad variety of AAL approaches reaching from sensors and

L. A. Maciaszek et al. (Eds.): ICT4AWE 2021/2022, CCIS 1856, pp. 103–122, 2023.
https://doi.org/10.1007/978-3-031-37496-8_6

actuators, over smart interfaces to artificial intelligence can be integrated into the living environments and lives of older people (in need of care) to detect and prevent severe situations such as falls as well as to support the participation and maintenance of activities of daily living [1,5]. Within the broad range of AAL applications, wearable or ambient installed sensors can be used for lifelogging which summarizes the recording, storage, analysis, and interpretation of physiological and behavioural data in order to digitally track and document a person's individual everyday life [6]. Research on the acceptance of lifelogging applying AAL technologies identified positive evaluations of the potential and the advantages the usage of AAL applications brings along (e.g., [4]). However, existing barriers and concerns regarding the usage of AAL applications, in particular focusing on possible invasions of the own privacy, still impede a sustainable acceptance and adoption within the everyday life (e.g., [7]). Here, an identification and detailed analysis of the specific mental models of privacy, privacy concerns, and respective requirements of potential AAL users are so far missing, but are necessary in order to expand the understanding of future users needs and to enable a user-tailored technology development. Therefore, this paper presents a two-step empirical approach investigating mental models of privacy as well as privacy concerns and requirements in the context of using AAL technologies in older age. Within the next Sect. 2, the theoretical background of the empirical approach is presented. Then, Sect. 3 describes the methodological approaches of the first qualitative interviews study as well as the subsequent quantitative online survey study. Based on that, Sect. 4 presents the results of the qualitative and quantitative study according to the thematic focal points. Finally, the results and insights of both studies are discussed related to the current state of research including derived implications as well as limitations and ideas for future research (Sect. 5).

2   Acceptance of AAL Technology and the Role of Privacy

Diverse empirical studies on the acceptance of AAL technologies revealed that generally most AAL applications are perceived positively by diverse user groups who especially acknowledge the advantages of an improved independence and increased feeling of safety (e.g., [8–11]). However, other previous research identified an invasion of privacy, the lack of personnel contact, fear of data misuse as well as perceived control and surveillance to be relevant barriers and expressed concerns in the context of using AAL technology at home in older age (e.g., [12–15]). In addition to technology-related benefits and barriers, previous research identified an increased need for care [16, 17] as well as care experience as influencing parameters on the acceptance of AAL technologies. Thereby, the results indicate that emotional aspects are more relevant for care-experienced compared to inexperienced individuals [18]. Real decisions to use or not to use AAL technology depend on trade-offs between the perceived benefits and barriers. Here, previous research [18] revealed that data access and privacy are the most relevant factors when people in need of care and caregivers have to decide to use AAL technologies. Several other work confirms that privacy concerns represent a main barrier to the acceptance and sustainable adoption of AAL [4,7]. These concerns rise particularly when the actual level of privacy does not match the desired amount [19]. Privacy invasion can be seen as the the most extreme case of mismatch between desired and actual level of privacy and happens when "another gains access to facts more personal than is deemed appropriate for one of his/her level of intimacy" ([20], p.94).

Previous investigations revealed that personal characteristics and attitudes as well as the specific context impact both, the desired amount of privacy and the trade-off between sharing and protecting individual data [19,21,22]. These insights suggest that privacy concerns are always newly weighted according to specific situations and circumstances. In more detail, previous findings found that older adults are willing to exchange privacy for safety when their autonomy is strengthened [23]: this suggests that the users' willingness to lower their privacy changes especially when they feel to be in control of the situation. Further parameters that potentially decrease privacy concerns are positive contributions to health and well-being, an easy use of the assisting applications as well as preventing stigmatization [23]. Beyond that, previous studies also recognised other privacy-related parameters in the sense that the locations where assisting technology is applied influences the users' acceptance [24]: thereby, using assisting applications in rather private rooms, e.g., bedroom or bathroom, is less accepted compared to less private rooms, such as living room or kitchen. Besides the described circumstances and situations, entities or person groups can have a considerable impact on privacy evaluations and may even be more relevant for privacy preferences for ubiquitous technologies than the context [25]. Ourlasvita and colleagues [26] studied long-term effects of ubiquitous surveillance through among other video camera and network traffic in homes of ten volunteers. As part of a post-implementation interview participants mentioned that they would least willingly share video data to authorities, public media, friends and acquaintances, companies and employers as well as the police. Regarding networking data participants added commercial actors, criminals and insurance companies to their list of entities they would avoid sharing data. In the field of unobtrusive home monitoring such as AAL or lifelogging the ones monitored (i.e., older adults) want to decide and are selective about who sees and receives the data [10,27]. In this context especially the willingness to share data with doctors, family members and friends was examined showing that data access by doctors and family members is quite accepted [28,29] and data access by friends is least tolerated [29]. Other research has applied a social identity approach [30,31] to study acceptance of surveillance and privacy infringement [32]. Social identity is defined as "that part of an individual's self-concept which derives from his knowledge of his membership of a social group (groups) together with the emotional significance attached to that membership" ([33], p.69). Across theories of the self an implicit distinction is made between two levels of social identities (1) the ones originating from interpersonal relationships and interdependence with typical intimate dyadic relationships like parent-child, lovers or friends but also membership in small face-to-face groups and (2) the ones that are built up from membership in larger, more impersonal collectives or social categories where personal contact is not required [34]. Based on these theoretical implications, O'Donnell and colleagues [32] report that surveillance was perceived less of an invasion of privacy the more the one supervising the surveillance shared identity with the person being surveyed. Privacy invasion was perceived as highest when the identity with the surveillance supervisor was not shared and the group order categorization was higher (i.e., more abstract and impersonal). In addition, perceptions of surveillance in terms of privacy invasion decreased the more the purpose of surveillance (i.e., safety) was perceived and the more levels of identity where shared between the supervisor and the one being surveyed [32].

Summarizing the insights and results of previous research, privacy can be characterized to be a multi-faceted and multi-dimensional construct. Moreover, also the role of privacy within the AAL context is not one-dimensional: it can be represented in concerns, in a desired state, and it can be a part of a trade-off with health-related advantages (e.g., autonomy), being always influenced by diverse individual as well as contextual parameters. The multifaceted nature of privacy impedes the definition of privacy and leads to many different approaches to define privacy. Based on several previous definitions of privacy, Burgoon [35] distinguishes four dimensions of privacy accounting for the complexity of privacy in the context of AAL applications [27]: the four dimensions include social privacy (i.e., control over social contacts, interaction, and communication), physical privacy (i.e., the degree of physical inaccessibility), psychological privacy (i.e., the degree of inaccessibility to thoughts, feelings, and intimate information), and informational privacy (i.e., control over personal information). Applying the assessment of mental models represents one way to study the multifaceted construct of privacy and its diverse dimensions.

In previous work, mental models have been applied to assess older adults' understanding of privacy in diverse (non-)digital contexts [36, 37], laypersons' general conceptualization of privacy [38], or older adults' privacy expectations when assisting technologies are used [39]. However, the mental conceptualizations of privacy still require further investigations, in particular in the context of ageing and living with AAL.

In the following, the approach of using mental models in empirical research is introduced and respective research results are described. First of all, mental models are cognitive representations of the external reality guiding people to interact with the world around them [40, 41]. People create a cognitive structure shaping the basis of reasoning and decision making based on their personal life experiences, their perceptions, as well as their understandings, ideas and concepts of the world. These cognitive structures or maps affect the kind of information individuals focus on and the perception of this information; thus, the cognitive maps have a leading role with regard to the integration and interpretation of new information [42]. Previous research revealed that people resort to familiar mental models resembling the unknown in order to explain unknown domains [43]. In more detail (e.g., [44]), people tend to explain phenomena that are not directly perceivable in the external reality in the same way as unfamiliar domains. Based on that, cognitive maps are described and understood as mental models depicting the scheme of individuals' cognitive representation of specific situations or problems [42]. Here, the pattern has been identified that the most important, significant, and relevant contents of a cognitive map are what quickly comes to mind [45]. To date, there is still no agreement on the definition of a mental model [46] and confusion about the nature of cognitive maps [47]. Nevertheless, there is a broad variety of methodological approaches to identify and analyze people's individual cognitive representations. One approach lies in the open-ended 3CM (conceptual content cognitive map) method, representing a corroborated method to assess the cognitive representation, processes, and structures of individuals [45]. This method has already been applied aiming at an understanding of individual perception, opinions, and concerns of people, e.g., in the case of people with a diagnosis of lung cancer [48] or with regard to nurses' perceptions of children's pain [49]. Overall, this methodological approach is appropriate for a measurement of people's representations and perspectives on complex domains [45]. As the usage, interaction, and support with AAL technologies and systems represents a complex domain, this approach is suited to be applied in this specific field of technology (acceptance) research. The open-ended version of the 3CM method is particularly suited for in depth explorations and to be applied in small samples.

Therefore, this method is applied in the present study to gain deeper insights about people's perspectives on privacy within a personal healthcare scenario using assistive technology. On the one hand, the effective use of the described methodological approach within the complex healthcare and AAL context is exploratorily tested through a semi-structured interview study. Beyond that, the present study aimed at an deeper understanding of thought processes, perspectives, and opinions related to the role of the individual privacy when AAL technology is applied for support, assistance, and care in older age. Thereby, the study will focus on a diverse sample (all age, diverse levels of care experience and technical understandings) of participants from two different European countries. Based on the previous theoretical explanations, the participants receive a scenario where people are confronted with using AAL technology in their own home for the first time, expecting them to immediately think of, possibly reveal and weigh core contents of their individual existing mental representations in light of the described scenario. Furthermore, in older age assistance, help, and support from many different stakeholders are necessary. These stakeholders are involved in providing care and therefore certain private information has to be shared with them to some extent. This means that it is of utmost importance to investigate who has the authorization to enter privacy in aging and care contexts and who not.

3 Methods

Within this chapter, the empirical design of the mixed-method approach is presented, describing the specific qualitative and quantitative procedures, their analyses, as well as the respective characteristics of the interview and the questionnaire participants.

3.1 Empirical Design

This was a mixed-method study that involved the use of both quantitative and qualitative components. The qualitative measures consisted of semi-structured interviews with the aim to understand thought processes of privacy while being supported by AAL technology and to exploratory understand conceptualizations of privacy for a subsequent quantitative assessment. Based on these qualitative findings, a quantitative questionnaire was developed assessing privacy. The quantitative part taken from this questionnaire will focus on the evaluation of various AAL related stakeholders and to what extent these entities are authorized to enter personal privacy (see Fig. 1).

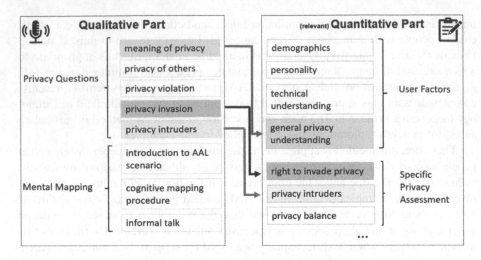

Fig. 1. Mixed-methods study design.

3.2   Procedures

Qualitative. Participants were welcomed to the interview with a general introduction into the topic of privacy and AAL technologies and where told that the interview was divided into two main parts. The first part of the interview consisted of four main questions regarding the meaning of privacy, privacy behaviour, and feelings of privacy violation and intrusion which were later used to conduct the quantitative study. The second part of the interview started with the description of a scenario in which participants were encouraged to picture themselves as an eighty-year-old healthy but frail person living alone at their own home with having AAL technology installed as a support to counteract frailty. Then participants were guided to create their mental representation of this scenario based on the Conceptual Content Cognitive Map (3CM) method described by [45]. Participants answers of three related questions were written down in boxes to create a visualization of their thoughts (each box representing another mental object). These three questions addressed participants' first impression of the scenario, connections they could draw to privacy and their ideal imagination of this technology in line with their privacy preferences. Each topic was discussed extensively and only when participants clearly signalled that the visualization map was complete for them, the interviewer proceeded. In this way the number of objects included in each map varied depending on participants' personal understanding of the scenario. As for the subsequent task participants were asked to sort the answer boxes into meaningful groups of statements in order to code each group or statement according to how important they would consider each of their statements in terms of privacy. Participants were encouraged to name whether there was any adequate replacement for the statement rated as the most important aspect. Lastly, the interview ended with an informal talk about participants' demographics and their experiences in care as well as regarding technology.

Quantitative. Based on the previously described preceding qualitative study, a questionnaire was developed which was delivered online through the social media channels of one of the researchers and addressed participants of all age. First, demographics such as age, gender, educational level, as well as living situation and place of living were assessed. Then, information about their subjective health status and care were asked. Regarding care experience, participants were asked if they had ever cared for another person, either professionally or informally. Subsequently, additional user factors such as technical understanding (four items) [50,51] and general privacy attitudes (16 items) were measured. The theoretical foundation of these items were the four privacy dimensions elaborated by [35], namely physical, informational, social and psychological privacy as well as items taken from the previous qualitative study. The subsequent questions addressed privacy from different angles. Participants were asked on a six-point Likert scale (1 = completely disagree, 6 = completely agree) to what extent a selection of ten different entities, have the authorization to enter their privacy. The selection of entities was on the preceding qualitative study and including public institutions, professional groups or person groups. The subsequent evaluation regarding privacy involved privacy violation and respective concerns regarding such a violation. Items were again taken from the previous qualitative study. At last, several possible invaders into privacy (previously identified through qualitative assessment) were presented and participants had to rate on a six-point Likert scale (1 = not bad at all, 6 = very bad) how bad it would be if these actors really did invade privacy in a way that was inappropriate to their role and powers. The questionnaire ended with assessing several attitudes regarding video based AAL technology.

3.3 Data Analysis

Qualitative. The interviews were audio-taped and transcribed verbatim. The theoretical foundation of the analysis was the thematic qualitative text analysis as outlined by [52]. The study was carried out in both German and Italian. The selected quotes were translated into English for this publication.

Quantitative. In the quantitative part of the study, reliability analysis ensured measurement quality of all constructs (Cronbach's $\alpha > .7$). The measured constructs are reported by means of descriptive statistics such as means (M) and Standard Deviations (SD) and percentages (%) of the examined sample.

3.4 Participants

Qualitative. The qualitative interview study was carried out between June and July 2021 with twelve participants who were interviewed with semi-standardized questions through videophone. The interviews lasted approximately one hour and were conducted with German and Swiss (Swiss-Italian) participants of a broad age range differing in their level of technical understanding and care experience who were recruited from the personal network of the authors and volunteered to take part in the study. The interviews (N = 12 participants, ranging in age between 23 and 82 years: M = 52.67; SD = 22.49) were conducted and analysed. Gender was balanced with half of them being females (50% males). Totally, five Swiss and seven Germans were interviewed. As their highest educational level, seven out of all participants stated to hold an academic degree, among them one participant holding a doctorate, whereas four completed vocational training and one person holding an A-level certificate. Roughly more than half of participants (i.e., seven participants) stated having (professional or informal) care experience, three among them reported working in the medical or care sector. High levels of technical literacy were attributed to four participants whereas three were classified as having low technical literacy. The remaining five participants ranged in between. No participant reported hands-on experience and knowledge of AAL technologies. All participants were transparently informed about the use of the collected data as well as the purpose of this qualitative research and agreed to take part in it. No compensation was given for participation.

Quantitative. Data collection took place in Germany in December 2021, convenience sampling was applied with the aim to reach people from all age. Completing the questionnaire took about 20 min. Overall, N = 134 completed the entire questionnaire. Participants' age ranged from 17 to 69 (M = 31.15; SD = 14.75) with 67.2% females (N = 90), 32.1% males (N = 43; one person indicated being divers). Asked for participants' highest educational degree, 26.9 % (N = 36) indicated to have obtained a university degree or promotion, among the remaining 73.1%, slightly more than half i.e., 55.2% (N = 74) indicated having an A-Level Degree. Overall, it was a very healthy sample as 98.5% of all participants considered their health as good or better. The numbers of people with chronic illnesses reflects this trend, indeed, only 20.9% (N = 28) specified to suffer from a chronic illness such as asthma, mental diseases, diseases concerning internal organs, or migraine. No participant indicated to need care. Regarding the experience of having cared for another person it shows that 24.6% (N = 33) have had either professional or informal care experience or both remaining with 75.4% (N = 101) with no care experience at all. Technical understanding could be considered as decent (four items; M = 4.19; SD = 1.03; Cronbach's α = .85; min = 5 and max = 24 scores). General understanding of privacy was quite high (sixteen items; M = 4.57; SD = 0.51; Cronbach's α = .74; min = 46 and max = 92 scores) and especially informational privacy seemed to be well understood (M = 4.97; SD = 0.70).

4   Results

First results from the qualitative mental mapping procedure are reported, followed by the quantitative results regarding privacy invasion of various stakeholders.

4.1   Privacy in an AAL Scenario

Descriptive Results. In total, maps of eleven participants were examined (P2–P12). Their maps differed in the number of objects included in the map and on average participants included M = 14.36 (Median = 12; Mode (bimodal) = 7,12) objects. Interestingly, the most care experienced participant (P3, 59 years, MA. Nursing and health sciences, 22 objects) conceptualized the most complex map with the highest number of objects included followed by the youngest, technically highly skilled participant (P6, 23 years, 21 objects). Among the participants who created the least complex map were the two oldest participants (P11 and P12 both aged 81, low-medium technical literacy,

P12 informal care experience, both 7 objects). Participants with more complex maps (P2, P3, P4, P5, P6, P9, P10) were able to group their objects into two to six categories, whereas this was not possible for the less complex maps of P7, P8, P11, and P12. Seven participants were able to select one most important object of the map and five among them could name an adequate replacement (See Fig. 2).

Qualitative Findings. Results from the thematic analysis of the single maps revealed three major categories, "General Aspects of the AAL Scenario", "Privacy Aspects of the AAL Scenario" and "Ideal Conceptualization of AAL Technology". These three broad classifications were further divided into several major and minor subcategories.

Overall, across participants general positive thoughts on the AAL scenario prevailed compared to general negative thoughts. In fact, all participants but one (P4) mentioned some positively connoted thoughts as part of their the first impression. Several positive aspects even revealed excitement for the entire AAL system, such as: *"I am enthusiastic, [...] it lights my thoughts. Without the technology no one knows about my health, and I can only guess if I am not well. Just thinking that with this technology there is someone, is a great relief" (P10).*

As what can be identified as general negative aspects or concerns regarding the AAL technology, only a few were mentioned. Participants feared that interaction with AAL devices would make them particularly aware of their frailty or in the extreme case be the cause of further health decline and frailness, indeed: *"I am afraid that I am no longer challenged. Basically, it is like diminishing self-esteem from the outside" (P4).*

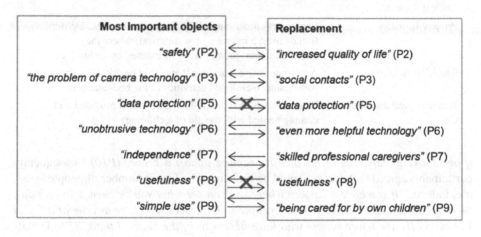

Fig. 2. Participants' most important objects and their replacements for it.

The emerging privacy aspects could be subdivided into three major themes such as Handling Data, Handling Technology and Critical Aspects (adapted from [53]). Each of these themes could be further divided into several sub-themes (See Table 1). The theme Handling of Data comprises participants worries, preferences and thoughts on how data should be treated. The fear that data may be used for non-authorized purposes was prominent, for instance: *"I wouldn't want many others to know that I have a certain illness. I mean inappropriate dissemination of data. You have to understand who is on the other side, [...] if one looks for a specific purpose regarding health okey, but*

Table 1. Privacy Aspects of AAL Scenario.

Theme	Description
Handling of Data	
Data Misuse	Participants were aware that the AAL technology records highly sensitive data (e.g., everyday activities, health information) and feared that this data could be misused for wrong purposes
Data Storage	How data is stored was only a matter for participants with high technical understanding who understood the implications different storage options have for data security
Data Control and Access	Participants agreed that the fewer people have access and control of the data, the better. However, some preferred giving access to a small circle of trusted people others favoured a care service
Handling of Technology	
Autonomy and Independence	Participants answers were determined by the meaning they assigned to autonomy and independence in old age considering values and views on life
Maintenance of Control	Participants thoughts were driven by the fear of losing control over technology which may lead to losing control over oneself
Critical Aspects	
Privacy Invasion	Participants mentioned daily life situations (e.g., having friends over, a moment of withdrawal) where they considered their privacy to be threatened by technology
Sensitive Activities	Among sensitive activities that would be critical to monitor participants mentioned activities in the bed- and bathroom
Technological and Human Care	Participants hoped that human care is still provided and complemented with the aid of technology

if one looks to make fun of me then it becomes almost a crime."(P10) Consequently participants agreed that access should be limited to the fewest number of people possible, indeed: "If you have a camera where you can see what you've been doing all day, then of course I don't want so many people to have access to it or anyone at all. [...] But basically, the fewer people who have access to it, the better, I think."(P6) Details regarding the storage options where mentioned only by a few technologically skilled participants who provided detailed insights about their preferences: "For me, it would be positive if the data were stored locally, i.e. not in a cloud. And the analysis of the data also happens locally. So the artificial intelligence is also on site, so to speak (...). And only if an irregularity is detected, yes, that one then no longer works locally, so to speak, but communicates externally" (P5).

The theme Handling of Technology summarizes how participants imagined the interaction with the technology and especially to what extent the use of these devices would have an effect on their autonomy and independence discovering this aspect might be two folded: "On one hand something is taken over but then you keep your indepen-

dence longer [...]. On one hand deactivated, on the other hand, increased autonomy. It is perhaps a paradox." *(P4)* Additionally, participants discussed the amount of control over the own life once AAL is installed in the own home which should be warranted in the best way possible: *""When you are so old that you no longer know how to operate this device you even feel more controlled by the device. [...]. Then, it would be important that the device is hidden so that you don't notice it or that the device helps you to operate it to give you the feeling that it doesn't control you"* (P6).

Lastly, Critical Aspects regarding privacy where identified from participants answers and comprised situations and activities where privacy is of particular importance and prone to be threatened. As such for instance sensitive activities in the bath- and bedroom: *"What I don't feel comfortable with is, for example, when I go to the toilet, knowing that I am being watched, or other intimate acts that I don't like to do in public. As long as I understand this cognitively, I can accept it, even if reluctantly. But I think it becomes difficult when the mind can no longer grasp it. Then it becomes a burden."(P4)* Participants critiqued the lack of human support and shared their hope that AAL technology might be complemented and combined with regular human care: *"The technology is there but maybe one day a human being will come by. That is what I hope. [...] Even if everything is okey every two days, once a week, you can talk to a person about these things that were recorded or about your wishes, that would be good. It doesn't matter if all the values are good, you still want to talk to someone when you are alone"* (P3).

Furthermore, participants shared how technology should ideally be designed to be in line with their personal privacy preferences as well as their general wishes regarding functionalities, appearance, and interaction. Findings are summarized in Table 2 and adapted from [53].

Table 2. Ideal Conceptualization of AAL Technology [53].

Ideal Conceptualization	Description
Simply manageable	straightforward, easy interaction even for non experts
Adaptive	capable of learning about users' habits and health conditions
Customiseable	adaptive to users' life rhythms including customized functions
Rejectable	refusing technological help is possible anytime
Turning on-off	switching on or off is possible anytime
Adequate appearance	either a subtle, discreet and almost invisible device or design object

4.2   Privacy in Different Situations with Particular Entities

Authorization to Enter Privacy. Regarding the question which entity is authorized to enter one's personal privacy, it seems participants attributed less authorization, the more abstract and less personal an entity (see Fig. 3). Indeed, among other not accepted to enter privacy are Public Institutions (M = 2.19; SD = 0.93) which represent the least accepted entity overall and Legal Instances (M = 3.47; SD = 1.17).

However, according to participants also close relatives (M = 3.15; SD = 1.11) should not be allowed to enter privacy. The fact that there are entities that may be allowed to enter privacy shows the evaluation of no one (M = 3.40; SD = 1.46). Accordingly, listed from least to most accepted entity, Life Partner (M = 3.88; SD = 1.14), Parent/Guardian (M = 3.90; SD = 0.99), Police (M = 3.98; SD = 1.27), Tutor of a person in need of care (M = 4.07; SD = 1.12), Medical Doctor (M = 4.26; SD = 1.12) are the ones that have the right to enter privacy. Participants were free to name other possible entities that would have the right to invade privacy and rate them, however no one specified other entities.

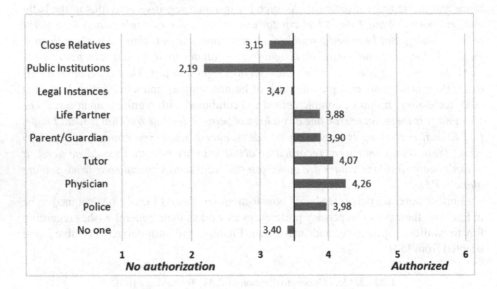

Fig. 3. Evaluation of entities and their right to invade privacy.

Privacy Invasion. Participants had to evaluate several entities according to how bad it would be if they invade privacy in a way that is inappropriate in terms of their role. Here, the previous trend that more abstract and impersonal entities are least accepted to enter privacy prevails and seems to be even more pronounced. In fact, critical invaders would be Insurance (M = 4.37; SD = 1.07) which is seen as the "worst possible intruder", followed by Medical Device Manufacturer (M = 4.17; SD = 1.20), Health Insurance (M = 4.11; SD = 1.05), Ministry of Health (M = 4.07; SD = 1.17), and RKI (German federal government agency and research institute responsible for disease control and prevention) (M = 3.75; SD = 1.26). Friends (M = 3.51; SD = 1.26) as possible intruders into privacy were seen as controversial with a marginal tendency to be among the critical ones of possible intruders. The only rather impersonal entity which was evaluated less critically was the Hospital (M = 3.25; SD = 1.09). Even less critical or even uncritical were concrete person groups such as Medical Personnel (M = 2.80; SD = 1.032), Care Personnel (M = 3.15; SD = 1.07) and the least critical Family Members (M = 3.22; SD = 1.40). Results are also visualized in Fig. 4.

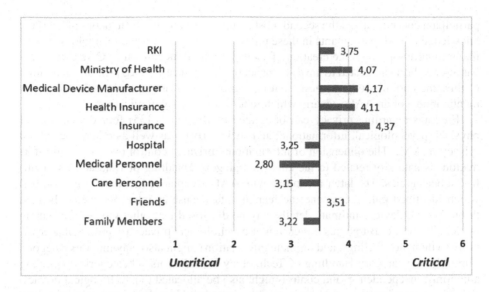

Fig. 4. Evaluation of possible privacy intruders.

5 Discussion

This mixed-methods approach aimed at understanding thought processes regarding privacy when in need of care due to age-related frailness and being supported by AAL technology. The paper presented cognitive maps of potential users of AAL technology and the resultant findings regarding their opinions on living with such assistive devices. Furthermore, the quantitative part aimed at understanding privacy dynamics regarding the interplay of authorized and unauthorized invasion of privacy of different AAL related stakeholders.

5.1 General Findings and Privacy Criteria

Generally, participants had a positive impression of themselves using AAL technology at home in older age and raised more positive than negative aspects which is in line with existing literature in that domain (e.g., see [8–11]). Through the cognitive mapping procedure consisting of the qualitative part of this study, participants' were encouraged to share their viewpoints of the AAL scenario. According to literature experts of a given field tend to include stronger and more objects [45]. This was also the case in this study where map complexity varied depending on participants previous knowledge in related fields. The least complex maps were created by the two oldest participants (both 81 years) both with limited technical understanding and no professional care experience. Perhaps older adults generally lack experience with technology compared to younger adults. The latter could be one explanation why these person groups have less developed mental models of how to use technological devices and especially AAL [54]. Contrarily, the most complex map was done by the most care experienced, technically skilled adult (59 years, MA. Nursing and health sciences). The youngest technically highly skilled participant conceptualized the second most complex one. In line with theory [43,44] the knowledge of both participants in these related domains of care and technology is very likely to have supported the creation of such compound mental maps. Care experience has already been suggested to have an impact on acceptance of AAL [16,18]. In relation to this, the current study suggests that care experiences are strongly reflected in the mental model of an AAL scenario which focuses on privacy implications.

Findings regarding privacy can be related to Burgoon's [35] four dimensions of physical, psychological, informational and social privacy as well as other research on privacy in AAL. The dimension of informational privacy (control over personal information) is naturally related to the emerged category Handling of Data and its identified subcategories. The latter are in line with AAL acceptance literature (e.g., [14,18]) which identified data access and the fear of data misuse as relevant aspects. In fact, through AAL devices intimate details may be disclosed that otherwise would remain hidden. Therefore, Burgoon's dimension of psychological privacy (degree of inaccessibility to thoughts, feelings, and intimate information) might also play into this category. Similarly, the category Handling of Technology including its subcategories regarding autonomy, independence, and control might also be allocated to psychological privacy. Psychological privacy needs to be particularly preserved in order to maintain autonomy and independence. For older adults the feeling of autonomy and independence is important during the interaction with technology as previous studies show (e.g., [10,23]). Within the subcategory Maintenance of Autonomy and Independence, several participants concluded that despite being intrusive into intimate daily life AAL technology would strengthen independence and autonomy. In literature, this is known as trade-off between autonomy and privacy (e.g., [10]). Closely related to autonomy and another core aspect is the aspect of control. More in particular, the feeling of being in control when using AAL (e.g., [23,27]) which is represented with the subcategory Maintenance of Control. The latter resumes participants' requirements to keep control over their data as well as the AAL hardware which includes being able to reject technological offers and being able to turn devices off completely. For the category Critical Aspects all privacy dimensions may be of relevance. Regarding the subcategory Sensitive Activities the psychological as well as the physical dimension of privacy may be prevalent. Sensitive activities such as showering or sleeping are typically done in the bath and bedroom. These locations were mentioned by some participants and are consistent with findings from [24]. Additionally, as known from the literature and as remarked by participants of this study, technology should not replace human care (e.g., [10]). In the subcategory Technological and Human Care participants share their desire to discuss their well-being with actual humans which in itself is an important contribution to their well-being. The subcategory Privacy Invasion and several ideal conceptualizations (i.e., "Able to learn", "Customiseable") show that privacy within an AAL scenario is a very personal matter and customisation and individual support can be an important leverage to overcome privacy concerns.

Turning towards the quantitative results and the potential intrusiveness of several AAL stakeholders, there is a clear trend for both evaluations that the less personal an entity the more sensible participants' reactions regarding privacy. Abstract entities are given less authorization and are described as being the worst intruders. Similarly, there was a tendency that entities providing direct social support are more authorized to enter privacy and are seen as less critical intruders. Especially in the evaluation of authorization to enter privacy, public institutions are strongly not authorized to enter privacy whereas physicians is given the most authorization. Generally, participants would give authorization to social and health care providers such as police or healthcare personnel, tutors or guardian/parents. In essence, all entities whose overall purpose of entering privacy consists in providing any sort of assistance to most vulnerable groups of society such as kids, people with special needs or people suffering from any sort of illness. Regarding the evaluation of intrusiveness, insurance was evaluated as being the worst potential invasion whereas the most uncritical invasion would be medical personnel, followed by hospital, family members, and care personnel. Friends are somewhat on the edge. For most entities a similar trend has been reported before, stating that the willingness to share monitoring data is highest for entities like a family doctor and family members [28, 29] compared to being low for among other authorities, governments, insurance companies as well as friends and acquaintances [26]. Considering findings regarding surveillance and theoretical implications of social identity [30–32], entities which clearly imply a collective relationship such as public institutions, legal instances, ministry of health or health insurance where always rated more critically compared to entities where interpersonal relationships are possible for instance, with a life partner, a physician, or with medical and care personnel. As control is a decisive aspect in AAL [10,23,27], one reason for this trend may be that identity management and privacy is easier to control in face-to-face interactions and relationships. Furthermore, O'Donnell's [32] findings suggest that the purpose of surveillance mitigates perceptions of privacy infringement. In this assessment, the purpose of privacy infringement was not openly communicated to participants. However, entities with a supporting role in society were shown to be considered as less harmful. Lastly, findings can also be interpreted jointly with qualitative results of the category Handling of Data. For instance, in the subcategory Data Misuse participants feared that data could get in wrong hands. Participants mentioned the importance of knowing the purpose of why others access the own mostly sensitive data. Participants would be less worried if the access was related to health which naturally happens through entities and people working in the social and healthcare sector. Additionally, in the subcategory Data Control and Access participants specified that the fewer people have access the better. This is also in line with the trend that more impersonal entities are rated more critically. Data flow and access by a company or institution is definitely less controllable and who is accessing is unobtrusive.

5.2 Pracitcal Implications

AAL is a multidisciplinary field by its nature which benefits from close inter-and transdisciplinary exchange and communication. Therefore, the reported findings may be informative for engineers, designers, and lawmakers working on aspects of AAL. In particular, other disciplines and professional groups may be interested in the perception of an "Ideal" Conceptualization of AAL Technology in terms of expectations and requirements of potential users. From the results, some key principles can be summarized:

Usability. Usability is one of the most crucial aspects. It implies simple and easily explainable interaction with AAL devices which enhances users' feeling of control over the devices. This feeling would further be supported by an on/off switching modality and technological management with minimal technical knowledge.

Interaction Style. Technological support should be provided as subtle as possible and avoid assertive ways of interaction. If devices can adapt to personal life rhythms through customisation and personalisation, acceptance of AAL becomes more natural for users. Preferences can range from technological functioning, interaction modality, and data sharing to the actual design and visibility of AAL.

AAL and Interior Design. Besides users' life rhythms, AAL needs to fit their own home and the interior structure in a way so users feel at home. The own four walls are a place of refuge, creativity, and well-being and not a healthcare facility. Despite its purpose of care and health monitoring, the AAL hardware should be designed to reflect standards of home interior.

Legal Framework and Users' Perception of Control. Participants as potential users strongly prefer to be in control of both their technological devices and the data captured. Thus, the notion of control is very important and potential AAL users are concerned about data misuse and hacking. Generally they want to know and decide with whom, how, and when data is accessed and distributed. Data elaboration methods should be adaptable to users preferences while ensuring ways of strict legal prosecuting in case of data misuse.

Overall, user aspects should be considered and integrated already during early design stages to maximize the potential that technology will be accepted and adopted by a broad range of users. Especially those key features should be integrated in future professional education not only for care personnel but also for technical designers and persons that are in charge of providing legal frameworks. In the AAL context camera technologies are an essential parts where privacy perceptions are particularly critical. Thus, based on current research [29], future studies should focus on the specificity of privacy perceptions of visual technologies at home.

5.3 Limitations and Future Research

The present mixed-method study evaluated implications of privacy in the AAL context. The applied qualitative method including the 3CM Method was effective in making participants share their thoughts and reflections about the given AAL scenario as well as their preferences and concerns regarding privacy. However, due to the scenario-based character of the study, neither actual technology nor real-life experience with AAL was evaluated. Additionally, the AAL scenario used for the mental mapping procedure was very generic in order to explore participants opinions about a broad range of devices, services and functions. Future work studying cognitive maps should ideally provide opportunities for participants to test the technology or provide a more specific and detailed explanation of a concrete technology and its functions. The timing of the mental mapping procedure was not ideal as the task was done towards the end of a one-hour semi-structured interview. This circumstance might have caused concentration loss specifically among older participants. Future studies attempting to study mental conceptualizations should put this cognitively demanding task towards the beginning of the assessment. The qualitative study took place in Germany and Switzerland while the quantitative study was conducted solely in Germany. Hence, the context of study was limited to central Europe which prevented to generalize results to other non-European contexts with different healthcare systems and other cultural- as well as political structures. The study approach should be applied in other non-European countries to compare mental conceptualizations of privacy within AAL as well as privacy infringement by various stakeholders of AAL in different contexts.

Acknowledgements. The authors would like to thank all interview and survey participants for sharing their opinions, wishes, and needs in the context of privacy and acceptance of AAL technologies. We also thank Sophia Otten and Alexander Hick for research support. This work resulted from the project VisuAAL "Privacy-Aware and Acceptable Video-Based Technologies and Services for Active and Assisted Living" and was funded by the European Union's Horizon 2020 research and innovation programme under the Marie Skłodowska-Curie grant agreement No 861091.

References

1. Blackman, S., et al.: Ambient assisted living technologies for aging well: a scoping review. J. Intell. Syst. **25**(1), 55–69 (2016)
2. Muñoz, A., Augusto, J.C., Villa, A., Botía, J.A.: Design and evaluation of an ambient assisted living system based on an argumentative multi-agent system. Pers. Ubiquit. Comput. **15**(4), 377–387 (2011)
3. Pollack, M.E.: Intelligent technology for an aging population: the use of AI to assist elders with cognitive impairment. AI Mag. **26**(2), 9–24 (2005)
4. Peek, S.T.M., Wouters, E.J.M., van Hoof, J., Luijkx, K.G., Boeije, H.R., Vrijhoef, H.J.M.: Factors influencing acceptance of technology for aging in place: a systematic review. Int. J. Med. Inform. **83**(4), 235–248 (2014)
5. Calvaresi, D., Cesarini, D., Sernani, P., Marinoni, M., Dragoni, A.F., Sturm, A.: Exploring the ambient assisted living domain: a systematic review. J. Ambient. Intell. Humaniz. Comput. **8**(2), 239–257 (2017)
6. Selke, S.: Lifelogging: Digital Self-tracking and Lifelogging - Between Disruptive Technology and Cultural Transformation, 1st edn. Springer, Heidelberg (2016). https://doi.org/10.1007/978-3-658-13137-1
7. Yusif, S., Soar, J., Hafeez-Baig, A.: Older people, assistive technologies, and the barriers to adoption: a systematic review. Int. J. Med. Inform. **94**, 112–116 (2016)
8. Garg, V., Camp, L.J., Lorenzen-Huber, L., Shankar, K., Connelly, K.: Privacy concerns in assisted living technologies. Ann. Telecommun./Ann. Telecommun. **69**(1–2), 75–88 (2014)
9. Gövercin, M., Meyer, S., Schellenbach, M., Steinhagen-Thiessen, E., Weiss, B., Haesner, M.: SmartSenior@home: acceptance of an integrated ambient assisted living system. Results of a clinical field trial in 35 households. Inform. Health Soc. Care **41**(4), 430–447 (2016)
10. Lorenzen-Huber, L., Boutain, M., Camp, L.J., Shankar, K., Connelly, K.H.: Privacy, technology, and aging: a proposed framework. Ageing Int. **36**(2), 232–252 (2011)
11. Wild, K., Boise, L., Lundell, J., Foucek, A.: Unobtrusive in-home monitoring of cognitive and physical health: reactions and perceptions of older adults. J. Appl. Gerontol. **27**(2), 181–200 (2008)

12. Beringer, R., Sixsmith, A., Campo, M., Brown, J., McCloskey, R.: The "acceptance" of ambient assisted living: developing an alternate methodology to this limited research lens. In: Abdulrazak, B., Giroux, S., Bouchard, B., Pigot, H., Mokhtari, M. (eds.) ICOST 2011. LNCS, vol. 6719, pp. 161–167. Springer, Heidelberg (2011). https://doi.org/10.1007/978-3-642-21535-3_21

13. Demiris, G., et al.: Older adults' attitudes towards and perceptions of "smart home" technologies: a pilot study. Med. Inform. Internet Med. **29**(2), 87–94 (2004)

14. Kirchbuchner, F., Grosse-Puppendahl, T., Hastall, M.R., Distler, M., Kuijper, A.: Ambient intelligence from senior citizens' perspectives: understanding privacy concerns, technology acceptance, and expectations. Ambient Intell. AMI **2015**(9425), 48–59 (2015)

15. van Heek, J., Himmel, S., Ziefle, M.: Caregivers' perspectives on ambient assisted living technologies in professional care contexts. In: Proceedings of the 4th International Conference on Information and Communication Technologies for Ageing Well and E- Health, pp. 37–48 (2018)

16. Offermann-van Heek, J., Schomakers, E.-M., Ziefle, M.: Bare necessities? How the need for care modulates the acceptance of ambient assisted living technologies. Int. J. Med. Inform. **127**, 147–156 (2019)

17. van Heek, J., Himmel, S., Ziefle, M.: Helpful but spooky? Acceptance of AAL-systems contrasting user groups with focus on disabilities and care needs. In: Proceedings of the 3rd International Conference on Information and Communication Technologies for Ageing Well and e-Health, pp. 78–90 (2017)

18. Offermann-van Heek, J., Ziefle, M.: Nothing else matters! Trade-offs between perceived benefits and barriers of AAL technology usage. Front. Public Health **7**, 1–16 (2019)

19. Altman, I.: Privacy a conceptual analysis. Environ. Behav. **8**(1), 7–29 (1976)

20. Marshall, N.J.: Privacy and environment. Hum. Ecol. **2**(1), 93–110 (1972)

21. Bergström, A.: Online privacy concerns: a broad approach to understanding the concerns of different groups for different uses. Comput. Hum. Behav. **53**, 419–426 (2015)

22. Nissenbaum, H.: Privacy in Context: Technology, Policy, and the Integrity of Social Life. Stanford University Press (2010)

23. Ulrich, F., Ehrari, H., Andersen, H.B.: Concerns and trade-offs in information technology acceptance: the balance between the requirement for privacy and the desire for safety. Commun. Assoc. Inf. Syst. **47**, 227–247 (2020)

24. Himmel, S., Ziefle, M.: Smart home medical technologies: users' requirements for conditional acceptance. I-Com **15**(1), 39–50 (2016)

25. Lederer, S., Mankoff, J., Dey Anind, K.: Who wants to know what when? Privacy preference determinants in ubiquitous computing. In: CHI 2003 Extended Abstracts on Human Factors in Computing Systems, pp. 724–725 (2003)

26. Oulasvirta, A., et al.: Long-term effects of ubiquitous surveillance in the home. In: Proceedings of the 2012 ACM Conference on Ubiquitous Computing (UbiComp 2012), pp. 41–50. Association for Computing Machinery, New York (2012)

27. Schomakers, E. M., Ziefle, M.: Privacy perceptions in ambient assisted living. In: Proceedings of the 5th International Conference on Information and Communication Technologies for Ageing Well and e-Health, pp. 205–212 (2019)

28. Boise, L., Wild, K., Mattek, N., Ruhl, M., Dodge, H.H., Kaye, J.: Willingness of older adults to share data and privacy concerns after exposure to unobtrusive in-home monitoring. Gerontechnology **32013**(11), 428–435 (2013)

29. Wilkowska, W., Offermann-van Heek, J., Florez-Revuelta, F., Ziefle, M.: Video cameras for lifelogging at home: preferred visualization modes, acceptance, and privacy perceptions among German and Turkish participants. Int. J. Hum.-Comput. Interact. **15**(37), 1436–1454 (2021)

30. Tajfel, H.: The achievement of inter-group differentiation. In: Tajfel, H. (ed.) Differentiation Between Social Groups, pp. 77–100. Academic Press, London (1978)
31. Tajfel, H., Turner, J.C.: An integrative theory of inter-group conflict. In: Austin, W.G., Worchel, S. (eds.) Organizational Identity: A Reader, 56(65), 9780203505984-16, pp. 33–47. Brooks/Cole, Monterey (1979)
32. O'Donnell, A.T., Jetten, J., Ryan, M.K.: Who is watching over you? The role of shared identity in perceptions of surveillance. Eur. J. Soc. Psychol. 40(1), 135–147 (2010)
33. Tajfel, H.: Social identity and intergroup behaviour. Soc. Sci. Inf. 13(2), 65–93 (1974)
34. Brewer, M.B., Gardner, W.: Who is this "we"? Levels of collective identity and self representations. J. Pers. Soc. Psychol. 71(1), 83 (1996)
35. Burgoon, J.K.: Privacy and communication. Ann. Int. Commun. Assoc. 6(1), 206–249 (1982)
36. Ray, H., Wolf, F., Kuber, R., Aviv, A.J.: "Woe is me": examining older adults' perceptions of privacy. In: Conference on Human Factors in Computing Systems - Proceedings, pp. 1–6 (2019)
37. Ray, H., Wolf, F., Kuber, R., Aviv, A.J.: "Warn them" or "just block them"?: investigating privacy concerns among older and working age adults. Proc. Priv. Enhanc. Technol. 2021(2), 27–47 (2021)
38. Oates, M., et al.: Turtles, locks, and bathrooms: understanding mental models of privacy through illustration. Proc. Priv. Enhanc. Technol. 2018(4), 5–32 (2018)
39. Hamidi, F., Poneres, K., Massey, A., Hurst, A.: Using a participatory activities toolkit to elicit privacy expectations of adaptive assistive technologies. In: Proceedings of the 17th International Web for All Conference, W4A 2020 (2020)
40. Craik, K.J.W.: The Nature of Explanation. Cambridge University Press, Cambridge (1943)
41. Johnson-Laird, P.N.: Mental Models. Cambridge University Press, Cambridge (1983)
42. Kaplan, S., Kaplan, R.: Cognition and Environment: Functioning in an Uncertain World. Ulrich Books (1982)
43. Collins, A., Gentner, D.: How people construct mental models. In: Holland, D., Quinn, N. (eds.) Cultural Models in Language and Thought, pp. 243–268. Cambridge University Press, Cambridge (1987)
44. Rickheit, G., Sichelschmidt, L.: Mental models: some answers, some questions, some suggestions. In: Rickheit, G., Habel, C. (eds.) Mental Models in Discourse Processing and Reasoning, pp. 9–40. Elsevier, Amsterdam (1999)
45. Kearney, A.R., Kaplan, S.: Toward a methodology for the measurement of knowledge structures of ordinary people: the conceptual content cognitive map (3CM). Environ. Behav. 29(5), 579–617 (1997)
46. Thagard, P.: How brains make mental models. In: Magnani, L., Carnielli, W., Pizzi, C. (eds.) Model-Based Reasoning in Science and Technology. Studies in Computational Intelligence, vol. 314. Springer, Germany (2010). https://doi.org/10.1007/978-3-642-15223-8_25
47. Kitchin, R.M.: Cognitive maps: what are they and why study them? J. Environ. Psychol. 14(1), 1–19 (1994)
48. Lehto, R., Therrien, B.: Death concerns among individuals newly diagnosed with lung cancer. Death Stud. 34(10), 931–946 (2010)
49. Van Hulle Vincent, C.: Nurses' perceptions of children's pain: a pilot study of cognitive representations. J. Pain Symptom Manage. 33(3), 290–301 (2007)
50. Beier, G.: Locus of control when interacting with technology (Kontrollüberzeugungen im Umgang mit Technik). Rep. Psychol. 24(9), 684–693 (1999)
51. Beier, G.: Locus of control when interacting with technology: a personality trait with relevance for the design of technical systems (Kontrollüberzeugungen im Umgang mit Technik: ein Persönlichkeitsmerkmal mit Relevanz für die Gestaltung technischer Systeme), dissertation (2004)

52. Kuckartz, U.: Qualitative Text Analysis a Guide to Methods, Practice Using Software. SAGE Publications (2014)
53. Maidhof, C., Ziefle, M., Offermann, J.: Exploring privacy: mental models of potential users of AAL technology. In: Proceedings of the 8th International Conference on Information and Communication Technologies for Ageing Well and e-Health (ICT4AWE 2022), pp. 93–104 (2022)
54. Ziefle, M., Bay, S.: Mental models of a cellular phone menu. Comparing older and younger novice users. In: Brewster, S., Dunlop, M. (eds.) Mobile HCI 2004. LNCS, vol. 3160, pp. 25–37. Springer, Heidelberg (2004). https://doi.org/10.1007/978-3-540-28637-0_3

An Attempt to Counter Agism in Gerontechnology Through the Engagement of Older Adults in the Development of Wisdom of Age

Katja Antonia Rießenberger[1]([⊠]) [iD], Sabina Misoch[1] [iD], Samira-Salomé Hüsler[1] [iD], Damian Hedinger[1], Leen Stulens[2], Bogdan Gherman[3] [iD], and Sanne Broeder[2] [iD]

[1] Eastern Switzerland University of Applied Sciences, Rosenbergstrasse 59, St. Gallen, Switzerland
katja.riessenberger@ost.ch
[2] In4care - Happy Aging, Interleuvenlaan 10, Leuven, Belgium
[3] Technical University of Cluj-Napoca, Memorandumului 28, 400114 Cluj-Napoca, Romania

Abstract. The Wisdom of Age (WoA) project aims to develop a matchmaking mentoring platform with specialized knowledge from older adults to help them remain active while also supporting industrial businesses and students in their respective endeavors. Engaging older adults in technology development is crucial to enable and facilitate equal exchange between retirees and companies. Even more, it can contribute to bridging the digital divide among older adults. We explored the use of an online survey to assess the background and needs of the targeted future user-base of the WoA platform. The survey involved older adults with a background in engineering or IT in one of the early development stages and ensured that the necessary features were implemented o increase the potential usefulness of the platform. Overall, older adults showed a positive attitude towards spending time on the platform. They indicated that the platform can provide older adults an opportunity to support society as well as make them feel useful and engaged. In sum, we were able to collect quantitative data and assign a leading role to a larger sample of end-users in the early stages of the WoA development process. The WoA platform has the potential to address the age-related brain drain in industrial companies while supporting the individualization of retirement.

Keywords: Active aging · Digital divide · Participatory design · Brain drain · Ageism · Individualization of retirement process · Gerontechnology

1 Demographic Change, Retirement, and Digitalization

1.1 Activity Theory and Retirement

The transition to retirement is believed to be a major milestone in an individual's life [1, 2]. Although some enjoy their newfound freedom that allows them to focus more on family and volunteer activities, other retirees are challenged with the fact that they will

L. A. Maciaszek et al. (Eds.): ICT4AWE 2021/2022, CCIS 1856, pp. 123–137, 2023.
https://doi.org/10.1007/978-3-031-37496-8_7

no longer pursue their usual work activities [3]. Furthermore, in Europe the declining birth rate and still increasing life expectancy are resulting in a general change in society's age structure [4]. The effects of this demographic change, particularly regarding the retirement of the boomer generation (people born between 1946 and 1964), are associated with many social challenges such as loss of economic security, challenges in the health sector (e.g., shortages in experienced health care professionals), and maintaining quality of life, the latter often being related to concerns about individual choice, (independence), and dignity [5, 6]. This will affect both individuals and their life planning as well as modern work practices. These effects are especially impactful due to the new age composition of the labor market [7]. Thus, not only do the images of ageing need to be reconceptualized [8], but the economy itself needs to reorient and adapt as well.

To cope with this paradigm shift retirees might like to pursue activities related to their background and experience. This can be attributed to the fact that (un-)paid work may provide daily structure, maintain, or establish a social network, and offer a sense of purpose and achievement. The lack of such can have a negative impact on the individual's mental health and reduce their perceived quality of life [9, 10].

First coined by gerontologist Robert J. Havighurst in 1961, the activity theory of ageing proposes that older adults thrive most when staying active and maintaining social interactions. It assumes a positive relationship between activity and perceived life satisfaction [11]. Therefore, by maintaining an active lifestyle, older adults' benefit from long-lasting mental and physical health [12].

According to Coupland (2009), retirement is not just a category or status; it is a socially driven and linguistically produced idea that is influenced by peoples' lived experiences and shifting cultural meanings [13]. A previous study described that for the boomer generation "there is not one dominant normative pattern for retirement but rather a diversity of experiences, expectations and trajectories" [3]. As a result, retirement evolving into a series of transitions, boomers oftentimes choose to move into phased retirement, bridge jobs, second careers, or part-time employment. The sharp distinction between full-time employment and full-time leisure has faded among their generation and they no longer view retirement as a distinct event or stage in life [3]. Retirement decisions are heavily influenced by a variety of individual, professional, and societal issues [3, 14]. Instead of being a predetermined plan, retirement appears to be a contingent choice made in reaction to shifting personal, family, health, and employment circumstances. Being able to individually influence and control how and when (soon-to-be) retirees work and retire based on their changing living circumstances, seems to be protruding for this generation. The preferences and identities of the individual, albeit frequently bound by the social, cultural, and workplace contexts in which they are rooted, determine how older persons wish to spend their retirement [3]. In order to develop proactively, our society must respond to the needs of retirees individually and create ways for them to construct and create their retirement and older age according to their own wishes and needs.

1.2   Brain Drain of Deep Smarts

Together with the changes in individual retirement planning, a crisis is developing on the industry's side of things as a result of the demographic change. Valuable know-how in companies is disappearing with the boomer generation reaching the retirement age. The boomer-generation is taking their tacit knowledge and human information networks, which leads to an extensive knowledge and capability shortage in the industry [15–17]. The eventual consequence will be a brain drain of experts on what Dorothy Leonard and Walter Swap (2004) refer to as "deep smarts"—the tacit and explicit knowledge that is founded on experience and enables individuals to comprehend problems, put patterns together, and draw accurate conclusions with remarkable speed [15, 16]. Those experts are a major source of value creation within firms and are people who have deep specialized knowledge of a subject and who are tested and trained, primarily by experience. This comprises the reasons behind the organization's operations, prior achievements and setbacks, and the reasons why particular strategies or techniques per-form better than others. In general, those older employees are well-versed in the respective company, its clients, and its product lines. Also, they exhibit higher levels of efficiency, complete work with greater accuracy and cost effectiveness, and possess a vast understanding of methods and procedures as well as how to handle challenges and novel situations [15, 17].

What exacerbates this knowledge loss is that a large portion of those employees' knowledge and experience is neither preserved nor articulated when they leave the company [15]. As a result, as those boomer professionals - particularly technical ones - retire, we approach a retirement bubble. Networks, knowledge, skills, and experience disappear [16]. Calo (2008) as well as Hilsen and Ennals (2005) argue that organizations must take action to transfer the knowledge of older workers to avoid suffering an unprecedented loss of human capital [18, 19].

To counteract this brain drain due to retirement, a more flexible adjustment within the labor market needs to take place. Mentoring or similar services can help to facilitate knowledge transfer between current employees and people who are already retired or will soon do so. Small and medium-sized enterprises (SMEs), that make up 99% of companies in Europe [20], could benefit from these types of services.

1.3   A Subsection Sample

Currently, several online providers (social platforms, media, or apps) are available that try to meet two requirements respectively – the desire to stay active in retirement and on the company's sides the demand for life and work experience. However, despite some of them having older adults as their target group, the majority of these online providers answer to the needs of younger users and seem indifferent to the needs of older users – especially in terms of design and marketing. For instance, they contain complex error messages, have hard to read font size, color, and style, display aggressive advertising, and SPAM. Even more so, older people are too often excluded from marketing strategies [21].

These are only subaspects of the broader challenge of the growing digital divide. "With the digital transformation advancing, the digital divide is generally distinguished by a social disintegration that derives from an unequal distribution of access to technologies" [8]. With this divide largely being influenced by the social categories of age, gender, and education (in the sense of laymen and professionals), older adults often end up being pushed to the margins of participation [22, 23].

With ageism being "a process of systematic stereotyping of and discrimination against people because they are old" [24], older adults are perceived as less healthy, mentally slower, and not willing to learn new things [25, 26]. Despite ageism being a societal challenge long before, it become even more evident within the fourth industrial revolution. Here, older adults both exclude themselves in terms of the digitalization, while also getting excluded from product developers and researchers [27–29]. By adding the factor age in theorizing about the digital divide, it has become clear that the "grey digital divide" crystallizes itself to be a much bigger societal challenge.

The marginalization of older adults in digitalization also extends to all stages of technology development. Here, said marginalization is further aggravated by a diverse set of phenomena, including but not limited to design paternalism and age-scripting. With design paternalism appearing to be a mirror of societally held stereotypes, e.g., regarding age/ing, it is oftentimes implicitly assumed that older adults should not be disrupted or unsettled by technologies in their everyday life or when using them. The reciprocal nature of these two phenomena becomes clear when looking at the user's appropriation processes of technologies as well as their autonomy and freedom in using technologies [30–34].

Ageist attitudes can be present in both socially and personally held stereotypes, and still be implemented in new technologies. The public perception of aging is thus maintained by these representations, as are older persons' internalized beliefs [34–39]. To enable and facilitate an equal exchange between (soon-to-be) retirees and companies, the wishes and needs of older generations must therefore be given greater consideration in the development of online platforms. The goal of the WisdomOfAge (WoA) project is to develop an online platform that acts as a bridge between companies and individuals over 50, mainly in technology-related fields [21, 39]. Within the WoA community, older adults will share their experience with businesses in order to help them overcome specific difficulties. This will be done within a project-based framework through online courses, training, project management, mentorship, and more. The WoA project therefore intends to develop a new mentoring platform based on participatory, interdisciplinary research. Hence, the platform is aspiring to not only be socially inclusive but also developmentally [8, 21].

2   Participatory Design in the Development of Wisdom of Age

2.1   Involving Older People in Early Development Phases

Older individuals may be excluded as a result of the aforementioned and other deeply ingrained preconceptions and attitudes in western societies, particularly in the field of technology development and innovation creation [40]. The "grey digital divide" is negatively impacted by this lack of inclusion [41]. The economy and the technology industry will eventually need to include older individuals in their development strategies due to the rise in the number of people 65 and older. However, including older people only as consumers is insufficient; their participation in technology development is just as crucial. Increased age variety in the labor market as a result of older people's integration is advantageous for businesses. Most older people have faced a variety of business challenges throughout their careers, allowing them to approach issues with a more realistic perspective [42].

To counter the abovementioned challenges the WoA project team aims to include older adults from the earliest stages of development until the very final development steps. Older persons are not viewed as less capable within the project, but rather as knowledgeable and experienced. Their real-world expertise will be especially helpful for the conception and creation of innovative ideas. Older individuals are the knowledge providers and keepers in this setting. Thus, it is most important to assign our end-users a leading role, especially at the early stages of the development process of digital innovations. Their opinions and objections regarding concepts, user-friendliness, and the design must be considered [8].

The WoA project follows Spinuzzi's (2005) approach in participatory design. According to him, it is possible to use a variety of strategies and techniques as the development process progresses, using participatory design methods [43]. It involves the inclusion of individuals who are potential members of the platform in both qualitative as well as quantitative research in an iterative approach. This will enhance the engagement of the target group as well as ensure the implementation of required functionalities increasing the potential utility of the platform [43–45].

In the first stage of the WoA-project, four co-creation workshops with older adults ($n_{total} = 29$ participants) were conducted between September and November 2021 in Belgium and Switzerland. These first end-user workshops at the earliest project stage showed that the business model and network options needed to be examined in more detail. Therefore, in the second stage an online survey was developed to effectively understand the requirements and needs of potential WoA members (in this case older adults). More specifically, the survey, which is available upon request, assessed the availability of older adults as well as reasons for signing-up and staying engaged on the platform. Based on the feedback from these workshops and the survey results, a prototype version is being developed.

2.2 Exploring the Use of Online Survey Methods

The Online Wisdom of Age Survey – Aims, Participants, and Methods. To assess the needs, design, and market opportunity of the WoA project, the online survey explored the opinion of potential mentors regarding the attractiveness, credibility, and specific requirements of the WoA platform. By using a survey to explore the background and needs of the targeted future user-base of the WoA platform, we were able to collect quantitative data and assign a larger sample of end-users a leading role in the early stages of the development process.

Our sample included adults with a minimum age of 50 years, particularly with a background in engineering or IT – both currently working and retired to identify differences in their perspectives. To meet these criteria and to consider the specific context and target groups of the WoA platform, a non-probabilistic, purposive sampling strategy was applied. More specifically, participants were contacted via a personal approach in community groups and social media (i.e., email and direct messages) in Belgium, Romania, and Switzerland. The original version of the survey was developed in English and translated to Dutch, French, German, and Romanian. This way, the end users could answer the questions in their native language. All survey questions were digitally collected via Google Forms and participants could choose to complete the survey in a confidential or anonymous manner. The first section of the survey consisted of general questions regarding the background of the participants (gender, age, years of expertise, and employment status) as well as three multiple choice questions about their self-perceived availability. To assess the requirements for developing the WoA platform, participants were asked to rate 18 statements on a five-point Likert scale (Fig. 1). Data were collected over a five-week period, from May to June 2022.

The data were checked for inconsistencies, missing values, and outliers. All analyses were performed using SPSS Version 28 or GraphPad Prism version 9.0 and included descriptive statistics and one sample independent t-tests to assess significance. For the analysis of the Likert-scales (scores from 1 to 5), statements with an average score significantly greater than the neutral value (3) were considered as important. The values that were not statistically different from 3 suggested a neutral stance. The significance level was set at $p < 0.05$.

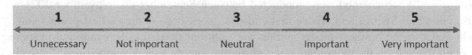

Fig. 1. Five-point Likert-scale, used in the survey section where requirements for developing the WoA platform were assessed by predefined statements.

Survey Results – Background and Availability of Participants. In total 120 persons completed the online survey. Two participants were excluded due to their age. The distribution of the participants according to their country was as follows: Belgium n = 45 (37.5%), Romania n = 30 (25%), and Switzerland n = 45 (37.5%). Full descriptive statistics of the demographic questions showed a well distributed sample of seniors across age but not for gender (i.e., remarkably more males). In total, 66 seniors were still working (55%) and the majority had more than 20 years of professional experience (88.3%). All frequency distributions of the demographics are reported in Table 1.

Table 1. Characteristics of the online survey participants (means ± standard deviations).

	Total (n = 120)	Belgium (n = 45)	Romania (n = 30)	Switzerland (n = 45)
Gender (M/F/O)	99/20/1	40/5/0	23/6/1	36/9/0
Age (years)	65 (±7)	63 (±6)	66 (±6)	66 (±9)
Employment status (R/W)	54/66	24/21	11/19	19/26
Experience (<5/5–10/10–20/ > 20 years)	1/3/10/106	0/0/2/43	0/0/1/29	1/3/7/34

Abbreviations: F = female, M = male, O = other, R = retired, W = working

To implement the principles of the activity theory, it is important to understand the self-perceived availability of older adults. In other words, how much time and when during the week and day are older adults available for additional activities such as mentoring on the WoA platform. To explore the perceptions of retired adults compared to those who are still working, the detailed data for this part of the survey were analyzed separately. Results showed that 36% of the retired participants are willing to be available 'once every few weeks' and 35% 'several times a week'. Of the participants that are still working, 46% are willing to be available 'once every few weeks' and 29% 'several times a week'. The older adults prefer to be available on weekdays and this applies to both retired (77%) and working participants (76%). Furthermore, results show that participants that are retired slightly prefer the morning (28%), whereas the seniors that are still working are mostly available during the evening (20%). However, differences between the two groups were not considerable. Figure 2 presents the availability distributions for both groups. Thus, overall, the older adults had generally positive attitudes towards spending time on the platform which will contribute to the maintenance of an active lifestyle.

Survey Results – Requirements for Developing the WoA Platform. The highest rated aspects of the WoA platform were that it gives retired older adults an opportunity to support society, to contribute in building the future as well as make them feel useful (all $p < 0.001$). Other aspects such as networking, being part of a community and recognition were also significantly considered as important (all $p < 0.05$). Interestingly, factors as financial compensation, awards or incentives, and certificates were in general considered as neutral (all $p > 0.05$) (Table 2). For participants that are still working, all suggested aspects were considered as important (all $p < 0.002$) (Table 3). Except towards awards given by the platform the attitude was neutral ($p = 1.00$). Thus, the platform should provide older adults an opportunity to support society as well as make them feel useful and engaged. Retired older adults would not join the platform to increase their income for a better life.

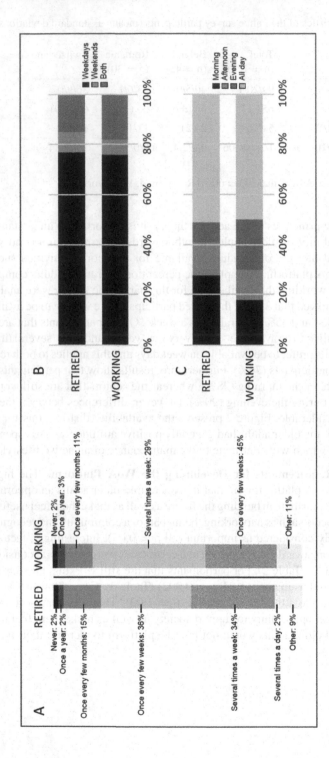

Fig. 2. The preferred availability of the survey participants in percentages: (A) the general availability per year, (B) the availability during the week, and (C) the availability during the day.

Table 2. Reasons for retired older adults to start and keep using the WoA platform. Higher mean scores are considered as more important.

		mean (± st.dev)	p-value
1	Support the society	4.0 (±1.0)	<0.001
2	Feeling useful	3.9 (±0.9)	<0.001
3	Take part in building the future	3.9 (±1.0)	<0.001
4	To stay engaged/active	3.8 (±0.9)	<0.001
5	To have a community of mentors/mentees	3.7 (±0.8)	<0.001
6	Being confident and satisfied	3.7 (±0.9)	<0.001
7	Meet other top consultants	3.6 (±0.8)	<0.001
8	Receive reviews and testimonials	3.6 (±0.9)	<0.001
9	Networking with companies/institutions/students	3.6 (±1.0)	<0.001
10	Being appreciated by leading companies	3.4 (±0.8)	0.001
11	Networking with other mentors	3.4 (±1.0)	0.002
12	The platform will direct 10% of the revenues to senior organizations	3.4 (±1.0)	0.002
13	Interacting globally from your home	3.4 (±1.1)	0.006
14	Recognition of your knowledge and expertise	3.4 (± 0.9)	0.007
15	Incentives	3.2 (±0.9)	0.051
16	Certification by the platform (i.e., proof of your proficiency as a mentor)	3.2 (±0.9)	0.066
17	Financial compensation	3.0 (±1.0)	0.388
18	Bonuses/awards for the most active mentors	2.9 (±1.1)	0.184

Table 3. Reasons for older adults that are still working to start and keep using the WoA platform. Higher mean scores are considered as more important.

		mean (± st.dev)	p-value
1	To stay engaged/active	4.1 (±0.8)	<0.001
2	Being confident and satisfied	4.0 (±0.8)	<0.001
3	Feeling useful	4.0 (±0.7)	<0.001
4	Networking with companies/institutions/students	4.0 (±0.7)	<0.001
5	Take part in building the future	4.0 (±0.8)	<0.001

(continued)

Table 3. (*continued*)

		mean (± st.dev)	p-value
6	To have a community of mentors/mentees	3.9 (±0.8)	<0.001
7	Support the society	3.8 (±0.7)	<0.001
8	Meet other top consultants	3.6 (±0.8)	<0.001
9	Interacting globally from your home	3.6 (±0.9)	<0.001
10	Networking with other mentors	3.6 (±1.0)	<0.001
11	The platform will direct 10% of the revenues to senior organizations	3.6 (±1.0)	<0.001
12	Being appreciated by leading companies	3.5 (±0.8)	<0.001
13	Recognition of your knowledge and expertise	3.5 (±0.9)	<0.001
14	Certification by the platform (i.e. proof of your proficiency as a mentor)	3.5 (± 1.0)	<0.001
15	Financial compensation	3.4 (±0.8)	<0.001
16	Receive reviews and testimonials	3.4 (±0.9)	<0.001
17	Incentives	3.3 (±0.9)	0.001
18	Bonuses/awards for the most active mentors	3.0 (±1.1)	0.500

3 Opportunities and Challenges in Participatory Design of Digital Innovation for Older Adults

3.1 The Role of Wisdom of Age in Bridging the Digital Divide

Participatory design that aims to bridge the digital divide, which itself can be considered multifactorially influenced (e.g., by age, gender, and education), should contemplate an inclusive approach [22, 23, 46]. The WoA project aims in the first instance to develop a platform for older adults with a background in engineering and IT. These sectors are not only known as the most male dominated working fields, but they also require specific knowledge and experience often obtained by long education trajectories [47]. The utilized non-probabilistic, purposive sampling strategy, focusing on this specific group of potential users, was justified for the purposes of WoA since it included the current target group of the platform. Though consequently, current results only contribute to bridging the 'digital divide' for older adults within this specific social category and are not generalizable. Furthermore, results from the survey are possibly biased. For instance, the finding that monetary compensation was not regarded as crucial may be related to the greater financial stability of adults with higher education in the technology sector in average. By using participatory design in the WoA project, a first attempt towards bridging the digital divide has been made and the platform has the potential to further contribute to this in the future. More specifically, the interest and digital capabilities of older adults with a background in engineering or IT in an online tool such as WoA will probably be higher than the one of the average older person. This increases the chances of successful implementation of the platform and provides opportunities to broaden the target group in later market introduction phases.

However, for upcoming development processes it is important to consider that even older adults that are experienced in technology usage suffer more often than younger users from physical decline and impairments, such as visual impairment or tremor in the hands [48]. Participatory design with larger samples of end users will provide valuable general insights regarding the needs of older adults and are implemented in the WoA project. Secondly, results from the online survey showed that a key motivator to be part of the WoA community is the opportunity to be actively engaged in the society through the platform, particularly for the retired participants. This may suggest that the WoA target group believes that this form of online mentoring can contribute to the social engagement of older adults.

As described by the activity theory, the maintenance of physical activities as well as staying interested and engaged in society play a crucial role in aging well [12]. However, evidence regarding the availability of older adults for additional activities, such as online mentoring, in their daily life schedule is limited. Therefore, the online WoA survey aimed to gain insights in the self-perceived availability of both, older adults that are retired and those that are currently still working. Results showed that in general the attitude of the participants was positive towards spending time on the WoA platform and there were no obvious differences between these two groups.

Since retirement is a socially driven concept, multiple ideas evolve around how the individual wants to create their own respective retirement. Boomers frequently decide to transition into phased retirement, bridge jobs, encore careers, or part-time employment as a result of the retirement process growing into a series of transitions. WoA tries to facilitate these transitions by e.g., allowing the older adult to individually determine their availability, amount, and frequency of mentoring sessions. One of WoA's key objectives is to enable people to personally manage how and when they work based on their changing living circumstances. Since their retirement decisions are greatly influenced by several professional, societal, and individual aspects, WoA wants to establish avenues for them to design and shape their retirement in accordance with their own needs and preferences. The results of the online WoA survey will be used for these purposes, however further involvement of older adults in later development phases will take place.

With the boomer generation retiring, organizations need to take action to transfer valuable knowledge of older workers [18, 19]. The aforementioned new wave of retirements leads to and extensive knowledge and capability shortage in companies. Resulting in an extensive brain drain of workers with 'deep smarts', which is amplified by the aspect of said knowledge not being preserved and articulated [15, 16]. WoA may be able to support countering the retirement-related brain drain in companies. For example, almost all survey participants expressed their willingness to share their knowledge regularly, therefore making it not only more quantifiable for companies, but also available to younger generations of workers. The in the survey stated availabilities of older workers furthermore indicate that it is possible to create and maintain a mentoring relationship – at least regarding time factors.

Finally, through both the implementation of participatory design in the development phase as well as by its future potential in society, WoA has a considerable role in bridging the digital divide amongst older adults. Even more so, potential users of the platform are willing to use the platform on a regular basis, contributing to increased activity of older adults.

3.2 Strengths and Limitations of the Online Survey as a Participatory Design Method

The current findings have to be interpreted against the drawback that we used a purposive sampling approach. Despite the international study set-up (i.e., representation of three nationalities), this resulted in a limited diversity of our participants, especially regarding gender, education level, and work experience. The results of the online survey are not representative and cannot be generalized to the population of older adults as a whole due to this sampling approach, the pre-experimental study design, and the homogeneity of the cohort regarding important social factors of the digital divide - age, gender, and education (see Sect. 1.3) Furthermore, the (anonymous) self-administrative character of an online survey has the drawback of respondents not being able to seek clarification if they do not understand a question [49]. On the contrary, ensuring anonymity or confidentiality of participants contributes to higher response rates in general and may lead to less social pressure, thus increasing the tendency to give honest rather than socially acceptable answers [50].

The current sample of 120 participants can be considered as small in typical quantitative social research, though is justifiable when taking the explorative character of this study design into account [51]. Depending on the applied approach, future participatory design investigations should consider larger and more heterogenous samples to improve the power and generalizability of results.

Participatory design is a research methodology with its own theoretical and methodological foundation [43]. Nonetheless there are still some research gaps that have not been filled yet, e.g., regarding the actual outcomes of the participatory design approach, as Merkel & Kucharski's systematic literature review from 2019 has shown [52]. As of right now it is widely used as value in and of itself and less because it has proven effective in delivering the expected results of a higher acceptance rate of older users. Therefore, it needs to be noted that it can be challenging to evaluate participatory design projects especially in terms of the research design (including sample sizing), as the research on it is insufficient to establish a gold standard.

3.3 Conclusion

WoA has a considerable role in bridging the digital divide amongst older adults by implementing participatory design in the development phase as well as by its future potential within the society. The attitude of potential users of the platform appears to be positive and both retired and working older adults are willing to spend their time on the platform as a way to stay engaged in society. With this outlook, it can be assumed that WoA can gain the capacity to play its part in counteracting the age-related brain drain in industrial companies while at the same time supporting the individualization of retirement.

References

1. Schmitt, A.: Übergang in und Anpassung an den Ruhestand als Herausforderung aus psychologischer Perspektive. Organisationsberat Superv Coach **25**, 337–347 (2018)
2. Yemiscigil, A., Powdthavee, N., Whillans, A.V.: The effects of retirement on sense of purpose in life: crisis or opportunity? Psychol. Sci. **32**(11), 1856–1864 (2021)
3. Kojola, E., Moen, P.: No more lock-step retirement: Boomers' shifting meanings of work and retirement. J. Aging Stud. **36**, 59–70 (2015)
4. Eatock, D.: Demografischer Ausblick für die Europäische Union 2019 (2019). https://www. europarl.europa.eu/RegData/etudes/IDAN/2019/637955/EPRS_IDA(2019)637955_DE.pdf
5. Mossburg, S.E.: Baby boomer retirement: are you up to the challenge? Nurs. Manag. **49**(3), 13–14 (2018)
6. Dennis, H., Migliaccio, J.: Redefining retirement: the baby boomer challenge. Generations J. Am. Soc. Aging **21**(2), 45–50 (1997)
7. Cedefop: Future skill needs in Europe: critical labour force trends. Publications Office of the European Union, Luxemburg (2016)
8. Rießenberger, K.A., Hüsler, S., Bruggmann, A., Eicher, S., Stulens, L., Misoch, S.: WisdomOfAge: developing a seniors digital platform for knowledge transfer through participatory design. In: Proceedings of the 8th International Conference on Information and Communication Technologies for Ageing Well and e-Health - ICT4AWE, pp. 261–267 (2022)
9. Boss, V.: Psychische Gesundheit bei älteren Menschen. In Blaser, M., Amstad, F.T. (eds.) Psychische Gesundheit über die Lebensspanne, Grundlagenbericht, pp. 107–116. Gesundheitsförderung Schweiz, Bern (2016)
10. Patel, R.P.: A study of impact of post-retirement work on psychological well- being of elderly. Indian J. Mental Health **5**(1), 63 (2018)
11. Havighurst, R.J.: Successful aging. Gerontologist **1**(1), 8–13 (1961)
12. Rupprecht, R.: Psychologische Theorien zum Alternsprozess. In Oswald, W., Fleischmann, U., Gatterer, G. (eds.) Gerontopsychologie, Grundlagen und klinische Aspekte zur Psychologie des Alterns, pp. 13–25. Springer, Vienna (2008). https://doi.org/10.1007/978-3-211-783 90-0_2
13. Coupland, J.: Discourse, identity and change in mid-to late life: interdisciplinary perspectives on language and ageing. Ageing Soc. **29**(06), 849–861 (2009)
14. Robertson, A.: "I saw the handwriting on the wall": shades of meaning in reasons for early retirement. J. Aging Stud. **14**(1), 63–79 (2000)
15. Leonard, D., Swap, W.: Deep smarts. Harv. Bus. Rev. **82**(9), 88–97 (2004)
16. Aiman-Smith, L., Bergey, P., Cantwell, A.R., Doran, M.: The coming knowledge and capability shortage. Res. Technol. Manag. **49**(4), 15–23 (2006)
17. Joe, C., Yoong, P., Patel, K.: Knowledge loss when older experts leave knowledge-intensive organisations. J. Knowl. Manag. **17**, 913–927 (2013)
18. Calo, T.J.: Talent management in the era of the aging workforce: the critical role of knowledge transfer. Public Pers. Manag. **37**(4), 403–416 (2008)
19. Hilsen, A.I., Ennals, R.: An action research approach to work ability, health and well-being of ageing workers. In: International Congress Series, vol. 1280, pp. 365–370 (2005)
20. Gischer, H., Herz, B.: Aktuelle Herausforderungen für KMU und Regionalbanken in der Europäischen Union. Institute of European Democrats, Brussels (2021)
21. Pisla, D., et al.: Development of a learning management system for knowledge transfer in engineering. Acta Technica Napocensis Ser. Appl. Math. Mech. Eng. **64**(3), 361–368 (2021)
22. Van Dijk, J.: Digital divide research, achievements and shortcomings. Poetics **34**, 221–235 (2006)

23. Buchmüller, S., Joost, G., Bessing, N., Stein, S.: Bridging the gender and generation gap by ICT applying participatory design process. Pers. Ubiquit. Comput. **15**, 743–758 (2011)
24. Butler, R.N.: Why Survive? Being Old in America. Harper and Row, New York (1975)
25. Swift, H., Steeden, B.: Exploring representations of old age and ageing. Centre for Ageing Better, Whitfield (2020)
26. Allen, J.O., et al.: Experiences of everyday ageism and the health of older US adults. JAMA Netw. Open **1**, 5(6) (2022)
27. Friemel, T.N.: The digital divide has grown old: determinants of a digital divide among seniors. New Media Soc. **18**, 313–331 (2016)
28. Knowles, B., Hanson, V.L.: The wisdom of older technology (non)users. Commun. ACM **61**(3), 72–77 (2018)
29. Schwab, K.: The Fourth Industrial Revolution. Crown Business, New York (2017)
30. Peine, A., Rollwagen, I., Neven, L.: The rise of the "innosumer" – rethinking older technology users. Technol. Forecast. Soc. Chang. **82**, 199–214 (2014)
31. Peine, A., Neven, L.: Social-structural lag revisited. Gerontechnology **10**(3), 129–39 (2011)
32. Peine, A., Moors, E.H.M.: Valuing health technology – habilitating and prosthetic strategies in personal health systems. Technol. Forecast. Soc. Chang. **93**, 68–81 (2015)
33. Neven, L.: 'But obviously not for me': robots, laboratories and the defiant identity of elder test user. Sociol. Health Illn. **32**(2), 335–347 (2010)
34. Neven, L.: Representations of the Old and Ageing in the Design of the New and Emerging: Assessing the Design of Ambient Intelligence Technologies for Older People. University of Twente, Enschede (2011)
35. Peine, A., Neven, L.: The co-constitution of ageing and technology – a model and agenda. Ageing Soc. **41**(12), 1–22 (2020)
36. Vines, J., Pritchard, G., Wright, P., Olivier, P., Brittain, K.: An age-old problem: examining the discourses of ageing in HCI and strategies for future research. ACM Trans. Comput.-Hum. Interact. **22**, 1–27 (2015)
37. Joyce, K., Mamo, L.: Graying the cyborg: new directions in feminist analyses of aging, science, and technology. In: Calasanti, T., Slevin, K. (eds.) Age Matters: Realigning Feminist Thinking, pp. 99–121. Taylor & Francis; Routledge, New York (2006)
38. Cozza, M., De Angeli, A., Tonolli, L.: Ubiquitous technologies for older people. Pers. Ubiquit. Comput. **21**(3), 607–619 (2017). https://doi.org/10.1007/s00779-017-1003-7
39. Gherman, B., Nae, L., Pisla, A., Oprea, E., Vaida, C., Pisla, D.: WisdomOfAge: designing a platform for active and healthy ageing of senior experts in engineering. In: Pissaloux, E., Papadopoulos, G.A., Achilleos, A., Velázquez, R. (eds.) ICT for Health, Accessibility and Wellbeing. IHAW 2021. Communications in Computer and Information Science, vol. 1538. Springer, Cham (2021). https://doi.org/10.1007/978-3-030-94209-0_2
40. Mannheim, I., Schwartz, E., Xi, W., Buttigieg, S.C., McDonnell-Naughton, M., Wouters, E.J.M., van Zaalen, Y.: Inclusion of older adults in the research and design of digital technology. Int. J. Environ. Res. Public Health **16**(19), 3718 (2019)
41. McDonough, C.C.: The effect of ageism on the digital divide among older adults. Gerontol. Geriatr. Med. **2**, 1–7 (2016)
42. Fischer, J.: Age Diversity bringt Mehrwert (2020). https://www.zwk.ch/de/wirtschaft-politik/agediversity-bringt-mehrwert-n1941
43. Spinuzzi, C.: The methodology of participatory design. Tech. Commun. **52**, 163–174 (2005)
44. Lindsay, S., Jackson, D., Schofield, G., Olivier, P.: Engaging older people using participatory design. In: Proceedings of the SIGCHI Conference on Human Factors in Computing Systems, Austin, TX, USA, pp. 1199–1208 (2012)
45. Hakobyan, L., Lumsden, J., O'Sullivan, D.: Participatory design: how to engage older adults in participatory design activities. Int. J. Mob. Hum. Comput. Interact. (IJMHCI) **7**(3), 78–92 (2015)

46. Pasick, R.J., Burke, N.J.: A critical review of theory in breast cancer screening promotion across cultures. Annu. Rev. Public Health **29**, 351–368 (2008)
47. Corbett, C., Hill, C.: Solving the Equation: The Variables for Women's Success in Engineering and Computing. American Association of University Women. 1111 Sixteenth Street NW, Washington, DC 20036 (2015)
48. Colón-Emeric, C.S., Whitson, H.E., Pavon, J., Hoenig, H.: Functional decline in older adults. Am. Fam. Physician **88**(6), 388–394 (2013). PMID: 24134046; PMCID: PMC3955056
49. Zutshi, A., Parris, M.A., Creed, A.: Questioning the future of paper and online survey questionnaires for management research. Paper presented at the 21st ANZAM Conference, Sydney, Australia (2007)
50. Ong, A.D., Weiss, D.J.: The impact of anonymity on responses to sensitive questions 1. J. Appl. Soc. Psychol. **30**(8), 1691–1708 (2000)
51. Hill, R.: What sample size is "enough" in internet survey research. Int. Comput. Technol. Electron. J. 21st Century **6**(3–4), 1–12 (1998)
52. Merkel, S., Kucharski, A.: Participatory design in gerontechnology: a systematic literature review. Gerontologist **59**(1), e16–e25 (2019)

Rescuing Relevant Features from Active Aging Surveys: A Data Mining Perspective

Juan-Fernando Lima[1] , Priscila Cedillo[2] , María-Inés Acosta-Urigüen[1,3] ,
Marcos Orellana[1]([⊠]) , and Alexandra Bueno-Pacheco[1]

[1] Laboratorio de Investigación y Desarrollo en Informática - LIDI, Universidad del Azuay,
Cuenca, Ecuador
{flima,macosta,marore}@uazuay.edu.ec
[2] Departamento de Ciencias de la Computación, Universidad de Cuenca, Cuenca, Ecuador
priscila.cedillo@ucuenca.edu.ec
[3] Facultad de Informática, Universidad Nacional de La Plata, Bueno Aires, Argentina
maria.acostau@info.unlp.edu.ar

Abstract. Within the psychological currents, several proposals on active aging
have been defined, conceptualizing it as a perspective or differentiated way of
aging satisfactorily. These proposals generate indicators that assess the level of
physical health, psychological well-being and adequate social and spiritual adaptation. The indicators are quantified based on active ageing surveys whose are
differs for each ageing proposal and collects different features of active aging
such as: health, cognition, activity, affection, fitness, and satisfaction levels. This
methodology is focused on rescuing the relevant factors (features) facilitating the
interpretation of the data, avoiding the non-required characteristics. The methodology proposes a set of data mining techniques for different types of data that
could be present in the forms of active aging, and seeking to make a concrete
proposal, the features of an active aging survey are evaluated, determining a subset of features where their weights make them more relevant in data collection,
and finally, this methodology is positively evaluated as a model of acceptance by
geriatric psychologists.

Keywords: Active ageing · Data mining · Features relevance · TAM ·
Methodology

1 Introduction

When old age concept was analyzed, until not long ago it was considered to be only
related to illness, memory problems, senility, dementia, poverty and depression [35].
The World Health Organization, in 2015 presented the World Report on Aging and
Health, which covers aging as the sum of several changes; biologically, aging is associated with the accumulation of a wide variety of molecular and cellular damages that
gradually reduce physiological reserves, increase the risk of many diseases, and generally decrease the individual's capacity [59]. In addition, it defines Active or Healthy
Aging as the process of promoting and maintaining the functional capacity that allows

L. A. Maciaszek et al. (Eds.): ICT4AWE 2021/2022, CCIS 1856, pp. 138–156, 2023.
https://doi.org/10.1007/978-3-031-37496-8_8

well-being in old age, quantifying it through variables that include personal characteristics, health characteristics, genetic inheritance, functional capacity and intrinsic capacity of being human; as well as variables of the environment in which the person develops, such as identity, relationships, the possibility of enjoyment, autonomy, security and the potential for personal growth [5,59].

The World Health Organization (WHO) considers that there are three main periods of healthy aging: a relatively high and stable capacity, a diminished capacity, and a significant loss of capacity. It also identifies that these there are different approaches to quantify the active ageing, but all of them keep the same purpose of promoting and maintaining the human intrinsic capacity, so that people with reduced functional capacity can continue to carry out activities that are important to them [59]. Trajectory that does not depend on chronological age and that is not uniform among the individuals of a population.

Worldwide, the concept of active aging has gained interest; for example, the European Union has focused on issues related to a transition from the perception that older adults are only recipients of a retirement to an active orientation in which they are active subjects at the family, community, work, educational level, etc. [57] Another example is observed in China, Japan, and South Korea; they have proposed an integrated, composite index for measuring the contribution of older people to the society, to their communities and their families, considering the percentage of older population aged 60 or more. This index is compound of metrics that identify the staying in labor market longer, the contribution or participation in the community, society and family activities, the capacity of living independently, and the promotion of individuals' capacities [56].

Although identifying active aging in a people is relevant, for governments, it is even more relevant to generate population indicators that allow them to build policies with a view of improving the reality of this segment of the population. In this context, data mining techniques is useful to quantify, tabulate and obtain results oriented to active aging, where the generation of datasets and the application of various techniques becomes an attractive option to evaluate and interpret the concept of active aging among a wide range of variables and their combinations [40,41,54]. Prediction, detection of outliers (anomaly detection), clustering and decision making are some of the most used techniques in the data mining field [38,47].

According to the above descriptions, active ageing definitions such as by the WHO, European, and Oriental have some similar characteristics among them, but also differs on multiples definitions and variables to measure the active ageing, this obstruct the way to create a general framework to evaluate the active ageing surveys designed by psychologists basing on the definitions that they believe proper. Thus, it is required to propose a data mining methodology to evaluate variables collected by active ageing surveys. The perspectives of data scientists are base to communicate the relevant techniques and tools to face and overcome the most important barriers for each data analysis stage. A previous work presented the first steps to discover insights among active ageing variables and the method was embodied as a business process notation [2]. Based on it, this paper presents the methodology for surveys guided by a software engineering specification, deep into the data mining techniques, and shown an instance of the method analyzing variables of an active ageing survey.

The paper is organized as follows: In Sect. 2, in form of background, the active ageing definitions are presented allowing to give context to readers. In Sect. 3, The methodology to face the evaluation of active ageing variable is shown. In Sect. 4, the evaluation by psychologists of this method is presented. In Sect. 5, the conclusions and viable applications of this method are shown.

2   Related Work

While the concept of active ageing is analyzed, the WHO highlight that old ageism refers to creating stereotypes, discrimination and prejudice against old people [59]. Since at the end of the 60s of the 20th century, various sociological perspectives have been proposed as theoretical objectives focused on distinguish the "good" and "bad" ways of aging. However, models of aging based on exact psychological indicators have now been developed, although these models have a great common basis, each of them represents a different perspective of aging successfully, below the most relevant perspectives are shown.

2.1   Successful Aging

This concept presents a model based that measure the capacities of elderly taking into account the absence and risk reduction of disease and disability; the high functional capacities, and active engagement with life. This term was introduced by Robert J. Havighurst (1961) [39] in order to classify aging patterns in two groups, normal and pathological capacities; and according to authors such as [23] or [45], it is necessary to distinguished heterogeneity within elderly groups, each of them having different stereotypes, experiences and expectations. Thus, the Rowe and Kahn model (1997) establishes three key indicators to characterize successful aging related to the probability of suffering diseases or disabilities, the function of cognitive and physical capacities and the engagement to life. The model of successful cognitive ageing compares an elderly individual to other groups, the approach compares the cognitive performance of an specific person with data obtained of the same chronological age and establishes an index on relative homogeneity in young adulthood but heterogeneity thereafter [35].

2.2   Optimal Aging

The concept of optimal ageing can be described in the manner an elderly spends his life and the opportunities he has including not only aspect related to the biological, medical and socioeconomic environment, but also including a form of life that can be optimized and cultivated [46]. It measures satisfaction despite the presence of adverse medical conditions that can alter the life of an older adult [10]. The concept of optimal ageing includes the decision of an individual to optimize different stages of his life, depending on his goals, his projection or his environment. The concept includes, in addition to the level of health, the mental health and the social functioning as major elements that determines plasticity in aging. In [3], where the selection, optimization and compensation are mandatory to adjust proper goals and objectives related to that age [6]. The concept includes the analysis of aspect related to the effect of physical activity, nutrition, and social as elements to determine the physical functioning, the mental/cognitive functioning, the active social functioning, and an overall health indicator [37]. Brummel-Smith considered the social environment and support system as elements that influences the process in adaptation to changes and also prevents individuals from pathologies caused by stress [9].

2.3   Active Aging

The WHO in 2002 raised the concept of active aging. This proposal, from the beginning, included health, participation and safety as basic components, although later this work was taken up again and learning was included as a fourth component of this concept [8]. In this way, active aging has been defined as "... the process of optimizing opportunities for health, participation and safety in order to improve the quality of life as people age" [28], proposal that can be approached from a public policy perspective. The first pillar, health, refers to preventing diseases and promoting healthy habits that promote well-being on a physical, mental and social level [28]. The pillar of physical level depends on peace, security, food, income, ecosystem, and other variables that constitute the individual's system [28]. Active aging has a third pillar, the safety, since insecurity of any kind could have harmful effects on health and well-being. At the individual level, the risks of illness, death, unemployment for long periods; food insecurity, economic and cultural insecurity [8]. The latest and newest pillar in active aging is the learning. This is seen as a resource that improves the ability to remain healthy, by allowing different knowledge and skills to be acquired and updated to maintain people's capacities and also to better reinforce personal safety [28].

2.4   Positive Aging: European Model

Fernández - Ballesteros points out that this concept integrates what has been defined as optimal, successful, active, productive, healthy aging, and other nomenclatures that express, in short, an aging that entails the integral well-being of the subject. The author points out that three main aspects are grouped under all these concepts, a) successful aging is multidimensional, since it encompasses biophysical, emotional, cognitive and social aspects; b) they cannot be reduced to purely biological domains in terms of health and disease, nor to subjective conditions; and c) there are no great intercultural differences in this construct. Thus, it is determined, through exploratory factor analysis, that there are 5 factors that affect this type of aging, and they are: a) health, cognition, activity, affect, and fitness [20].

2.5   New Proposals for Successful Aging

A recent proposal states that successful aging is determined by four aspects: physical, psychological, social and pleasant activities [34]. The psychological factor refers to the existence of a lower stress level, as well as a generalized sense of psychological well-being, which implies self-acceptance, positive relationships with others, autonomy, mastery of the environment, purpose in life and personal growth [49]. Regarding the social factor, social support (availability of people that one can count on), religion and commitment to life are mentioned as essential points that help people face the adversities of life [51]. Pleasant activities include actions like exercise or vacations. In order to evaluate this factor, questions were asked that inquired about the frequency with which the person traveled outside the city or the frequency with which they carried out exercise. This model was tested using structural equations, and had a very good fit showing that these factors make up the successful aging construct [34].

2.6 Psychosocial Models of Successful Aging

Carver and Buchanan's proposal seeks to highlight non-biomedical aspects that are considered in other models. This would allow to speak of a good or optimal aging even in those older adults who have some disease. Their approach considers, as a main point, leaving aside biomedical constructs so that more older adults can be included. In this case, several aspects need to be considered: commitment to life, optimism or positive attitude, resilience. In addition, the factor of spirituality or religiosity is included, and can be beneficial. It is understood as the fact of getting involved in contemplative or altruistic activities. Finally, self-efficacy and self-esteem are indicated as significant in the model, as well as gerotranscendence, which refers to the older adult being able to see his life in retrospect and give it meaning and purpose, as well as understand it coherently [13].

In Sweden another model established that successful aging has to do with a subjective and retrospective assessment of overall quality of life. From this point, they affirm then that the commitment with life is the main factor to have a good aging [52]. This concept is based on the theory of activity, specifically related to the participation in pleasant or leisure activities. In this sense, a person who presents higher levels of activity in this type of dynamism will be opposing the so-called lack of productivity that comes with retirement, thus guaranteeing their successful aging. In [26] a model for activity domain includes culture-entertainment, productive-personal growth, physical-outdoors, recreation-expressive, friendship, and formal group. Those items remark the importance of participation and the commitment that they generate. As it has been analyzed, these models in general have something in common: they all seek the integral well-being of people. They show the interest in the deep human being, beyond the only visible and objective, it considers the person in all its facets.

3   Methodology

Based on the Software & Systems Process Engineering Metamodel (SPEM) specification, the proposed methodology is an instance of the six stages of the Cross-Industry Standard Process for Data Mining (CRISP-DM) [58], and it is shown in Fig. 1. The active ageing context is fundamental providing: roles, concepts, and artefacts such as codebooks and the raw datasets. Several datasets has to be transformed to ordinal types, therefore, data dictionaries are essential to accomplish this task. And after that, the model can be build according the data quality, the feature selection model has to support different data types.

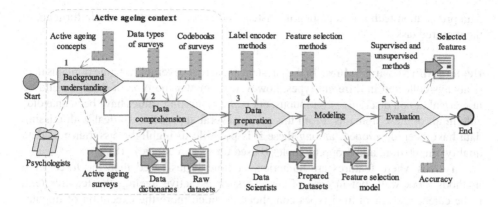

Fig. 1. Methodology for select the relevant features among active ageing surveys.

3.1 Data Comprehension

The different approaches focused on evaluate the active ageing seen in the above section collect several variables and data types making hard the interpretation if collected data, it inclusive for only one ageing survey. In this context, grateful to the web page of Institute for Research on Ageing it is possible to confirm the several approaches and waves for ageing analysis, the institute collected and opened multiple datasets seeking to improve the research on this knowledge domain [27].

To address this propose, one survey collected in the study by the Advanced Cognitive Training for Independent and Vital Elderly carried out in United States since 1999 until 2001 [55] is used as an input example to detect the relevant features and discard the others without lose the weight of the input data for a machine learning algorithm. In order, from the 43 collected forms in the study, seeking proof but also simplify this whole methodology, we selected the data of the DS0027 folder related to the form 618-Medication Audit. This dataset is conformed by 38 features and 5156 records by people aged between 65 and 94 years. Each feature is a medicament, the description of each feature is stored in the respective codebook, and the referent value indicates how many the person forgot to take the medicine.

3.2 Data Preparation

In a data mining process the data preparation stage wastes more than the 50% of the whole process, this is caused by one or multiple techniques are applied until to get a proper dataset to be used as input in a data mining algorithm. The processes inside of the data preparation stage commonly are: normalization, label encoder, missing values treatment, data discretization, dimensional reduction; in addition, surveys require extra techniques due to the text existence, in these cases, techniques such as: lower case, quantities parsing, punctuation treatments, stop words, stemming, and lemmatization are indispensable prior to extract relevant information from the active ageing forms collected in textual mode. This subsection aims to describe the more relevant data preparation techniques among the listed, and according to the sample form apply the required tasks.

Dealing with Missing Values. In the latest years, across several academic domains data is always collected in different types, however, no matter the type of data, it could be numerical or not, discrete or continuous, but perhaps missing values have been unavoidable in all of these domains. From this point, several approaches to deal with missing data have been developed, among these it is possible to highlight: assurance of data quality, imputation, and dropping tuples (based on its percentage) [18].

In cases where features are numerical or time series-based then the forecasting methods work well, but in case of surveys such as active ageing, the features tend to be categorical, or ordinal types complicating much more the execution of imputation approaches. Works such as Swindell [54] shows how to deal with continuous and categorical features, proposing to fill in missing data with the "Imputation approach" method. The missing data are imputed based on the average value between the $k = 20$, but the credibility of the imputed data is low. In psychology domain, the choice about missing data relapses on the opinion of experts and on the amount of data collected [18], if there are missing fields, the Neuropsychologists experts prefer to backup up and drop the records and all the linked records to avoid the noise in the results [41].

Transforming by Data Discretizacion. According to [41], a challenge to face in surveys is the standard for peoples' ages transformation, who are part of the group to be analyzed. Ages are indispensable across studies for healthy. The Research of Adult Learning and Development Handobbok address the guidelines for treatment of these age groups [53]. A simple way is to transform ages focused on standardize the age in groups as: childhood, adolescence, emerging adulthood, average adulthood, and late adulthood. In complement to it, the ordinal encoders can give support to these age groups making possible to include in numerical data mining algorithms [61]. In the same way, Ethnicity can be categorized [42] but label encoders can be used instead of ordinal encoders [61]. The encoders are trained to allow transform nominal to numerical types, but also these algorithms execute the inverse task facilitating to trace the data discretization and transformation.

Dealing with Likert Scales. In the same way, satisfaction and comfortable feedback levels are part of active ageing surveys, commonly these levels are based on the Likert scale. Both ways to deal with this scale are present, on the one hand, ordinal encoders can transform and make these appropriate for a data mining process, but on the other hand, special algorithms for deal with this scale are available increasing the power of data mining process improving the goodness in the results [30].

Dealing with Texts. In data containing words or phrases, it is necessary to identify words that will contribute or not to a mining process [38]. Text mining is considered a huge topic inside data knowledge retrieval, perhaps to develop a Natural Language Processing (NLP) perspective over surveys can fit as a specific papers to address the treatment. However, in this point, it is presented a overview of the main techniques for a text mining process. In an initial description, we highlight that it has the same six steps than a data mining process [58]. According to [24], the text preparation includes the following techniques:

Nonalphabetic Characters Removal. The preprcessing technique allows to remove numbers, punctuation, special characters. However, depending of the domain understanding, number can be transformed to words to avoid loss information. For example, A question in survey related to number of pill administration per patient.

Text Conversion. Lowercase and uppercase conversions are used to standardize the inputs, and reduces the vocabulary, therefore, it decreases the number of dimensions. It is necessary highlight that inside NLP each word is a dimension (feature).

Spelling Correction. Due to manual writing could contain wrong words or personal styles, the spelling is used for correct these issues. Also, this technique helps to increase the statistical power and avoid the capture of styles.

Contractions and Abbreviations. It uses a dictionary to transform the abbreviations (both formal and informal) and get the complete words.

Stop Words. It is a list of word contains common words to be removed without value in the analysis, for example, the sentence connectors.

Lemmatization and Stemming. These techniques are focused on get a root among words wrote in different tenses. The first one uses a dictionary to get the simple root of a word, for example: *"wrote"*=> *"write"*. On the other hand, stemming seeks to truncate the word through rules, for example: *"speaking"*=> *"speak"*, however, it does not consider the tenses, for example, *"funnier"*=> *"funnier"*.

3.3 Modeling

Reveal the features whose characterize the active aging is the main interest of this work, several feature selection approaches could be take into account to resolve the objective, however, only a select group of approaches have support for the multiple data types collected in the related surveys of active ageing how is shown in the above. The most simple approach is determine the influence of variables using the algorithm "Select by weights" that selects only those whose weights satisfy a criterion concerning the input weights [36].

Clustering. The selection or removal of features depends of the input data, therefore, in some cases it is need to apply filters or a deeper filter analysis for discovering some groups of individuals with similar patterns, hence, when this requirement floated out, the clustering technique is justly focused on divide data onto subgroups of interest, incorporating a unsupervised approach as part of the analysis. The application of unsupervised methods has been used in similar works focused on data segmentation, the work of [43] evidences the predictive value of different measures of cognition, clustering found that girls with the high socioeconomic status trend to higher academic achievement in science stream, and boys with low socioeconomic status had trends higher academic achievement in general. The application of clustering over social domains has been widely used as an unsupervised technique for human activity recognition [4], this leads to take it as part of a possible segmentation case.

When it is clear how clustering will solve it, it is necessary to select the proper technique among the multiple algorithms such as: hierarchical, k-means, random sampling, randomize search, condensation based, densityBased, grid-based, probabilistic model-based, clustering graphs, or network data [44]. The goodness of data is proportional to the fulfilment of its purpose, normally, the technique creates groups mutually exclusive based on three possible conditions: a) Defining the maximum cluster distance and minimizing it, b) Compute the sum of averages of the distances and minimizing it, and c) Compute the total cluster distance and minimize it [44]. The problem defines two segments: proper or no proper values for active aging. Therefore, k-means algorithm is proposed to generate the two segments [30], clustering gives another advantage related to the responses of likert scale due to its nature of losing information and data distortion.

Feature Selection and Dimensional Reduction. The above points aim to create a validated and structured input to be used in this stage. However, a concern is data with redundant variables [25], and also the unstructured data collected from interviews or tests such as cognitive diagnostics or clinical treatments are also an issue to overcome [11], in both cases, high dimensional treatment is the gap to overcome, therefore, two ways are visible to accomplish to task.

Feature Extraction. In this method algorithms are focused on transforming a set of features (variables) to a new dataset, with low dimensions using mathematical functions, some of them can revert the process, but there is some loss in precision of the output values. These techniques are widely used in the neuropsychological domain as a dimensionality reduction to deal with data collected from digital machines as function of Magnetic Resonance Images [19,29], or Electroencephalograms images (EEG) [1,7,17]. The principal component analysis (PCA) or its variants is the common method to perform this task.

Feature Selection. This approach selects only the relevant variables from a dataset. Unlike feature extraction which transform data, this method keeps the understanding of the variables. This approach requires a better data pre-processing, and finally, an evaluation process to ensure the quality of the output features. The evolution of feature selection has granted multiple vias or methods such as: Filter Methods. A ranking mechanism is used to grade the features (variables), and based on a value as a threshold, the features are removed. The methods are based on relevance and redundancy. The common methods are: variance, information measure, correlation measure, distance measure, consistence measure, fuzzy set theory, and rough set theory [14]. Wrapped Methods, this method uses the predictor performance as an objective function to evaluate the variable subset, suboptimal subsets are found by employing search algorithms, the algorithms start with an empty dataset and then add features (or by full dataset and removing features) until to obtain the maximum objective function [60]. Evolutionary Computation Paradigms, some authors of consider the evolutionary computation into the wrapped methods, however, a more recent study [60] details the importance of split these methods, the heuristic search evaluates different subsets until it optimizes the objective function, multiple subsets are created by searching in a searchspace, the used algorithms by this method are genetic algorithms, genetic programming, particle swarm optimization, ant colony optimization, and differential evolution. The feature selection process is shown in Fig. 2.

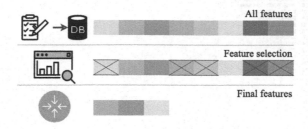

Fig. 2. The overview of feature selection for active aging forms.

Case of Rescue Relevant Features. Using as input the data of the survey 618 explained in Sect. 3.1, The objective is to evaluate relevance among features (X axes), therefore, the feature selection has to be applied. As preprocessing operations: the AID, OTHERMED, and NUMMEDS features were dropped, and the VISIT feature was transformed using an ordinal encoder and set itself as evaluation predictor known also as a target.

In order, in the modeling stage, to evaluate the weight of each feature, a filter method was used due to the absence of a target feature, how we have seen the wrapped method uses a predictor to evaluate each variable. The chi-square test evaluates the relationship among the features, its main advantage is the support for nominal, ordinal, and numeric values. The test compares the features against the normal distribution, the distribution is described as $x^2 = \Sigma Zi^2$, where $z1, z2, .., z(n)$ are standard normal variables. In feature selection the test aims to select the features which are highly dependent on the response. For null hypotheses (H0) the two variables are independent, and for alternative hypotheses (H1) two variables are not independent. The python package for machine learning provides an API for feature selection, and it can be used by the method $SelectKBest(chi2, k = n)$ simplifying the analysis. In Fig. 3 is possible see the $p - value$, the null hypotheses is rejected if the value falls in the error region (alpha from 0 to 0.05). In this survey, 12 features are independents due to these fall into the alpha range, and the rest of features are not independent.

In this case, one of the surveys was analyzed, but the rest of these can to follow the guidelines described in the above subsection. Therefore, evaluate the relevance among: successful, optimal, active, positive, psychological proposals described in Sect. 2.

3.4   Model Evaluation

The main advantage models based on a predictor analysis is itself validation due to its precision values, as we have seen, the p-values are fundamental for evaluating the

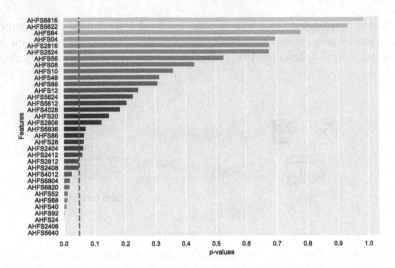

Fig. 3. Rescuing relevant features from the Form 618-Medication Audit, $alpha = 0.05$.

weight among features. On the other hand, If clustering was used prior the feature selection, a simple way is verify the grouped data is related is through multidimensional graphs. Generally, 2D or 3D dimensional plots are used to display the groups [31], the visual analytics is a recent strategy in which the human capabilities are used to interpret the data behavior. The interpretation is executed over popular visualization methods as: Bar charts, Line charts, Pie charts, and Scatter plots. In this case, the scatter plot is a standard method to describe a clustering application, while the human can evaluate according to the dispersion of data. However, this method is hard to assess if clusters are very closed [15]. In this case a mathematical indicator is required to improve the verification of goodness. Two indicators are proposed by the literature, the elbow analysis and the silhouette indicator are viable to increase the confidence of the generated groups [50].

4   Evaluating the Feature Selection of Surveys

In the same way as the previous work [2], This section presents a case study seeking to evaluate the acceptance of this methodology. In this context, Runeson in 2012 proposed a set of activities to evaluate a product [48], the activities to be tracked are: 1) design, 2) preparation for data collection, 3) collecting evidence, 4) analysis of collected data and reporting, and 5) threats of validity analysis. The results of this evaluation represent an essential knowledge for data engineers who work in factors associated with active aging in the proposed methodology. To achieve this evaluation experts in active aging evaluate the inputs used in the proposed methodology according to Runeson.

4.1   Designing the Evaluation

Seeking to obtain a degree of agreement among the experts, this evaluation analyzes regarding the variables in a survey of healthy aging. Besides, this case study is focused on evaluate the perceptions among health personnel regarding the usefulness of the results derived from the stages of the data method.

The evaluation and the scope were addressed by the Goal-Question-Metric (GQM) approach proposed by Basili et al. in 1994 [12]. The GQM scheme is structured as follows: a) The analysis of the inputs for the methodology proposed by the data engineers, b) What is the purpose of the objective measures the agreement among active ageing experts against each activity regarding the usefulness of the information resulting from the methodology, c) From the point of psychologists, and d) In the health context where this study is carried out.

Analyze. The evaluation analyzes the inputs for the methodology proposed by the data engineers.

With the Purpose of. reach a degree of agreement among health experts, and evaluate their perceptions regarding the usefulness of the information resulting from the methodology.

From the Point of View of. Clinical psychologists.

In the Context of. a real execution of feature evaluation.

And, in this context, the research questions are:

1. What stage(s) are not avoidable in the health domain?.
2. What the perception of health personnel on the usefulness of a methodology that allows selecting active aging variables collected utilizing data mining techniques?.

Based on Runeson et al. [48] recommendations, this case study method is holistic-multiple, and the units of analysis are presented in Fig. 4.

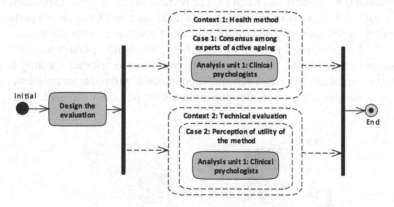

Fig. 4. Process for evaluation the acceptance of this work.

4.2 Preparation for Data Collection

Two surveys were designed to achieve the objectives of this case study. For Context 1, a form was developed based on Lak, Rashidghalam, Myint, and Bradaran [32] (see https://n9.cl/iwle), who propose a list of active aging characteristics based on the study of related work. The purpose of this first form is to reach a consensus of experts in the gerontological health area of the variables that should be considered for the characterization of healthy aging through data mining.

Next, seeking to evaluate the Context 2, a form was created based on the technology assessment model (TAM) proposed by Davis [16]. However, to limit its application, we only analyze the constructs of the Perceived Utility (PU) and the Intent to Use (UIT) in the future, therefore, the final product of the methodology is analyzed. Hence, data mining experts designed the form with its respective explanation based on the likert scale, it is shown in the following URL: https://n9.cl/qcmb4.

4.3 Data Analysis and Reporting of Results

Both questionnaires were explained, then were filled by two Clinical psychologists with experience in the gerontological domain, they are experts due to their experience both in academic degree and also in practical field.

Next while the results were interpreted, it was found that in Case 1, Fleiss' Kappa statistical measure used for assessing the reliability of agreement between a fixed number of raters when assigning categorical ratings (likert) to several items or classifying items. The action is scored between 0 and 1 (0 means low agreement, and one refers to a high deal). Fleiss' Kappa also is used to validate the process of inclusion/exclusion of variables presented in Appendix 1 of the form (see https://n9.cl/iwle). Finally, the selections of each reviewer was checked and some discrepancies were resolved with consensus among they.

For the both two raters, the Fleiss's Kappa for agreement on inclusion in the active aging resulted 0.83, Landis and Koch [33] provide a table to evaluate and interpret the resulting values, thus, values between 0.81 and 1.00 are considered almost perfect. The average of the responses obtained for the two TAM constructs analysed was calculated (see Fig. 5). It is concluded that clinical psychologists mention that this technological contribution can reduce the time and effort to evaluate the relevance among features. Also, the experts recall that it is a valuable input since it will allow an excellent characterization of the study variable to develop intervention plans in different levels.

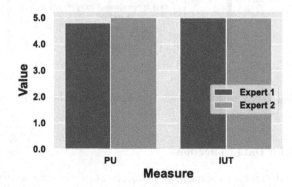

Fig. 5. Results of the case study - Perceptions of the clinical psychologists.

In comparison with the previous work, the results of the evaluation of this TAM does not change, the psychologists maintain their responses. It could be due to the simplicity to fill the forms and the experience of the raters. The values obtained in the previous works of 0.82 and 0.83 in this work do not change the results of this case study.

4.4 Threats of Validity

The evaluation of threats to validity in a case of study is a critical task focused on secure the quality of empirical studies in Software Engineering (SE), this includes the systems and methods for data treatment and analysis due to these are part of information systems. Threats to validity normally is understood by four categories: construct, internal, and external validity, and conclusions [62].

Construct Validity: focuses on identify the correct use of operational measures for the concepts being studied. In context 1, the work by Sutano [22] as a list of active ageing features collected in a systematic literature review. In order to compare the degree of experts agree seeking to not fall into personal subjectivities the Fleiss Kappa scale was used. For context 2, the questionnaire proposed and validated by the Cronbach's alpha is ideal. Thus, constructs were interpreted in the same way by the researcher and the interviewees.

Internal Validity: is focused on establish a causal relationship, whereby certain conditions are believed to lead to other conditions, in this case, how the participants were selected. The knowledge and experience of participants about data mining could influence the responses and perceptions when using the proposed solution. To avoid this threat, the participants have a similar professional profile.

The External Validity: defines the domain to which the findings can be generalized. in this case, selecting the sample of individuals who participated was made at convenience; for this reason, the results have to be analysed carefully because they are not generalizable due to the specific requirements of each data mining technique.

The Conclusion Threat: demonstrates that the operations of the case of study such as the data collection procedure can be repeated, with the same results, this threat is avoid due to the use of general forms, the first one based on literate, and the second one validated by the Cronbach's alpha value. Moreover, the qualitative responses were quantified using a Likert scale to avoid introducing interpretation bias.

5   Conclusions and Further Work

This paper in determine the relevance among features of surveys providing by active ageing evaluation. In perspective of data scientists, the data mining techniques are fundamental to achieve a proper data evaluation identifying among features are strongly associated with the topic discarding the others. Data recollected from different sources in the psychological tests as mental, physical, social, policy health, and personal behavior [21], these variables commonly are collected based by models proposed by the international organizations and according to the neuropsychologists perceptions [41].

The multiple data mining techniques for measuring variables have allowed creating this method to rescue the most relevant variables among different data types, therefore, evaluating the relevance of these it is possible to focused on the proper variables for active aging. Moreover, the proper techniques to analyze them into each data mining process: Likert scale values treatment, listwise deletion or missing values imputation for missing values dealing, standardized data discretization of continuous values, and ordinal and label encoders for sociodemographic variables.

Then, according to the objective evaluation, a clustering technique could be used as part of the analysis to split data in subgroups and then evaluate the features weight. However, the use of clustering has to perform a performance evaluation of groups using indicators or visual analytics to get the best precision in the generated groups, after getting the results, we seek to report results seeking to apply different data mining techniques to evaluate the features. The critical premise is to evidence the existence of a target feature as predictor. According to the application case shown in Sect. 3.3.3, this predictor allow to compare among features and rescue the most relevant. On the other hand, when there is not a predictor, feature extraction techniques such as PCA can be used although the original structure of features has to change. If the data analysts want to maintain the original values among features, filter methods are candidates to execute this task, the information measures will be generated by techniques such as correlation or variance among the popular techniques.

In our application over the survey 618-Medication Audit, we detect 12 features are independent among them, rescuing this features as the relevant to be interpreted by clinical psychologists and gerontology experts. The evaluation of this method as a TAM is positive among the experts. Further efforts are mainly centered on evaluate features between the feature selection and the feature extraction techniques. The perspectives to create this method are fundamental and were well received by experts who do not part of the data science domain, this paper grants several tools and theoretical applications of techniques over survey collected by active ageing evaluations. Based on these evidences, it will be possible to detect the most relevant features among the surveys and contrast them with the base proposal and its principles of ageing to verify the application of the active proposal.

Acknowledgements. The authors wish to thank the Vice-Rector for Research of the University of Azuay for the financial and academic support and all the staff of the Laboratory for Research and Development in Informatics (LIDI), and the Department of Computer Science of Universidad de Cuenca.

References

1. Abdulhay, E., et al.: Computer-aided autism diagnosis via second-order difference plot area applied to EEG empirical mode decomposition. Neural Comput. Appl. **32**(15), 10947–10956 (2020). https://doi.org/10.1007/s00521-018-3738-0
2. Acosta-Urigüen., M., Cedillo., P., Orellana., M., Bueno., A., Lima., J., Prado., D.: Finding insights between active aging variables: towards a data mining approach. In: Proceedings of the 8th International Conference on Information and Communication Technologies for Ageing Well and e-Health - ICT4AWE, pp. 268–275. INSTICC, SciTePress (2022). https://doi.org/10.5220/0011068100003188

3. Aldwin, C.M., Spiro, A., Park, C.L.: Five - health, behavior, and optimal aging: a life span developmental perspective. In: Birren, J.E., Schaie, K.W., Abeles, R.P., Gatz, M., Salthouse, T.A. (eds.) Handbook of the Psychology of Aging (Sixth Edition), pp. 85–104. Academic Press, Burlington (2006). https://doi.org/10.1016/B978-012101264-9/50008-2. https://www.sciencedirect.com/science/article/pii/B9780121012649500082

4. Ariza Colpas, P., Vicario, E., De-La-Hoz-Franco, E., Pineres-Melo, M., Oviedo-Carrascal, A., Patara, F.: Unsupervised human activity recognition using the clustering approach: a review. Sensors **20**(9) (2020). https://doi.org/10.3390/s20092702. https://www.mdpi.com/1424-8220/20/9/2702

5. Baldassar, L., Atkins, M.: Healthy active ageing rapid evidence review, heart foundation walkwise, pp. 978–1 (2020). https://doi.org/10.26182/zdh2-ej22

6. Baltes, P.B., Baltes, M.M.: Psychological perspectives on successful aging: the model of selective optimization with compensation. Successful aging: Perspectives from the behavioral sciences, pp. 1–34. Cambridge University Press, New York (1990). https://doi.org/10.1017/CBO9780511665684.003

7. Basterrech, S., Krömer, P.: A nature-inspired biomarker for mental concentration using a single-channel EEG. Neural Comput. Appl. **32**(12), 7941–7956 (2020). https://doi.org/10.1007/s00521-019-04574-2

8. Brazil, I.L.C.: Active ageing: A policy framework in response to the longevity revolution (2015)

9. Brummel-Smith, K.: Optimal aging, part ii: evidence-based practical steps to achieve it. Ann. Long Term Care **15**(12), 32 (2007)

10. Brummel-Smith, K.: Optimal aging, part i: demographics and definitions. Ann. Long Term Care **15**(11), 26 (2007)

11. Buendía, F., Gayoso-Cabada, J., Juanes-Méndez, J.A., Sierra, J.L.: Transforming unstructured clinical free-text corpora into reconfigurable medical digital collections. In: 2019 IEEE 32nd International Symposium on Computer-Based Medical Systems (CBMS), pp. 519–522 (2019). https://doi.org/10.1109/CBMS.2019.00105

12. Caldiera, V.R.B.G., Rombach, H.D.: The goal question metric approach. Encycl. Softw. Eng., 528–532 (1994)

13. Carver, L.F., Buchanan, D.: Successful aging: considering non-biomedical constructs. Clin. Interv. Aging **11**, 1623–1630 (2016)

14. Chandrashekar, G., Sahin, F.: A survey on feature selection methods. Comput. Electr. Eng. **40**(1), 16–28 (2014). https://doi.org/10.1016/j.compeleceng.2013.11.024, https://www.sciencedirect.com/science/article/pii/S0045790613003066. 40th-year commemorative issue

15. Chen, W., Guo, F., Wang, F.Y.: A survey of traffic data visualization. IEEE Trans. Intell. Transp. Syst. **16**(6), 2970–2984 (2015). https://doi.org/10.1109/TITS.2015.2436897

16. Davis, F.D.: A technology acceptance model for empirically testing new end-user information systems : theory and results (1985)

17. Devipriya, A., Nagarajan, N.: A novel method of segmentation and classification for meditation in health care systems. J. Med. Syst. **42**(10), 193 (2018). https://doi.org/10.1007/s10916-018-1062-y

18. Enders, C.K.: Applied Missing Data Analysis. Guilford Press, New York (2010)

19. Estella, F., Delgado-Márquez, B.L., Rojas, P., Valenzuela, O., Roman, B.S., Rojas, I.: Advanced system for automously classify brain MRI in neurodegenerative disease. In: 2012 International Conference on Multimedia Computing and Systems, pp. 250–255 (2012). https://doi.org/10.1109/ICMCS.2012.6320281

20. Fernández-Ballesteros, R.: Envejecimiento saludable. In: Congreso sobre envejecimiento. La investigación en España, pp. 9–11 (2011)

21. Fernández-Ballesteros, R.: Positive ageing: objective, subjective, and combined outcomes. E-J. Appl. Psychol. **7**(1), 22–30 (2011)

22. Fleiss, J.L.: Measuring nominal scale agreement among many raters. Psychol. Bull. **76**(5), 378–382 (1971). https://doi.org/10.1037/h0031619
23. Gutiérrez, M., Desfilis, E.S., Zacarés, J.J.: Envejecimiento óptimo: perspectivas desde la psicología del desarrollo. Promolibro (2006)
24. Hickman, L., Thapa, S., Tay, L., Cao, M., Srinivasan, P.: Text preprocessing for text mining in organizational research: review and recommendations. Organ. Res. Methods **25**(1), 114–146 (2022). https://doi.org/10.1177/1094428120971683
25. Houari, R., Bounceur, A., Kechadi, M.T., Tari, A.K., Euler, R.: Dimensionality reduction in data mining: a copula approach. Expert Syst. Appl. **64**, 247–260 (2016). https://doi.org/10.1016/j.eswa.2016.07.041, https://www.sciencedirect.com/science/article/pii/S0957417416303888
26. Hutchinson, S.L., Nimrod, G.: Leisure as a resource for successful aging by older adults with chronic health conditions. Int. J. Aging Hum. Dev. **74**(1), 41–65 (2012). https://doi.org/10.2190/AG.74.1.c. PMID: 22696843
27. Institute for Research on Ageing, McMaster University: Open access datasets from aging studies (2022). https://mira.mcmaster.ca/research/open-access-datasets-from-aging-studies. Accessed 15 Aug 2022
28. Kalache, A., Gatti, A.: Active ageing: a policy framework. Adv. Gerontology = Uspekhi Gerontologii **11**, 7–18 (2003). http://europepmc.org/abstract/MED/12820516
29. Kale, V.V., Hamde, S.T., Holambe, R.S.: Brain disease diagnosis using local binary pattern and steerable pyramid. Int. J. Multimed. Inf. Retrieval **8**(3), 155–165 (2019). https://doi.org/10.1007/s13735-019-00174-x
30. Kandasamy, I., Kandasamy, W.B.V., Obbineni, J.M., Smarandache, F.: Indeterminate likert scale: feedback based on neutrosophy, its distance measures and clustering algorithm. Soft. Comput. **24**(10), 7459–7468 (2020). https://doi.org/10.1007/s00500-019-04372-x
31. Kandogan, E.: Visualizing multi-dimensional clusters, trends, and outliers using star coordinates. In: Proceedings of the Seventh ACM SIGKDD International Conference on Knowledge Discovery and Data Mining, KDD 2001, pp. 107–116. Association for Computing Machinery, New York (2001). https://doi.org/10.1145/502512.502530
32. Lak, A., Rashidghalam, P., Myint, P.K., Baradaran, H.R.: Comprehensive 5p framework for active aging using the ecological approach: an iterative systematic review. BMC Public Health **20**(1), 33 (2020). https://doi.org/10.1186/s12889-019-8136-8
33. Landis, J.R., Koch, G.G.: The measurement of observer agreement for categorical data. Biometrics **33**(1), 159–174 (1977). http://www.jstor.org/stable/2529310
34. Lee, P.L., Lan, W., Yen, T.W.: Aging successfully: a four-factor model. Educ. Gerontol. **37**(3), 210–227 (2011). https://doi.org/10.1080/03601277.2010.487759
35. Lupien, S.J., Wan, N.: Successful ageing: from cell to self. Philos. Trans. R. Soc. Lond. Ser. B Biol. Sci. **359**(1449), 1413–1426 (2004)
36. Malik, H., Mishra, S.: Feature selection using rapidminer and classification through probabilistic neural network for fault diagnostics of power transformer. In: 2014 Annual IEEE India Conference (INDICON), pp. 1–6 (2014). https://doi.org/10.1109/INDICON.2014.7030427
37. McREYNOLDS, J.L., Rossen, E.K.: Importance of physical activity, nutrition, and social support for optimal aging. Clin. Nurse Spec. **18**(4) (2004). https://journals.lww.com/cns-journal/Fulltext/2004/07000/Importance_of_Physical_Activity,_Nutrition,_and.11.aspx
38. Moreira, L.B., Namen, A.A.: A hybrid data mining model for diagnosis of patients with clinical suspicion of dementia. Comput. Methods Programs Biomed. **165**, 139–149 (2018). https://doi.org/10.1016/j.cmpb.2018.08.016. https://www.sciencedirect.com/science/article/pii/S0169260718307569

39. Nassir, S., Leong, T.W., Robertson, T.: Positive ageing: elements and factors for design. In: Proceedings of the Annual Meeting of the Australian Special Interest Group for Computer Human Interaction, OzCHI 2015, pp. 264–268. Association for Computing Machinery, New York (2015). https://doi.org/10.1145/2838739.2838796

40. Nayak, R., Buys, L., Lovie-Kitchin, J.: Influencing factors in achieving active ageing. In: Sixth IEEE International Conference on Data Mining - Workshops (ICDMW 2006), pp. 858–862 (2006). https://doi.org/10.1109/ICDMW.2006.100

41. Nayak, R., Buys, L., Lovie-Kitchin, J.: Data mining in conceptualising active ageing. In: Li, J., Simoff, S.J., Kennedy, P.J., Christen, P., Williams, G.J. (eds.) Data Mining and Analytics 2006: Proceedings of the Fifth Australasian Data Mining Conference, pp. 39–46. Australian Computer Society, Australia (2006). https://eprints.qut.edu.au/14011/

42. Nerenz, D., McFadden, B., Ulmer, C.: Race, Ethnicity, and Language Data: Standardization for Health Care Quality Improvement. National Academies Press (2009). https://books.google.com.ec/books?id=JDOYmzQSUNsC

43. Pal, A.K., Pal, S.: Evaluation of teacher's performance: a data mining approach. Int. J. Comput. Sci. Mob. Comput. 2(12), 359–369 (2013)

44. Pandove, D., Goel, S., Rani, R.: Systematic review of clustering high-dimensional and large datasets. ACM Trans. Knowl. Discov. Data 12(2) (2018). https://doi.org/10.1145/3132088

45. Posada, F.V., Tur, M.C.T., Resano, C.S., Osuna, M.J.: Bienestar, adaptación y envejecimiento: cuando la estabilidad significa cambio. Rev. Multidiscip. Gerontol. 13(3), 152–162 (2003)

46. Poscia, A., et al.: Workplace health promotion for older workers: a systematic literature review. BMC Health Serv. Res. 16(5), 329 (2016). https://doi.org/10.1186/s12913-016-1518-z

47. Páez, D.G., de Buenaga Rodríguez, M., Sánz, E.P., Villalba, M.T., Gil, R.M.: Healthy and wellbeing activities' promotion using a big data approach. Health Inf. J. 24(2), 125–135 (2018). https://doi.org/10.1177/1460458216660754

48. Runeson, P., Host, M., Rainer, A., Regnell, B.: Case Study Research in Software Engineering: Guidelines and Examples, 1st edn. Wiley Publishing, Hoboken (2012)

49. Ryff, C.D.: Beyond ponce de Leon and life satisfaction: new directions in quest of successful ageing. Int. J. Behav. Dev. 12(1), 35–55 (1989). https://doi.org/10.1177/016502548901200102

50. SAPUTRA, D.M., SAPUTRA, D., OSWARI, L.D.: Effect of distance metrics in determining k-value in k-means clustering using elbow and silhouette method. In: Proceedings of the Sriwijaya International Conference on Information Technology and Its Applications (SICONIAN 2019), pp. 341–346. Atlantis Press (2020). https://doi.org/10.2991/aisr.k.200424.051

51. Seeman, T.E., Lusignolo, T.M., Albert, M., Berkman, L.: Social relationships, social support, and patterns of cognitive aging in healthy, high-functioning older adults: Macarthur studies of successful aging. Health Psychol. 20(4), 243–255 (2001). https://doi.org/10.1037/0278-6133.20.4.243

52. Silverstein, M., Parker, M.G.: Leisure activities and quality of life among the oldest old in Sweden. Res. Aging 24(5), 528–547 (2002). https://doi.org/10.1177/0164027502245003

53. Smith, M., DeFrates-Densch, N.: Handbook of Research on Adult Learning and Development. Routledge, Milton Park (2009). https://books.google.com.ec/books?id=HrWslN2zgL4C

54. Swindell, W.R., et al.: Indicators of "healthy aging" in older women (65-69 years of age). a data mining approach based on prediction of long-term survival. BMC Geriatrics 10(1), 55 (2010). https://doi.org/10.1186/1471-2318-10-55

55. Tennstedt, S., et al.: Advanced cognitive training for independent and vital elderly (active), United States, 1999–2001 (2010). https://doi.org/10.3886/ICPSR04248.v3

56. Um, J., Zaidi, A., Choi, S.J.: Active ageing index in Korea - comparison with China and EU countries. Asian Soc. Work Policy Rev. **13**(1), 87–99 (2019). https://doi.org/10.1111/aswp.12159

57. Walker, A., Maltby, T.: Active ageing: a strategic policy solution to demographic ageing in the European union. Int. J. Soc. Welf. **21**(s1), S117–S130 (2012). https://doi.org/10.1111/j.1468-2397.2012.00871.x. https://onlinelibrary.wiley.com/doi/abs/10.1111/j.1468-2397.2012.00871.x

58. Wirth, R., Hipp, J.: CRISP-DM: towards a standard process model for data mining. In: Proceedings of the 4th International Conference on the Practical Applications of Knowledge Discovery and Data Mining, vol. 1, pp. 29–39. Manchester (2000)

59. World Health Organization: World report on ageing and health. Technical report, World Health Organization (2015). Accessed 01 Aug 2022

60. Xue, B., Zhang, M., Browne, W.N., Yao, X.: A survey on evolutionary computation approaches to feature selection. IEEE Trans. Evol. Comput. **20**(4), 606–626 (2016). https://doi.org/10.1109/TEVC.2015.2504420

61. Zhang, H., Zheng, G., Xu, J., Yao, X.: Research on the construction and realization of data pipeline in machine learning regression prediction. Math. Prob. Eng. **2022**, 7924335 (2022). https://doi.org/10.1155/2022/7924335

62. Zhou, X., Jin, Y., Zhang, H., Li, S., Huang, X.: A map of threats to validity of systematic literature reviews in software engineering. In: 2016 23rd Asia-Pacific Software Engineering Conference (APSEC), pp. 153–160 (2016). https://doi.org/10.1109/APSEC.2016.031

Configuring Participatory Design of ICT for Aging Well as Matters of Care

Alina Huldtgren[1](✉) [iD], Holger Klapperich[1] [iD], and Cordula Endter[2] [iD]

[1] CoDe for Health, Faculty of Media, University of Applied Sciences Düsseldorf, Düsseldorf, Germany
{alina.huldtgren,holger.klapperich}@hs-duesseldorf.de
[2] Catholic University of Applied Sciences Berlin, Berlin, Germany
cordula.endter@KHSB-Berlin.de

Abstract. For good reason, a culture of user-centered and participatory design of technology has been established in the context of aging well in addition to the problem-solving approach for recent decades. We owe this shift in thinking not only to the collaboration of gerontologists, physicians, sociologists, and technology developers, but also to funding programs that explicitly call for user involvement and user studies in real life contexts. This is expected to lead to a better adaptation of the system requirements to the actual needs of the users and thus ensure a higher acceptance of the final product of technology. Finally, the approach should help to increase the subjective well-being of users and other stakeholders. This paper reports our own experiences and research on user-centered design and participation in the development of technology. From both an internal perspective as designers/developers and an external perspective as ethnographic researchers, we critically examine current practices of user integration in this paper. In doing so, we highlight and contextualize crucial aspects of reflexivity, reciprocity, and empowerment and provide the notion of configuring participation in the design process as matters of care. Moreover, we are convinced that participatory user-centered approaches should be at the center of future research on for ICT design in healthcare and thus also for the aging society.

Keywords: User-centered design · Participatory design · Subjective wellbeing · Ageing · AAL · eHealth

1 Introduction

The first author became involved in research in the field of information and communication technologies (ICT) for aging ten years ago. With her Scandinavian background in user-centered design (UCD) and her strong personal motivation to help older people live better and more independent trough the help of technology, she was highly motivated to start her first European project on ambient assisted living (AAL) using UCD. In parallel, she discussed, how UCD unfolds in AAL projects, with the last author of this article, who was trained in ethnography. Now, 10 years later, it is time for a joint reflection and roadmap for further research in this area including the perspective of the second author on designing for subjective wellbeing.

L. A. Maciaszek et al. (Eds.): ICT4AWE 2021/2022, CCIS 1856, pp. 157–176, 2023.
https://doi.org/10.1007/978-3-031-37496-8_9

In the past, we observed that technological innovation took up a large part of the development in the field of AAL and ICT for aging. Partially, the social innovation component, the goal of enabling the aging society to live well in old age, has taken a back seat. For example, technological advances in ICT, robotics, sensors, AR, and VR have been made to address the challenges associated with the aging population and to help people live at home longer and alleviate the shortage of caregivers. However, user-centered approaches although available, were initially used rather sparingly in development. This led to a variety of systems being developed, but few being adopted and accepted by potential users. Fortunately, this has changed in recent years and social innovation has also been further considered and has been able to complement technological innovation. First, a stronger positive attitude toward early user involvement in the design and development process emerged, so that funding programs today often mandate the use of user-centered or participatory design (PD). Involving individuals from the intended system's target population is meant to improve the match between system requirements and user needs to ensure that the outcome is usable by those individuals on the one hand and promotes or re-enables well-being on the other. Consequently, user acceptance could be increased. This kind of user participation is currently taking place in various forms in ongoing research projects. They are referred to as UCD (Norman and Draper 1986), co-design, or co-creation (Sanders and Stappers 2008), with some following the original Scandinavian approach to PD (Schuler and Namioka 1993). Many approaches are described in the literature as user-centered or participatory. However, the definition of these terms and the accompanying research activities are varied, ranging from selective moments of participation, e.g., through interviews during requirements analysis, to co-creative participation throughout the project, e.g., through regular focus groups or user workshops, iterative ideation sessions, and prototype testing.

Although it has been demonstrated (see, e.g., Bertelsmann Stiftung 2018) that continuous user participation can be beneficial for the acceptance of eHealth applications, a systematic analysis of the extent of participation, its impact on the people involved, and its value for project outcomes is lacking. Compagna and Kohlbacher (2015) emphasize that user integration primarily acts as a guarantor for receiving project funding. The extent to which people are successfully integrated is rarely evaluated or discussed. Nor is there much discussion of what successful integration means, how it might be measured, and for whom it benefits. However, as we argue, it is particularly important for the field of health and well-being to analyze and reflect on the forms and methods of user participation and their added value, as the outcomes have direct implications for the health and quality of life of the stakeholders involved. While this paper is neither about a systematic analysis of methods nor about success criteria of user integration, we provide experiences from our own research and raise several issues and accompanying research questions to be considered in future research in the field of UCD of ICT for aging well. In particular, we propose a way to see the configuration of participatory design (PD) of ICT for ageing well as matters of care, thereby providing a framework for the integration of users in the design process. This paper is based on our earlier work (Huldtgren et al. 2022) and provides additional empirical research from a current project as well as a more in-depth discussion of aspects regarding PD as matters of care.

2   Approaches to Integrate Users into Technology Design

Over the decades, a range of user-centered and participatory approaches have developed in different political and scientific contexts. User-centered design was coined first as a term by Rob Kling (1977) in the late 70s and adopted by Don Norman (1986), a psychologist working on the design of (IT) artefacts in California, USA. After the latter publication the approach experienced a major uptake. Interestingly, at about the same time in the 70s cooperative design emerged in Scandinavia, in a political setting where unions had a strong position and advocated for an involvement of the workers in the design of new (IT) systems. The notion of cooperation between workers and managers, e.g. meeting face-2-face, was far-fetched for the American context at the time. The term 'cooperative' was later changed to participatory design to better encompass other ways of participation beyond direct face-2-face cooperation. While participatory design encompasses democratic values strongly, other participatory approaches have arisen in the 2000s, such as co-design and co-creation, that focus less on these values. Generally, it is hard to pinpoint the historic development of co-design and co-creation and the terms are not clearly defined. While co-design can refer to creative processes, in which ICT designers and other stakeholders develop new ICT artefacts together, it can also refer to the simultaneous development of hardware and software in a project. In addition, the term Co-Creation is often used synonymously, and both terms have found resonance in a business context with a focus on the creation of business value between companies or between a company and its clients.

In this paper, we focus on the way human-computer interaction (HCI) researchers use the terms in the development of new ICT systems. Even though we present UCD, PD, Co-Design and Co-Creation separately in the next sections, research practice does not always subscribe to one methodology, but moves along a continuum of participation reaching from a focus on user needs being elicited to shared control of design decisions being made. In ICT for ageing well projects, combinations of methods from these approaches can be found and sometimes projects label their approach with a specific approach even though its original values are not fully embedded.

2.1   User-Centered Design

The most widely used umbrella term when it comes to IT development that involves people from the target audience, denoted as 'users', at certain points in the design process (e.g. requirements analysis or prototype testing) is UCD. As described earlier the term was made popular by Don Norman's (1986) work in the 1980s at the intersection of psychology and computer science. He developed design principles for user interface design that adapts to the user's cognitive and physical abilities. A strong focus of UCD lies in the usability and, more recently, the user experience of an artefact. As the term suggests the focus of the development lies on the users. This is reached by following an iterative design process that involves the four steps of context analysis, concept design/ideation, prototyping and user testing in each iteration. Intended users are mostly involved in the context analysis through interviews or focus groups that lead to a set of requirements for the system, and in the user testing of prototypes.

Throughout the last decade funding programs on assistive technologies (AAL) for older people have advocated for UCD as the main approach to enable participation in the design and development of ICT (Fischer et al. 2020; Merkel and Kucharski 2019; Ogonowski et al. 2018). One of the main objectives for using UCD in this particular context was to overcome the lack of market success of the early AAL systems. As these systems derived often from a technology push, they did not serve the needs of the envisioned users (Fachinger 2018; Greenhalgh et al. 2016).

2.2 Participatory Design

Participatory Design (PD) has recently become more popular in the context of integrating older people into the design of AAL and eHealth systems. PD goes a step further than UCD: It does not only put users at the center of technology development, but also involves them actively in the process and, consequently, transfers some of the decision-making power to them. Actually, PD also tries to involve other stakeholder to draw a bigger picture of user context from transdisciplinary perspectives. As briefly outlined above, the approach has its origin in the Scandinavian tradition of Cooperative Design that aimed at empowering later users and other stakeholders of ICT through giving them more control and possibilities to influence the design process (Kaptelinin und Bannon 2012). PD dates back to the 1970s when the digitalization of the workplace started. There was a strong demand by labor unions of a broad, societal participation of workers and emancipatory citizen engagement. Bringing together workers and managers was unique. PD followed humanistic and democratic values. Nowadays, PD is mainly seen as an approach to involve future users in the design process of technology (Bødker et al. 1988; Greenbaum und Kyng 1991; Muller und Kuhn 1993; Schuler und Namioka 1993).

Mackay et al. (2000) point out that the current practice of user participation in gerontechnology has little in common with the humanistic, democratic and utopian ideal of PD. Rather, users are considered as a "good thing" (2000, 738) because their participation would lead to an improvement of the technical artefact (Endter 2021).

It seems to be a paradox situation that technology could mean an enhancement to older people, even if cognitive impairments or a restricted mobility limits their abilities. For instance, digitality could empower them to organize their daily routines, such as making appointments at the doctor through an app or staying in contact with their relatives by using a video communication tool. Here the initial barriers seem insurmountable for older people. Especially for them it is important to include them in participatory processes to find out about those barriers and how to lower them, while understanding the added value of technology and digitality in their life. Often older people are surprised what possibilities could be initialized through technology, but they need to be informed, and they to be empowered to discuss their needs with people who develop technology for them.

2.3 Co-design and Co-creation

Further terms that are becoming more common in the HCI discourse on system design are co-creation and co-design. As mentioned above, there are no clear definitions and boundaries between these terms. This is partially due to the fact, that the terms are used in diverse contexts, e.g. business, software development, interaction design. Nevertheless, the shared creative process of developing innovations by a number of stakeholders from different disciplinary backgrounds seems to form a common ground in the definitions and uses of the terms. Co-Creation and Co-Design could be seen as an active form of participation in a design- or developing process. Again, co-creation involves diverse stakeholders in a creative process leading to shared innovation. In our perception, co-design is a specific implementation of co-creation focused on designing technology. As described by Sanders and Stappers (2008) the difference to UCD in its traditional form, is that PD or co-design do not see the user only as a source of information, but as an active designer, being involved through methods and toolkits, that empower her to voice her needs, but also decide on systems' functionalities and aesthetics. Co-design differs from PD as the focus on democratic and humanistic values is less, but the focus on creative activities mediated by a range of hands-on methods for designing prototypes is stronger. Ideally, participants identify with the envisioned tool, evaluate developments continuously, influence design, decide on functionality or even develop parts of the system themselves (Lieberman et al. 2006).

3   Challenges in the Integration of Users into ICT Design

Critical gerontologists argued that UCD fails to involve older people adequately (Endter et al. 2022; Lassen et al. 2015; Merkel and Kucharski 2019; Peine and Neven 2019). Main critique includes that participation is used to legitimize technological development or to foster market success through matching user requirements and systems (Endter 2016; Neven 2010; Peine et al. 2014). In addition, socially deprived or educationally disadvantaged older people are often left out of participatory processes (Biniok et al. 2016; Künemund and Tanschus 2013; Compagna 2012).

When funding programs demand the integration of users, developers are faced with involving people that they often know little of. Nevertheless, they must choose the right methods to let them participate while making sure that the project is not jeopardized. From our own experience, we can tell that balancing project objectives and the involvement of people into the design process is not easy. In the following sections we will describe some insightful experiences from selected research projects as well as a number of overarching challenges before we propose a new way of configuring the participatory design process in Sect. 4.

3.1   Care@Home Project

The Care@Home project (Fitrianie et al. 2013) was part of the EU AAL funding scheme and focused on the development of a smart TV platform for older people allowing them to access services of daily living (from a doctor's call to grocery shopping). The project initially hypothesized that older adults 1) are or may become less mobile and 2) are used to operating TV sets. Thus, the envisioned TV service platform seemed like an ideal technical solution to fix issues or mobility and to allow users to age in place. We engaged in a UCD process. Users were involved for the first time when we had paper versions of the UI ready and, later, when hi-fidelity prototypes required usability testing.

The first author of this paper led the tests in both phases. Reflecting on the first sessions, which were carried out at the homes of the older people recruited through a partnering senior organization, we realized that the test group was biased in terms of technology affinity and competence. Since several of them had taken part in previous studies they had acquired technologies like smartphones, tablets, and even smart TVs. Furthermore, they had a positive attitude to technology in general. In addition, since the sessions were at people's own homes, which was a conscious choice to mitigate barriers, we experienced that some test participants were acting as hosts, being explicitly polite. In our perception this, however, stopped people from giving the critical feedback that would have been helpful in this early project phase. Even though we explicitly asked for critique, the configuration of host-guest situation seemed to have hindered them. In addition, we had a young student with us who had hand-drawn the interfaces – also a conscious choice to avoid making it look like we had programmed the UIs already. The hand-drawn interfaces let to a situation during an interview where the participant exclaimed how impressed she was that the student drew so well. A nice compliment, but when asked about feedback to different designs she simply liked them all and called them "beautiful". While we could be happy as technology developers when people supposedly like the UI design, a situation during the prototype testing showed the pitfalls of involving people to "confirm" the usability of the design. This time the running system was set up in a community center to avoid the host-guest situation but to still allow for a familiar environment. A usability test with several tasks to be executed by participants by themselves was conducted using the prototype and concurrent think-aloud. This time we made sure to recruit a mixed group of older adults with various level of technology knowledge. One participant was a 70+ year old woman in a wheelchair – a seemingly perfect match to our target group. We were happy to see that she could navigate the UI. However, while it may confirm the good usability, which would probably be a result published in a paper, the post-test interview revealed that the person would never use the system. She told us that she did not need such a system and suggested that her 90+ mother could. She agreed that she was immobile but doing everything through the TV was clearly not desirable. While not being representative, this shows that even highly usable systems could be designed far from the lived world of the target audience.

3.2 Nutzerwelten Project

'Nutzerwelten' (English: User Worlds) was a project that followed a participatory app-roach focusing on the involvement of care givers, people with dementia, social workers, and relatives before having a pland of what would be developed (Huldtgren et al. 2017). The goal at the project start was to support people with dementia to communicate with caregivers and relatives mediated through the means of digital media. In the initial phase, we took our time to get familiar with the target audience, their lived world and commu-nication patterns. Later on, we developed several technology probes based on the gained insights, field visits and conversations with stakeholders. One such probe was a tangible world map (Huldtgren 2015) that was interactive and showed the places where a person with dementia had lived, as well as an audio line with recorded stories from the person about the place. In our perspective, the map was a means for a person with dementia to keep memories while the disease progresses, but also a means to give caregivers con-versation triggers. Interestingly, in an interview with the person the following situation unfolded:

"What are you going to do with the map? Will it be in an exhibition?" Mrs. Smith asks. My colleague is surprised and says that our intention was to improve the map and maybe give it to her, but Mrs. Smith likes her idea of making the map and her stories publicly available. "It could be interesting to other people to hear my stories," she says. Later in the conversation Mrs. Smith suggests that we could also give the map to her GP, who seems to be dear to her, after she passed away. "Then he can remember my stories." she says – her eyes filling with tears."

Clearly, the map had a very different purpose for her than what we had understood in the first place. Hence, we need the deeper engagement with the participants to fully understand their needs and motivations to participate beyond the goals of our projects.

3.3 MemoPlay Project

MemoPlay was a German state-funded technology development project which ran from 2012 until 2014. The goal was to develop an interactive online platform to enable older people suffering Mild Cognitive Impairment (MCI) to train their cognitive abilities by conducting the memory training. It was intended for individual use at home without the need for assistance from care givers or medical staff. The project followed a UCD process with people aged 60+, who were involved as interview partners or test users during the requirements analysis, the formative and summative evaluation of the prototype.

The last author of this paper conducted ethnographic fieldwork from March to November 2014 in this project. To do so, she accompanied project members at dif-ferent point in the UCD process, conducted interviews and participated as a participant observer in test sessions with older people in the laboratory and at their homes. In the following we provide only a short excerpt from a usability test session, for the detailed account, see (Endter 2020).

"[The researcher conducting the test] repeatedly emphasises how important it is that older people are involved in the development of technology that they will later use, hence why it is so important that the participants are here today and have agreed to participate in the study. She also appeals to their individual ambition and sense of responsibility when she describes the user test. No questions are asked during her presentation, everyone is listening carefully. Some take notes, but most of them follow [the researcher's] explanations and wait and see how things will unfold. In the further course of the test, they also only react when asked, they keep quiet, they complete the questionnaires without asking questions and they agree to the tests [the researchers] are doing with them, even if some mention later in a subordinate clause that they felt uncomfortable in the test situation they had to undergo during their visit. They want to

appear competent and informed and, as if their participation would be put to the test, they want to prove themselves as suitable candidates." (ibid, p.104).

Analysing the observed usability test one can find an asymmetrical relationship between the researchers conducting the usability test and the older test participants. The way the researchers conducted the study guaranteed that the participants behaved like test users. In addition, they were configured to develop a high level of compliance with the procedures to ensure that the evaluation was carried out successfully. The hierarchy between researchers and participants ensured that the uncertainty introduced by the participation of older people is kept under control, thereby serving the goals of the project rather than accounting for the true motivations and feelings of the participants. This contradicts recent approaches to genuine participation, which includes that the participants are involved "as themselves" instead of being forced into a role (Østergaard et al. 2018).

3.4 NaDiA Project

The NaDiA project (short for 'Nachgefragt! Digital im Alter', in English "Inquired! Digital in old age) aimed to involve older people (aged 60+) in the scientific process of fostering digital competence in older populations. Focus of the project is the involvement of citizens in a dialogue around the topic. A central activity is gathering questions from cititzens to us researchers. Those collected questions were categorized and built the foundation of the project for further engagements between older citizens, care workers, HCI researchers and students. In this context we tried to develop diverse formats for participation. They were designed to integrate people with different attitudes concerning technologies in their everyday life: For those with a negative view or rejection of technology, based on frustrations or fear, an experience space was created in which they could experiment with technology, such as the IKEA augmented-reality app, where you can place furniture in your own surroundings. This led to further discussions about the acceptance of those technologies. Moreover, a dialogue series called "coffee and cake – digital" was initialized. In a low-threshold interactive format we offered discussions and experiences around topics referring to the collected questions. Technology-interested older people took part. Another format was a video-box where people of every age could record their questions regarding digitality in old age, or answer questions asked by others.

On the one hand, the diverse formats lowered the barriers for participation, on the other hand we found that the majority of older people wants to participate spontaneously without liabilities and only if their personal interest is high enough. Especially when it came to longer-term participation in projects, older people tend to decline a continuous participation. Only few people with high motivation were participating continuously. Here the commitment was based on a high interest in the topic. They were already curious to know more about digitality, because the added value of technology in their everyday context was obvious to them. Despite only a few people could not relate to the topic and were not any more participating in dialog-event. Interestingly, we found that those who were especially critical about digitality and science could be convinced through direct communication with students and scientific staff. After those participants visited a couple of interactive events a trust building was in progress. This led to a motivation to visit the participation events constantly with the side effect that they also learned more interesting facts about digitality leading to a generally more positive attitude.

Within the NaDiA project we undertook eight semi-structured interviews to get a more detailed view of older people's motivations for participation in a technology development process. It was interesting to see that half of the participants (P2,P3, P4, P8) had the feeling of putting a lot of effort in the participation, besides all of them had joy doing so. Surprisingly the role within the co-creation process was not rather clear to the participants. One participant thought the scientific staff was not well prepared or had just a little knowledge in this field, P5 said "I sometimes had the impression that they were not so far advanced with the project and that I basically had more basic knowledge that they actually need for their platform [...]. Maybe they were technically more advanced, but [...] maybe they lacked a bit of everyday experience in dealing with people with dementia." (pos. 183). This shows that the participants were not aware about their role as experts with lived experiences in the co-creation process. Furthermore, the needs of older people in a participation process need to be regarded better. Interviewees did not want to put in much commitment, as P2 puts it "being in an organization and then being available to certain necessary ones is what you don't want at all as a retiree." (pos. 126). The motivations for participation were diverse so personal interests was mentioned from all participants. Moreover, seven of eight participants mentioned social relatedness as a motivation besides social responsibility reported by five of eight persons. Similarly, five of eight persons said experiencing something new and having a hand-on connection to the topic represented a motivation for them.

3.5 General Challenges

The excerpts above reveal a glimpse of our own experiences in the context of user involvement into ICT design. Despite the rather anecdotical evidence, they point to some interesting insights. They show that researchers configure the design process in a powerful manner that transform democratic ambitions into hierarchical power structures. People are invited into the process that fit the age group, and ideally match the defined user characteristics. They are involved at certain points in the process, typically as interview partners during requirements analysis, or as test persons to evaluate prototypes of various fidelities. However, they are rarely asked beforehand whether they intent to actually become users of the system or about their motivations to take place in the first place. Nevertheless, we call it 'user testing' and talk about 'users' in the scientific discourse. Both the Care@Home and the Nutzerwelten example showed that not all participants considered themselves users and NaDiA showed that motivations for participation can be diverse. In fact, we often heard that people enjoy "helping science" or "feeling needed" as motivations for becoming participants. This points to a consideration that participation can take other forms than being users, e.g. taking part as design partners or consultants (see 4.2). In addition, the NaDiA project showed that older people tend to enjoy selective engagements rather than being involved over longer periods of time and with more responsibility.

Another problem is that older or vulnerable people, for example people with demen-tia, are often seen as a homogenous group with certain skills, lifestyles or motivations. In projects with people with dementia the focus is often symptom-based and little research tries to see the people as full individuals (see Wallace et al. 2013 for a notable exception). This may not always be possible as it may counteract the project goals. Allowing real needs, feelings and motivations to surface may result in requirements that do not match the original project idea or do not even demand for technological innovation but for social innovation. This contradicts the way funding is organized, where the goals and envisioned system must be stated clearly in proposals. There is little room for changing direction during the project. Thus, as we saw in MemoPlay, user testing is mostly configured in a way that people are involved to confirm the system's usefulness. Hierarchies between researchers and participants ensure the compliance and keep uncertainties under control.

Another important issue lies with recruiting. There is a selection bias towards people who are generally interested and active, higher educated with good income and more technology savvy as we e.g., saw in the Care@Home project. While a more heterogenous group should be involved it is challenging to reach people who are not willing to volunteer. The NaDiA project shows that diverse formats of participation could help to engage users and that a trust building process is key. We need to constantly engage people and make clear to them that they are in a role of a co-researcher, which is a competence that needs to be built up during the participation process. This can be done by offering formats to the users that provide opportunities for competence building. User literacy is neither a self-evident quality that users bring with them nor something that they acquire exclusively themselves in the participation process. In addition, projects could benefit from an involvement of a broader stakeholder range, not only direct users. Limited resources and time constraints make this difficult. Nevertheless, a first step would be to make the biases more visible in publications, reflect on the implications of excluding groups (e.g. precarious elderlies, older migrants, disabled elderlies) and think of ways to motivate people to volunteer.

4   Configuring Participatory Design as Matters of Care

The problems and shortcomings of current approaches and practices outlined here make it clear that participation currently represents more of a continuum between non-participation and the full involvement of real users in their diversity and heterogeneity. As we have seen, current user-centered design approaches often lack to involve stakeholders adequately. The fact that we are still a bit away from the full involvement of users should motivate us to continue searching for tipping points that can help us shape the participation process in the sense of the users, without jeopardising innovation and the achievement of goals.

Critical gerontologists and technology researchers (Lassen et al. 2015; Merkel and Kucharski 2019), especially from the field of Science and Technology Studies and CSCW, have been pointing out for some time that the participation process does not represent genuine reciprocity (i.e. the human activity of mutual exchange, see chapter 4.1) and "genuine participation" (Østergaard 2018). To allow for actual reciprocity and a more genuine participation researchers and developers in the field of ICT for ageing well need to engage in a more reflective participation practice and develop co-design processes that empower participants in order to open up exploratory and experiential spaces. By reflective practice we refer to reflecting on (1) our own role as 'researcher participants' configuring the design and development process, (2) the selection of 'user participants', (3) their motivations and attitudes towards the system and towards participation, and (4) the effect of participation on the project outcomes.

We posit that a move has to be made from pure focus on eliciting needs and turning them into system requirements towards more self-design and world shaping (Kruse 2017) by the participants, i.e. the older adults. True reciprocity can only arise when people realize and to some extent learn that they can have a say in the shaping of society and the digital artefacts. Very often in our projects with older adults we notice a reluctance in people to voice their inputs and concerns. While HCI researchers talk about involving people as *experts of their own lived experience*, this role and expert status is often not clear to participants (see NaDiA project above). Instead, participants often see the researchers as more knowledgeable in general. To reach an emancipatory moment in the co-design process participants need to aware of their role and expertise.

Therefore, we consider a process of empowerment of the users throughout all phases of the design to be central. This requires a space for experience and experimentation in which the participants can take part according to their competences, familiarise themselves with the technical innovation process as well as with their role as users in a protected space and to develop a certain self-confidence in the content of their own statements. This space does not have to be a physical space, but it can be. Rather, it is a matter of designing the participation process in such a way that there are always opportunities for reflection, experience and discussion in formats that provide users with the opportunity to familiarise themselves with the often very fast and dynamic development process at their own pace. Such a space can give users the opportunity to experience themselves as a group and to discuss their own needs and requirements together.

At the same time, such a space also offers the researchers the opportunity to change roles or to become aware of their own role and the power positions associated with it, and to think about these when dealing with and addressing the stakeholders of the context (e.g. patients, caretakers, doctors), but also in the conception of the participation formats. In this sense, an experience-based experimental space is an offer of communication and reflection for all actors involved.

This democratic orientation is a prerequisite for a co-creative technology development process in the mode of reciprocity. At the same time this mode of reciprocity is the key for configuring participatory design as a matter of care. The concept 'matters of care' was introduced by Puig de la Bellacasa (2011), who expanded Latour's conception of technology as matters of concern by an affective dimension. "Caring in this sense is understood [...] as a reflexive practice that asks how the project members involved in the constitution of the technical artefact evaluate their actions of user involvement and to what extent they see themselves as responsible for the involvement of older people as users in the design of the technology." (Endter 2020, p.99) Part of this reflexive practice is also questioning the general notion of user participation as being a good thing. To understand what can be considered as good care, we turn to Tronto (1993). She conceptualized good care as characterized by attentiveness, responsibility, competence, and reciprocity. These aspects are required and fulfilled by caregivers to recognize the needs of others and to serve them, thereby building a mutual relationship between caregivers and people being cared for. Tronto's criteria can function as a "heuristic for examining the extent to which user-centred design actually empowers users to participate in the design process and fosters a fit between technology and user needs" (Endter 2020, p. 99).

In the following we concretise the components of such a mode of participation as matter of care, starting with a deeper dive into reciprocity first. Next, we will discuss our idea of configuring participation with care and the importance of the multiplicity of age in this respect. This leads to considerations of empowerment of the diverse participants and finally, we propose design methods that can help us towards a more genuine participation process.

4.1 Allowing for Reciprocity

Reciprocity refers to the human activity of mutual exchange. It is one of the four requirements for good care according to Tronto (1993), and it is also a core value in PD (Bødker and Iversen 2002) as well as in Gerontology. For example, Andreas Kruse (2017) emphasizes that older people aim at forming oneself and the world in a dynamic process. Providing older people with opportunities to form their individual ageing process in correspondence to their needs and values as well as giving them the chance to contribute their knowledge and competences to society is the best way in for an ethically framed good life in old age.

We pose that ability to form their life in correspondence to this interrelated demand as a key requirement for reciprocity. According to Dreessen et al. (2020) reciprocity is a mutual exchange that can either lead to a direct gain for the participants or can be characterized by acts with the interest of the other in mind regardless of direct gains. A reciprocal relationship can be open, closed, or dynamic over time. In their analysis of their own community-based participatory projects they describe a lack of felt reciprocity and provide four handles to foster reciprocity, e.g., the designers' competence of being embedded in the community of the participants, or their willingness to become engaged in the community in the long run. As we see, supporting reciprocity requires a deeper understanding of the people we envision as users, which in turn needs long-term engagement with these people in their own settings. Questions such as 'How can ICT researchers manage this involvement and the resulting complexity?' 'How can projects be initiated and closed within these mutual relationships of researchers and citizens?' arise and need to be addressed in future research. In addition, the strategies provided by Dreessen et al. focus merely on the researchers. However, 'What are the needs of developers and the responsibilities of participants to enable and foster mutual relationships?' Despite these open questions, we suggest that a reflective process and configuring users and participation with care, as a step forwards to reach reciprocity and genuine participation.

4.2 Configuring Users and Participation with Care

As the MemoPlay example showed, researchers conducting user studies in UCD configure older people as users. In a deeper analysis of the design case Endter (2020) describes how the researchers conducting the usability test employ powerful practices to configure the older adults as users in four ways, i.e., spatially, affectively, discursively, and materially. The way the seating is arranged in the room, the materials researchers give people and the ways they present the participants' involvement (e.g., in this case appealing to the people's competence and compliance) establishes a hierarchy and the presented case left the participants in a rather passive position, not acting 'as themselves' or 'with themselves', which are preconditions to genuine participation (see Østergaard 2018). In the Care@Home case, we saw a different scenario unfolding. When we interviewed people in their own homes we had little control over the environment. As it happened, we suddenly found ourselves in a host-guest relationship, in which participants were seemingly too polite to criticize our designs. Already 15 years ago, Redström (2006) pointed out that there is a predominant interest in HCI in fitting people to technologies – although at that point the discipline had already moved away from the notion of users as mere cognitive information processors and acknowledged their richness in terms of motivations, feelings, and culture. Indeed, employing words like 'users', 'user testing' implicates that we do focus on how people can become users of the things we present to them.

Using Redström's argument as a starting point Vines et al. (2013) have discussed several important aspects around how we configure not only users but participation. They consider a reflection on the forms of participation, initiators and beneficiaries of the participation as well as sharing control as central issues. They call for reflection on how participation can unfold, e.g., people can and already do participate in ways that are "witting, unwitting, spectator-like, as a reflexive commentator or as creator" (p. 433) and argue for more transparency regarding these engagements, and their beneficiaries. Especially when desiging for vulnerable people, we believe, the benefits of including these should be made clear. In addition, opening up to moving beyond involving people as users only, but also seeing them as commentators, or design partners and letting them transition between roles throughout the project will allow more genuine participation. This would also correspond better to the motivations of older people regarding their participation in projects as we found in the interview study in the NaDiA project. Older people were less likely to commit longer-term and take on responsibilities but were open to different roles (e.g. critic) at selective points.

Furthermore, as Endter (2020) put it „user participation is less a manifestation of the participation process of older people than of the powerful practices of establishing controllable users. If UCD should lead to an involvement of older users, it must become a matter of care for those responsible for the user involvement." (p. 109). This means developers and designers have to feel responsible for their technological innovation and their doings because they are responsible for the users.

4.3 Opening the Door to the Multiplicity of Age

As described, older people are integrated into the design of assistive technologies in a process mostly initiated and configured by researchers or developers. The images taken for granted about old age as a time of decline, loss and vulnerability and assistive technologies as generally being helpful for people in such a state, however, is problematic.

Ageing is a multidimensional, heterogeneous, diverse process that is characterized by a high level of diversity both in terms of the group of older people and the individual ageing process. And ageing is an ongoing process of gains and losses. Approaches that standardize ageing as a problem and thus fail to do justice to the complexity of the ageing process fall short accordingly. However, technological development is characterized by the idea of developing a technical solution for a problem. Accordingly, a conception of ageing as a problem, for which technology then offers the solution, is dominant. Such a narrowing perspective problematizes age and excludes the simultaneity of gains and losses to the benefit of the losses. This can lead to technologies missing the actual needs of older users.

However, the problem here is not only the lack of knowledge about lifeworld needs, but also the stigmatization of old age as a process of loss resulting from the focus on problems. No older person wants to use technology that is based on such an image of old age, although they often must because alternatives are missing.

To avoid such a problem-oriented path dependency and the narrowing of technology as a problem solver, which is criticized by gerontologists as technology fix (Neven and Peine 2017, Peine et al. 2021), it is necessary to be open to the heterogeneity of the target group, as well as to have appropriate formats in order to be able to correspond to this heterogeneity within the framework of the participation process. This also includes funding formats as a necessary prerequisite for conducting such a process with enough resources and time.

Another aspect is relevant: Certain facilitators are needed. So-called gatekeepers into the world of old age. Who could do this better than gerontologists? They have to bring their gerontological expertise to bear on technology development and, above all, ensure that the project conception is based on knowledge about old age from fundamental research. For it does not make sense to involve older people at all points; sometimes it also requires appropriate advocates who act as mediators between scientific knowledge and practical needs.

4.4 Empowering Older People to Participate

As we explained earlier, older people need to be empowered to participate to create a mutual relationship between researcher and participant. UCD tends to involve people at specific points in the process (e.g., to gather requirements, user test). However, if we want to reach a point where participants can benefit from the design process as well, and control is truly shared between researchers and participants, we have to move towards long-term engagement with citizens in the target group and employ more democratic, participatory methods is needed. Early PD (Greenbaum and Kyng 1991) provided such methods, as the focus was on democratic values and destabilizing power structures in times when workers and unions were faced with the introduction of new technology in the workplace. "[PD] emphasized the importance of providing these workers and union officials the knowledge and skills about the potential of computational systems so that their views would be better articulated when bargaining with management." (Vines et al. 2013, p.430) Thus, the focus of involving people should not be on how to get the information developers require out of them to design the system they have in mind, but to empower people with an understanding of the technologies that enables them to vocalize their concerns and needs as well as actively take decisions in the development of digital systems. We must be aware, that empowerment entails that informed participants and truly shared control may lead to a rejection of the envisioned designs or at least to major changes or uncertainties in the projects. Ideally, funding programs allow researchers to react on this. One way to deal with changing requirements is to employ an action research approach, e.g. the community-based participatory research approach by Kang et al. (2020).

In addition, approaches to participation, such as Co-Design and Co-Creation (Sanders and Stappers 2008) provide many creative tools to engage with people in user workshops. This is one step to provide people with boundary objects (i.e., objects that bridge between social worlds, in this case between designers and citizens, e.g., a model of a scenario) to understand the design space and communicate. Nevertheless, we argue that there is still a need for developing participatory methods that focus more on advanced user interface technologies such as AR, VR, or mixed reality as well as AI-based systems. Especially given the older target audiences are commonly less in touch with such advanced user interfaces, they need to be given space to experience and grasp the technologies – besides the specific system that is being developed in a particular project.

4.5 Designing for Wellbeing and Values

While the considerations outlined above are rather of a theoretical than practical nature, one could ask how to put into practice the considerations of reciprocity and genuine participation as well as seeing UCD or co-design as matters of care. To provide an entry point for ICT developers we propose a couple of design methods as starting points, design for wellbeing and value-sensitive design.

The terms 'positive computing' and 'design for wellbeing' [Calvo and Peters 2014, Pohlmeyer 2013] do not implicate only social aspects within a technology developing process, however, a social innovation besides a technological one takes center stage. Participation of future users and other stakeholders is regarded as a logical consequence to understand how to flourish subjective wellbeing in a technology-driven context. How does the abstract construct of subjective wellbeing differ for people of old age? As a matter of fact, a design and developing process needs to adapt to the conception of people's wellbeing of older age, if it is supposed to add value in people's lives.

First of all, it is important to find a common understanding of subjective wellbeing in general. Helpful might be Lyubomirsky's (2007) definition of happiness as the "experience of joy, contentment, or positive well-being, combined with a sense that one's life is good, meaningful and worthwhile" (p. 32). Thus, happiness occurs within our positive experiences in everyday life, besides an individual conviction of living a meaningful life. Usually, people decide on their own what activities could make them happy. In age, however, those decisions rely on one's ability based on health and mobility. Steptoe and colleagues (2015) argue that subjective wellbeing is influencing old people's health and vice versa. They point out that not only health is a factor for a positive subjective wellbeing but also "[…] material conditions, social and family relationships, and social roles and activities—factors that also change with age." (p.2). These factors are individual and complex and can only be recognized through the participation of a group of people with lived experience.

For a first impact it is important to record and analyze meaningful and positive activities or in other words 'social practices' of older people. Here Klapperich and colleagues (2018) suggest an interview tool to collect insights of positive social practices, which could be used to enrich a technology innovation process with lived experience. This tool is based on meaningful social practices which satisfy psychological needs or values [Sheldon 2001] such as 'security', 'stimulation', 'autonomy', etc. In our opinion, insights arising from this tool may be a meaningful possibility to open a co-creation process and sensitize every participating stakeholder for the context, but also for possible vulnerable groups inside this context.

Furthermore, it becomes clear, that psychological needs or values do not change in old age, but they are influenced through health issues caused by aging. Reduced mobility can lead to reduced autonomy. Cognitive impairment could shake one's security or self-determination. Limited social contacts limit social participation and the need for stimulation remains unsatisfied. Thereby social practices change, and methods used in the technology design process need to address such a change of wellbeing. However, empowering technology must be developed with people in a participatory way, otherwise the desired empowerment can quickly turn into paternalism. Here, value-sensitive design (VSD) can help to address challenges in participation that relate to paternalism.

Value sensitive design (VSD) "is a theoretically grounded approach to the design of technology that accounts for human values in a principled and comprehensive manner throughout the design process" (Friedman et al. 2013). In particular, the tripartite methodology focusing on iterations of conceptual, empirical, and technical investigations allows for a reflective practice in the design process and the co-creative methods open up spaces for experience, experimentation and reflection (e.g. the value sensitive action-reflection model, see Yoo et al.. 2013). Diverse stakeholders (i.e. designers, developers, users, etc.) are involved throughout the design process through methods that focus especially on uncovering the underlying values in the design space and addressing them proactively in a participatory design process to develop technology that supports certain values (and may also hinder unwanted ones). Special attention is drawn to the distinction of whose values are being considered, namely user values, designer values or explicitly supported values, the latter ideally being negotiated and decided upon in a discursive process by designers and users (or other stakeholders). As these values are not necessarily known by all stakeholders and often occur in a network of values, VSD provides reflective methods (e.g. Envisioning Cards, see Friedman and Hendry 2012) for becoming aware of one's values as well as finding value trade-offs, when values are in tension with each other (e.g. freedom and safety in a GPS-based monitoring system for people with dementia). Besides the helpful methods that VSD provides, the community of VSD researchers works closely with philosophers and involves reflection of their own roles and actions throughout the design, which makes it a suited methodology for designing ICT for ageing well by taking into account the aspects of reciprocity and genuine participation outlined above. In addition, it can be integrated or combined with other methodologies, e.g. design for wellbeing, UCD, co-design etc.

Besides the use of specific methodologies as suggested here, we advocate an additional approach to support the aspects discussed in the paper. We believe that accompanying social science research can act supportively, e.g. through supervision or mediation in technology development projects. By involving researchers that are not part of the development team an alternative perspective is provided to highlight value tensions, make thinking of different stakeholders more transparent or deepen the understanding of everyday knowledge and practices of the users. In doing so, the technical innovation process becomes a sociotechnical one. This will add another level of reflection, and ultimately provide new insights, also across the lifespan of single projects.

5 Conclusion

In this paper we have presented our reflection of user-centered design in the AAL/eHealth setting resulting from 10 years of experience in the field and from different backgrounds spanning HCI, gerontology and design. Starting from our own experiences to insights from the literature we have critically looked at challenges of including people as future users and given central research themes to be investigated in the future. First, we advocate more reflection and transparency on our own roles and practices on how we configure participation, on how participation can unfold and on who benefits, and second, we call for new methods to give people, in particular older adults, an understanding of new technologies, and third, we provided a theoretical frame for understanding participatory design as a matter of care, which is envisioned to lead to more reciprocity and genuine participation of older adults in technology development processes.

Acknowledgements. This research is funded by the German Federal Ministry of Education and Research (NaDiA project, 01WJ2227A and CoCreHIT project 16SV8796). Furthermore, we thank all our research participants and co-researchers.

References

Stiftung, B.: Stand der Digital-Health-Entwicklung in 17 untersuchten Ländern (2018). https://www.bertelsmann-stiftung.de/de/unsere-projekte/der-digitale-patient/projektthemen/smarth ealthsystems/standder-digital-health-entwicklung. Accessed 10 Feb 2021

Biniok, P., Menke, I., Selke, S.: social inclusion of elderly people in rural areas by social and technological mechanisms. In: Domínguez-Rué, E., Nierling, L. (eds.) Ageing and Technology: Perspectives from the Social Sciences, Bielefeld, transcript Verlag, pp. 93–117 (2016)

Bødker, S., Ehn, P., Knudsen, J., Kyng, M., Madsen, K.: Computer support for cooperative design. In: Proceedings of the 1988 ACM Conference on Computer-supported Cooperative Work, pp. 377–394 (1988)

Bødker, S., Iversen, O.S.: Staging a professional participatory design practice: moving PD beyond the initial fascination of user involvement, pp. 11–18. ACM (2002)

Compagna, D.: Lost in translation? the dilemma of alignment within participatory technology developments. Poiesis & Praxis: Int. J. Ethics Sci. Technol. Assess. 9(1–2), 125–143 (2012)

Calvo, R.A., Peters, D.: Positive Computing: Technology for Wellbeing and Human Potential. MIT press, Cambridge (2014)

Compagna, D., Kohlbacher, F.: The limits of participatory technology development: the case of service robots in care facilities for older people. Technol. Forecast. Soc. Chang. **93**, 19–31 (2015)

Dreessen, K., Hendriks, N., Schepers, S., Wilkinson, A.: Towards reciprocity in participatory design processes. In: Proceedings of the 16th Participatory Design Conference 2020-Participation (s) Otherwise, vol. 2, pp. 154–158 (2020)

Endter, C.: Skripting age – the negotiation of age and aging in ambient assisted living. In: Domínguez-Rué, E., Nierling, L. (eds.) Ageing and Technology: Perspectives from the Social Sciences, Bielefeld, transcript Verlag, pp. 121–140 (2016)

Endter, C.: User participation as a matter of care: the configuration of older users in the design of assistive technologies. TECNOSCIENZA: Ital. J. Sci. Technol. Stud. **11**(2), 93–116 (2020)

Endter, C.: Assistiert Altern. Die Entwicklung digitaler Technologien für und mit älteren Menschen, Springer, Wiesbaden (2021)

Endter, C., Merkel, S., Künemund, H.: The Configuration of Older Users as Drivers of Innovation in the Design of Digital Technologies. In "NOvation" (2022). (in press)

Fachinger, U.: Altern und Technik: Anmerkungen zu den ökonomischen Potentialen. In: Künemund, H., Fachinger, U. (eds.) Alter und Technik. Sozialwissen-schaftliche Befunde und Perspektiven, Wiesbaden, VS Verlag für Sozialwissenschaften, pp. 51–68 (2018)

Fischer, B., Peine, A., Östlund, B.: The importance of user involvement: a systematic review of involving older users in technology design. Gerontologist **60**(7), 513–523 (2020)

Fitrianie, S., Huldtgren, A., Alers, H., Guldemond, N.A.: A SmartTV platform for wellbeing, care and social support for elderly at home. In: Biswas, J., Kobayashi, H., Wong, L., Abdulrazak, B., Mokhtari, M. (eds.) Inclusive Society: Health and Wellbeing in the Community, and Care at Home, pp. 94–101. Springer, Heidelberg (2013). https://doi.org/10.1007/978-3-642-39470-6_12

Friedman, B., Hendry, D.: The envisioning cards: a toolkit for catalyzing humanistic and technical imaginations. In: Proceedings of the SIGCHI Conference on Human Factors in Computing Systems, pp. 1145–1148 (2012

Friedman, B., Kahn, P.H., Borning, A., Huldtgren, A.: Value sensitive design and information systems. In: Doorn, Neelke, Schuurbiers, Daan, Poel, Ibo, Gorman, Michael E. (eds.) Early engagement and new technologies: Opening up the laboratory. PET, vol. 16, pp. 55–95. Springer, Dordrecht (2013). https://doi.org/10.1007/978-94-007-7844-3_4

Greenbaum, J.M., Kyng, M. (eds.): Design at Work: Cooperative Design of Computer Systems. Lawrence Erlbaum Associates Inc., Hillsdale (1991)

Greenhalgh, T., et al.: SCALS: A fourth-generation study of assisted living technologies in their organisational, social, political and policy context. BMJ Open **6**(2), e010208 (2016)

Huldtgren, A., Vormann, A., Geiger, C.: Reminiscence map-insights to design for people with dementia from a tangible prototype. In International Conference on Information and Communication Technologies for Ageing Well and e-Health, vol. 2, pp. 233–242. SCITEPRESS (2015)

Huldtgren, A., Mertl, F., Vormann, A., Geiger, C.: Reminiscence of people with dementia mediated by multimedia artifacts. Interact. Comput. **29**(5), 679–696 (2017)

Huldtgren, A., Klapperich, H., Endter, C.: Next steps for user integration in ICT for aging well. In: Proceedings of the 8th International Conference on Information and Communication Technologies for Ageing Well and e-Health, pp. 291–298 (2022). ISBN 978–989–758–566–1, ISSN 2184–4984

Kang, Y.-S., Chen, L.-Y., Miaou, S.-G., Chang, Y.-J.: A community-based participatory approach to developing game technology to provide greater accessibility for children with intellectual disabilities. Syst. Pract. Action Res. **34**(2), 127–139 (2020). https://doi.org/10.1007/s11213-020-09519-8

Kaptelinin, V., Bannon, L.J.: Interaction design beyond the product: creating technology-enhanced activity spaces. Human-Comput. Interact. **27**(3), 277–309 (2012)

Klapperich, H., Laschke, M., Hassenzahl, M.: The positive practice canvas: gathering inspiration for wellbeing-driven design. In: Proceedings of the 10th Nordic Conference on Human-Computer Interaction, pp. 74–81 (2018)

Kling, R.: The organizational context of user-centered software designs. MIS Q. **1**(4), 41–52 (1977). https://doi.org/10.2307/249021.ISSN0276-7783.JSTOR249021

Künemund, H., Tanschus, N.: Gero-technology: old age in the electronic jungle. In: Komp, K., Aartsen, M. (eds.) Old Age in Europe, pp. 97–112. Springer, Netherlands (2013)

Kruse, A.: Lebensphase hohes Alter: Verletzlichkeit und Reife, Springer, Heidelberg (2017)

Lassen, A.J., Bønnelycke, J., Otto, L.: Innovating for 'active ageing' in a public-private innovation partnership: creating doable problems and alignment. In: Technological Forecasting and Social Change, vol. 93, pp. 10–18 (2015)

Lieberman, H., Paternò, F., Klann, M., Wulf, V.: End-user development: an emerging paradigm. In: End User Development, pp. 1–8. Springer, Dordrecht (2006)

Lyubomirsky, S.: The How of Happiness: A Scientiic Approach to Getting the Life You Want. Penguin Press, New York (2007)

Merkel, S., Kucharski, A.: Participatory design in gerontechnology: a systematic literature review. Gerontologist **59**(1), 16–25 (2019)

Muller, M.J., Kuhn, S.: Participatory design. Commun. ACM **36**(6), 24–28 (1993)

Neven, L.: 'But obviously not for me': robots, laboratories and the defiant identity of elder test users. Sociol. Health Illness **32**(2), 335–347 (2010)

Neven, L., Peine, A.: From triple win to triple sin: how a problematic future discourse is shaping the way people age with technology. Societies **7**(3), 26–30 (2017)

Norman, D.A., Draper, S.W. (eds.): User Centered System Design: New Perspectives on Human-Computer Interaction. Erlbaum, Hillsdale (1986)

Ogonowski, C., Jacobi, T., Müller, C., Hess, J.: PRAXLABS: a sustainable framework for user-centred ICT development. cultivating research experiences from living labs in the home. In: Wulf, V., Pipek, V., Randall, D., Rohde, M., Schmidt, K., Stevens, G. (eds.) Socio-informatics: A Practicebased Perspective on the Design and Use of IT Artifacts, pp. 319–360. Oxford University Press, Oxford (2018)

Østergaard, K.L., Simonsen, J., Karasti, H.: Examining situated design practices: nurses' transformations towards genuine participation. Des. Stud. **59**, 37–57 (2018)

Peine, A., Rollwagen, I. and Neven, L. (2014) The Rise of the "Innosumer"- Re-thinking Older Technology Users, in "Technological Forecasting and Social Change", 82, pp. 199–214

Peine, A., Neven, L.: From intervention to co-constitution: new directions in theorizing about aging and technology. Gerontologist **59**(1), 15–21 (2019)

Peine, A., et al.: Socio-gerontechnology: Interdisciplinary Critical Studies of Ageing and Technology. Routledge (2021)

Pohlmeyer, A.E.: Positive design: new challenges, opportunities, and responsibilities for design. In: Marcus, A. (ed.) DUXU 2013. LNCS, vol. 8014, pp. 540–547. Springer, Heidelberg (2013). https://doi.org/10.1007/978-3-642-39238-2_59

Puig de la Bellacasa, M.: Matters of care in technoscience: assembling neglected things. Social Stud. Sci. **41**(1), 85–106 (2011)

Redström, J.: Towards user design? on the shift from object to user as the subject of design. Des. Stud. **27**(2), 123–139 (2006)

Sanders, E.B.N., Stappers, P.J.: Co-creation and the new landscapes of design. Co-design **4**(1), 5–18 (2008)

Sheldon, K.M., Elliot, A.J., Kim, Y., Kasser, T.: What is satisfying about satisfying events? testing 10 candidate psychological needs. J. Pers. Soc. Psychol. **80**(2), 325–339 (2001). https://doi.org/10.1037//O022-3514.80.2.325

Schuler, D., Namioka, A. (eds.): Participatory Design: Principles and Practices. CRC Press, Boca Raton (1993)

Steptoe, A., Deaton, A., Stone, A.A.: Subjective wellbeing, health, and ageing. The Lancet **385**(9968), 640–648 (2015)

Tronto, J.C.: Moral Boundaries: A Political Argument for an Ethic of Care. Routledge, New York (1993)

Vines, J., Clarke, R., Wright, P., McCarthy, J., Olivier, P.: Configuring participation: on how we involve people in design. In: Proceedings of the SIGCHI Conference on Human Factors in Computing Systems, pp. 429–438 (2013)

Wallace, J., Wright, P. C., McCarthy, J., Green, D. P., Thomas, J., Olivier, P.: A design-led inquiry into personhood in dementia. In: Proceedings of the SIGCHI Conference on Human Factors in Computing Systems, pp. 2617–2626 (2013)

Yoo, D., Huldtgren, A., Woelfer, J.P., Hendry, D.G., Friedman, B.: A value sensitive action-reflection model: evolving a co-design space with stakeholder and designer prompts. In: Proceedings of the SIGCHI Conference on Human Factors in Computing Systems, pp. 419–428 (2013)

Gender Aspect in Online Health Information Seeking Behavior Among Estonians Aged ≥ 50 During the Covid-19 Pandemic

Marianne Paimre[1,2](✉) (iD) and Kairi Osula[1]

[1] Tallinn University, Narva Road 25, 10120 Tallinn, Estonia
mpaimre@tlu.ee
[2] Tallinn Health Care College, Kännu 17, 13418 Tallinn, Estonia

Abstract. Information and Communication Technology (ICT) tools are essential in accessing health information (HI) today, which has proven to be especially true under pandemic conditions. Since older people have been the most at risk of Covid-19 and many do not use new technology, this article focuses on older adults' online health information seeking behavior (OHISB) in the digitally advanced Eastern European country Estonia. A survey involving 500 people aged 50 and over was conducted in 2020. As expected, men reported better access to computers and smart devices and were also more willing to use digital health applications. However, women prioritized remote communication with medical personnel. The perceived need for HI and the frequency of searching for it were similar for men and women. However, in the older age group (≥65), female internet users claimed to search HI more frequently. Higher education among older men was associated with more intensive information seeking in the past 30 days. As expected, women tend to use a greater variety of HI sources. The fact that men were more eager to vaccinate against Covid-19 indicates that they may not be as oblivious to their health as commonly believed. The results of the study imply that older people in Estonia, well-educated men in particular, are enthusiastic digital technology users for health purposes. Men's interest in ICT devices and digital health applications should be considered more when developing health strategies and campaigns.

Keywords: Older adults · Gender differences · ICT · Health information seeking behavior · Covid-19 · Vaccination readiness

1 Introduction

Information and Communication Technology (ICT) tools create favorable conditions to cope independently in old age [1, 2]. Some technical solutions support managing at home alone while others enable monitoring health conditions or enable communication with relatives and caregivers. In addition, computers and smart devices also provide access to a wealth of health information (HI), which helps to shape people's responses to disasters and contribute to threat perception and act as a precursor of preventative behaviors [3–5]. Obtaining information from the internet has been particularly important during

L. A. Maciaszek et al. (Eds.): ICT4AWE 2021/2022, CCIS 1856, pp. 177–194, 2023.
https://doi.org/10.1007/978-3-031-37496-8_10

the Covid-19 crisis when distance communication was recommended by the authorities everywhere to avoid the virus [6]. Although the older generation need HI the most due to their deteriorating health status and being most at risk of contracting the corona virus, many of them do not use new technology at all, and those who use it face problems while online [7, 8]. Therefore, the HI seeking behavior (HISB) which is broadly an active need-fulfilment behavior by which people obtain on health, diseases and welfare from various sources, deserves greater scholarly attention, especially during the Covid-19 epidemic [3, 9]. Little is known about the gender difference in the online health information seeking behavior (OHISB) among older people and its relationship with their health behavior, for example with vaccination readiness. This article attempts to fill this gap by focusing on Estonian older adults in the wake of the corona pandemic's first wave in the summer of 2020.

The small country of Estonia in Eastern Europe has made a great digital leap over the last thirty years [10]. However, social welfare and the well-being of disadvantaged groups among the population (e.g., older people) have not yet caught up with the more developed Western countries in this respect [11]. For example, although Estonian pensioners tend to work longer and are better educated than their peers in many other European countries, they face the most significant poverty risk in the European Union [12, 13]. If in the whole EU, 20.4 per cent of people over the age of 65 are at risk of poverty, then the corresponding figure for Estonia is twofold (40.6%) [14, 15]. The rapid aging of the Estonian population will increase pension costs expenditure in the future, consequently depleting the resources in the healthcare and social support systems [16]. Digital services aimed at the elderly could be one possible solution to soften the blow [17]. For this, it is necessary to ascertain to what extent the elderly use technology for health purposes and search for HI online [18].

Gender differences emerge among Estonians in several aspects, e.g., there are considerably more women with higher education than men in Estonia [19]. As of 2021, an average of 36% of women aged 25–64 in the European Union have a higher education, while in Estonia the corresponding figure amounts to 53%, placing Estonia 3rd in this ranking [20]. As for men, the proportion of the highly educated is only slightly higher than the European average - in Estonia 34% of men aged 25–64 are highly educated. At the same time, 33% of men and 55% of women among old-age pensioners live in relative poverty. Over the past few decades, Estonia has witnessed a positive trend in various health ratings [21]. However, the gender gap in health indicators and life expectancy continues to persist to the detriment of men. Unfortunately, gender inequalities regarding health indicators and life expectancy are clearly evident putting women well ahead of men [22]. On average, Estonian men live eight years less than women and four years less healthy [23]. However, compared to the ladies of the same age, 65+ men report better health (17% and 19% respectively) perhaps due to certain misplaced confidence or simply an air of casual indifference [24].

During the Covid-19 pandemic, the health of Estonian people has taken a turn for the worse much in line with the global trend. In 2021, 2700 more deaths than in 2020 were recorded [25]. The number of patients per 100,000 population was 25 for those under 60 and 327 for those aged 60 and over [26]. Of all the hospitalized patients, 83% were aged 60 and older. The average age of a hospitalized patient is 67 for women and 63 for men whereas older people have the highest vaccination rate in Estonia [27]. This could partly be explained by the fact that seniors were the first group to receive a vaccine, yet the figure has remained constant since the vaccines became available to all adults. Women under the age of 60 have been more eager to vaccinate than their male counterparts while, conversely, the vaccination rate is higher among males aged 70 and older [27]. In countries like Estonia where the rapid aging of the population exerts unrelenting pressure on the health and care systems, the use of digital tools by the elderly for health purposes and the search for HI is particularly important.

This article is an extension of the article published in Spring 2022 in Proceedings of the 8th International Conference on Information and Communication Technologies for Aging Well and e-Health (ICT4AWE 2022). In contrast, this piece focuses on OHISB, also shedding light on relationships between different factors. The overview of literature has also been significantly expanded.

The following chapter of this paper outlines the older adults' use of ICT for health purposes and gender specificities in seeking HI. Thereafter, the applied methodology will be introduced followed by the principal outcomes of the study. The final part of the paper presents the findings together with the conclusions drawn from them.

2 Literature Review

2.1 Gender Differences in the Use of ICTs Among Older Adults

In developed countries, various health-related digital services and applications have been designed for older adults to support healthy aging and coping independently. The common problem so far has been that the target group's interest is not very high. Older people's lukewarm interest in digital HI and applications has been a shared concern among developed European countries for the past decade [28, 29]. The same goes for the internet, which is one of the primary sources of information (including HI) for large audiences due to its ease of use and speed today, yet many seniors prefer to stay offline.

In Estonia, people's health records are stored in an electronic register, and all drug information leaflets will soon be available only electronically, therefore, everyone must have access to ICT tools accompanied by adequate digital skills. Although Estonia is known for its digital success (e-government, e-residency, ID-card) 44% of the 65–74-year-olds never used the internet in 2018. The corresponding figure among 75-year-olds was 68% [30]. Since the state does not collect data related to the use of ICT among people aged 75 and older, no such recent indicators exist for this particular age bracket. Compared to younger age groups, internet use in Estonia declines among people in their 50s, which is why they are also included in this study. During the Covid-19 crisis, internet use among older people increased in Estonia. If in 2019, 69% of the 55–75-year-olds used the internet every week, then in 2021 the corresponding figure was already 74%. Among men, the growth in internet use has been more significant [31]. However, a study conducted in the UK indicates that the digital gap between the young and the old and also within the older population itself has actually increased during the pandemic [32].

Some studies suggest that men use digital devices more than their female counterparts [33–37]. Older women especially are seen as technophobes [38]. However, the gap between genders in ICT usage in Europe has not been that significant in the last few years. According to Eurostat, in 2020, an average of 87% of men and 85% of women aged 16–75 used the internet in Europe [31]. In Estonia, statistics indicate that while in the past (e.g., in 2005) men were more avid internet users, then by 2019 the gap had disappeared: 89% of men and 88% of women aged 16–74 used the internet. In 2020, the proportion of men and women using the internet was already on par (88%) [39]. Menéndez Alvarez-Dardet et al. have highlighted that the differences between older males and females do not seem to be unequivocal, instead they are related to other sociodemographic indicators, such as educational level [40]. As Anderson and Perrin note, older people who are more affluent and highly educated report owning and using various technologies at rates comparable to younger people. However, those seniors who are less affluent or with lower levels of educational attainment continue to have a distant relationship with digital technology. Whether or not a person starts using ICT tools depends on a number of psychological factors and previous experience with technology.

From the outset of Covid-19, little research has been done on ICT use among older people, and much is still unclear about ICT use by genders. In a rapidly aging country such as Estonia, it is especially important to study how ICT could generate public revenue so as to facilitate decent aging.

2.2 OHISB and Factors Influencing IT

Almost everywhere in the world, searching for HI has become a fairly popular online activity [40–42]. As seeking relevant information on the internet promotes digital skills and eHealth competence, online health information seeking (OHISB) has been deemed a helpful activity [19]. The internet substantially complements the so-called more traditional and interpersonal data providers (e.g., family members, friends, acquaintances), often indispensable for older people [6]. A limited number of information channels decreases the variety of information ranges; however, diverse sources reporting on the same issue provide different perspectives and levels of detail [3]. Certain resources (e.g., social media) tend to show a negative relationship with protective health behaviors and a positive one with Covid-19 conspiracy beliefs [43]. Obtaining relevant and reliable health information via different means is crucial during a crisis to form a more comprehensive picture of the risk factors and subsequently make the necessary decisions a (e.g., whether to get vaccinated or not) to protect oneself [3].

When researching HISB, it should be considered the relationship between information seekers' socioeconomic conditions, their information behavior, choices in health behavior, and other factors [43, 44]. It has been established that several factors, such as age, level of education, previous experience in searching for health information, computer self-efficacy, familiarity with internet searching, and outcome expectations regarding internet-based health information act as major determinants of an individual's intention to accept eHealth offerings and OHIS [42, 45]. Better education is associated with greater e-health literacy [46]. Older individuals are less likely to seek information related to their health conditions, share health information with others, or think about physical exercises needed to manage their health conditions [40, 42].

In the study of Eriksson-Backa et al. [4], gender closely affected both interest in information about health or illness (chi-square = 8.345, $p \leq .05$) as well as the actual information seeking activity (chi-square = 13.202, p ≤ .001). 80% of the female respondents compared to 65% of the male respondents claimed to be fairly or very interested in health information, and 71% of the women but only 50% of the men sought information fairly or very often. Enwald and her colleagues' study on OHISB among Finnish older people indicates that women were more likely to have shared information related to physical activity with others [5].

Several studies have found a positive correlation between Covid-19 risk perception and protective health behavior engagement [47, 48]. Likewise, a study demonstrated that certain communication styles (e.g., detailed information with positive educational messages) promoted more protective health behaviors [49]. Taken together, these previous studies have highlighted the importance of obtaining adequate information during public health crises such as a pandemic [3]. It has also been established that more exposures to news have direct implications for people's action, e.g., receiving timely and informative communication during uncertain times promotes public cooperation [50].

A study conducted by Chu et al. applied Carstensen's socioemotional selectivity theory to the context of Covid-19 in an attempt to understand a potential age difference [3]. In addition, this study investigated how obtaining information from more varied sources might be associated with psychological and behavioral outcomes relevant to the pandemic. Their concurrent and time-lagged analyses both revealed that older adults received information from a wider range of sources, and more frequently from traditional (e.g., newspaper and TV) and interpersonal sources (e.g., information shared by friends and families) compared to younger adults. Due to receiving information from a variety of channels, older adults were more worried about Covid-19 and consequently exhibited more protective health behaviors.

An earlier article by the authors of the current article determined that the most statistically significant relationships emerged in OHISB among Estonian older adults in respect of educational level and gender. Thus, the following subsection is devoted to gender differences in OHISB.

2.3 Gender Differences in OHISB

Although in the general population both men and women prefer the internet as a source of health information, previous studies indicate that women tend to seek HI online more often [51, 52]. Although women have been found to consult a greater variety of sources, men tend to be more concerned with the comprehensiveness and accuracy of the information [53]. Men also appreciate the ease with which they can access it and its familiarity, whereas women demonstrate greater interest in cognition, such as the ease with which they can read and understand the information. However, it has been established that younger, more active, and family-oriented males may be reached also with the help of online HI [54].

The results of a study conducted by Ek demonstrate that compared to men, Finnish women were keener on seeking health-related information, paid closer attention to potential worldwide pandemics and were much more curious as to how the goods they purchase in everyday life affect their health [52]. Women also reported receiving noticeably more informal health related information from close family members, next of kin, and friends/coworkers than men did. According to him, if we wish to successfully carry out health promotion activities, then gender differences in health information behavior should not be overlooked.to succeed in public health promotion and interventions the measures taken should be much more sensitive to the gender gap in health information behavior.

A study conducted by Nikoloudakis suggests that being a non-smoker and of younger age were also closely associated with online health information seeking for men and women alike. However, reporting poor health and the presence of two chronic diseases were positively associated with online health seeking for women only. Generally speaking, the correlates of seeking help online among men and women were not contingent on their health status. The results suggest that similar groups of men and women are likely to access health information online for primary prevention purposes, and additionally that women experiencing poor health are more likely to seek health information online than women who are relatively well [55].

Bidmon and Terlutter wanted to know why women use the internet more often for health-related information searches than men. They were also interested in gender differences in their research subjects' current use of the internet for communicating with their general practitioner (GP) and in their future intention to do so (virtual patient-physician relationship). Their results indicate that women use the internet for health-related information searches to a higher degree for social motives and enjoyment and they judge their information retrieval outcomes more profoundly than men. Women also reported higher health and nutrition awareness as well as a higher personal disposition of being well-informed as a patient. They concluded that women are driven by a stronger social motive for and experience greater enjoyment in health-related information searches most likely explained by their social role interpretations, suggesting that these needs should be met when offering health-related information on the internet. The authors also established that men were more open to remote consultations with their GP; therefore, they could be the primary target group for additional online services offered by GPs [56].

Little is known about how the health information behavior of men and women differed during the corona pandemic. Older people's OHISB, who clearly have been most affected by the virus, has remained relatively unexplored, including in Estonia.

In view of the above, it would be imperative to learn more about gender differences in OHISB among Estonian older adults and how this impacts their Covid-19 vaccination readiness since whether or not to vaccinate has been a momentous health decision for many people during the pandemic. As acceptance of ICT devices creates the much-needed prerequisites for successful online health information searches, access to digital tools and the keenness to make use of relevant technologies for health purposes has also been studied.

The overall aim of the study was to analyze the differences between genders regarding their willingness to use digital health-related solutions and communicate with medical staff remotely, OHISB, and vaccination readiness for Covid-19 among Estonian older adults.

The article makes the following hypotheses:

1. Men, especially the more educated ones with higher income, report better access to computers and smart devices and are more willing to use digital solutions for health purposes and remote communication with medical personnel.

2. Men have a lower need for health information and are less likely to seek information on health and diseases.
3. Men and women prefer different information sources; men use less diverse information sources from a more limited range.
4. Women exhibit better Covid-19 vaccination readiness.

3 Methodologies

Data for this study originates from a more extensive survey completed among Estonian older adults by the market research enterprise Norstat in 2020. The company drew a sample from a research panel of more than 20,000 people allowing them to carry out online, telephone and personal interviews. All the participants were randomly selected from other surveys (mainly phone interviews), thus ensuring that they represent various sociodemographic groups.

3.1 The Questionnaire

The whole questionnaire included 15 substantive multiple-choice questions as well as questions regarding the socio-demographic profile of the respondents (gender, age, nationality, education level, employed/unemployed) and monthly income. In this paper the following questions (11) were included (see Table 1).

Table 1. Questions asked and answer options.

Questions	Options
Do you have access to a personal computer or similar digital device which can be used for conducting online searches?	Yes/No
How would you rate your computer skills?	They are …. excellent/good/satisfactory/poor/I have never used a computer
Would you have any use for digital health solutions or services? (E.g., the kind that allow you to consult with medical personnel, monitor your blood pressure or sleep patterns, check your heart rate, remind you to take a pill or keep you company?	Yes/No/I don't know
During the Covid-19 lockdown, how important was it for you to have access to a doctor from a distance (e.g., exchanging e-mails, texting, video consultations)?	Important/not very important/rather unimportant

(continued)

Table 1. (*continued*)

Questions	Options
How often do you feel the need for information on illnesses or health in general?	Once a week or more often/2 to 3 times a month/2 to 3 times per 3 months/2 to 3 times a year or less often
When did you last conduct an online search on health, illnesses, or disease prevention?	In the past 7 days/In the past 30 days/In the past 6 months or less often/I don't look for information about health or illnesses on the Web
Did you come across health information…	by accident (e.g., while reading another article you also spot health news) or by conducting a relevant search (e.g., you submit the specific query)
What usually triggers your search for particular information?	How to stay healthy and prevent illnesses/About some illness or medical condition/About health facilities and doctors/About medicinal products and pharmacies/Personal medical records/Other
Most of the information on illnesses and health you find/obtain from … (you may select multiple answers)	TV and radio/print media (newspapers, magazines) and books/the internet/my GP/outpatient clinics, hospitals, pharmacies/Close friends and family members/Library/Social day care centers for seniors/Other;
The main online sources you obtain health information from include:	Designated e-health portals and websites on illnesses/Digital publications of mainstream media or online news portals and their health sections, health magazines/Social media platforms (Facebook, Twitter, YouTube, etc.)/Blogs/Wikipedia;/Alternative medicine websites/Internet forums and discussion groups where people share their experiences with medical professionals and illnesses/Alternative media/Official websites of international organisations, government offices and public agencies/Research databases and open access sites disseminating research outputs;/Films, videos/Any query results that Google displays first
Whether you would like to get vaccinated if the opportunity arose?	Of course/I doubt it/No

Socioeconomic indicators included gender, age, nationality, level of education, employment, and monthly income.

3.2 Participants

As the prevalence of internet use drops among Estonian people already in their 50s. Therefore, the study centers on adults aged 50 and above. The sample included 204 (40.7%) men and 297 (59.3%) women (see Table 2). The oldest participant was 94, the youngest ones 50 years old. The median age was 65. The survey had a representative sample regarding gender, age, and nationality.

Table 2. Sample composition.

(n = 501)	n	(%)		n	(%)
Gender			**Position at work**		
Male	204	(40.7)	Employee	58	(11.6%)
Female	297	(59.3)	Specialist	118	(23.6%)
Age			Manager	23	(4.6%)
50–54 years	88	(17.6)	Entrepreneur	26	(5.2%)
55–64 years	162	(32.3)	Pensioner	260	(51.9%)
65–74 years	134	(26.7)	Other	15	(3.2%)
75 +	117	(23.4)	**Monthly income (in euros)**		
Nationality			Up to 150	6	(1.2%)
Estonians	359	(71.7)	151–350	30	(6.0%)
Other nationalities	142	(28.3)	351–550	154	(30.7%)
Educational level			551–750	119	(23.8%)
Basic	26	(5.2)	751–1000	61	(12.2%)
Secondary	100	(20)	1001–1250	47	(9.4%)
Vocational	165	(32.9)	1251–1500	18	(3.6%)
Higher	210	(41.9)	>1500	19	(3.8%)
			Not willing to disclose	47	(9.4%)

3.3 Data Analysis

Cross-tabulation and chi-square tests were used to analyze the retrieved data. These methods were chosen because they are suitable for comparing groups of data measured on both the nominal and sequence scales, providing an overview at both the descriptive and general level. Chi-square tests were applied to compare all subgroups, but only statistically significant differences are addressed in this article subject to appropriate significance levels. SPSS 26.0 was used for data analysis.

4 Results

4.1 eHealth Readiness

Access to ICT Devices and Willingness to Use Technical Solutions for Health Purposes. 86.3% of men and 74.1% of women reported access to a computer or a smart device (p < .05, $\chi 2(1) = 10.87$). Men (39.5%) expressed greater interest in digital health gadgets and services than women (28.7%). The difference was statistically significant (p < .05, $\chi 2(3) = 9.64$).

Surprisingly more women (53.9%) than men (36.5%) deemed it essential to have access to a doctor from a distance (exchanging e-mails, texting, video consultations) during the Covid-19 lockdown. This can perhaps be explained by women's greater emotionality and need for communication on the one hand, and on the other hand by greater concern about their health. The difference was also statistically significant (p < .01, $\chi 2(2) = 13.87$).

In the case of men in the 65+ age group, education also played a role. A little more than one third of men with higher education (36%) were interested in remote communication with their GP. For men without higher education the corresponding figure was 25%.

In respect of different nationalities, non-Estonian women deemed it slightly more important (61.9%) to have the opportunity to communicate with a doctor remotely than Estonians (51.1%). The difference was statistically significant (p < .05, $\chi 2 (2) = 7.29$).

Self-Reported Computers Skills. There was no statistical difference between genders in computer self-efficacy ratings (p > .05, $\chi 2 (3) = 5.95$). In general, almost half of the respondents chose the response that they would not have any problems finding and interpreting information. A significant difference between men and women emerged only in the category "I don't know what to make of the information retrieved (e.g., should I believe the article/story or not)". Here, 41.8% of women and 31.3% of men chose this alternative. The difference was statistically significant (p < .05, $\chi 2 (1) = 4.68$).

4.2 Health Information Seeking Behavior (HISB)

The Need for Information. Nearly half (44%) of the respondents identified the need for HI a few times in a month or a quarter or more often and the need raised with age. However, only 10,6% of the respondents reported a need to look up information on health once a week or more often. The perceived need was similar for men and women alike, i.e., there was no significant difference (p > .05, $\chi 2 (3) = 3.01$). There was also no statistically significant difference as to education or nationality.

However, against the background of previous research, it was unexpected to learn that 65+ men claimed to feel the need for information slightly more often than women in this age group: 69% of men aged 65 and above and 59% of women of the same age said that they needed health information more than a few times a year.

In the age group 65–74, the information needs of people with higher education were higher than people without higher education (69% and 54% respectively). In the 75+

group, the opposite was true (63% and 85%). Nevertheless, the limited size of the 75+ age group does not allow firm conclusions to be drawn.

Search Goals. Respondents mainly strived for information about a disease or medical condition 327 (65.3%). There was less interest in how to remain healthful and how to prevent illnesses 219 (43.7%). Information was sought less on medications and drugstores 134 (26.7%), medical organizations and experts 124 (24.8%) and personal health data from digital records 120 (24%). There were no gender differences in this regard.

Frequency of Online Health Information Searches. In the ≥50 sample, 42.5% had searched for information on health, illness or disease prevention at least once in the last 30 days, and only a little over a fifth (22%) in the last 7 days. 12.1% answered that they had never searched the internet for information on health or diseases. There was no statistically significant difference between men and women regarding the last time they searched the internet. Both the chi square test and the distribution of answers in the table produced the same result.

While studying the OHIB of men with different levels of education, it appeared that 61.5% of men with higher education had searched for information within the previous month. In other groups, fewer men had looked for information during the preceding month, their percentage points ranged from 33% to 46.9%. The difference was statistically significant (p < .05, $\chi2$ (9) = 21.13). In the case of women, there was no difference.

As regards ethnicity, the difference was not significant. However, the age variable accounted for a statistically significant difference in the answers of women: during the previous month, women aged 55–64 had searched for more information than other females (68.1%). The difference was statistically significant (p < .05, $\chi2$ (9) = 18.30).

In ≥65 age group, female internet users in general search for more health information, however, more men than women aged with higher education had gone online to search for health information in the past 30 days (60% and 53% respectively). The level of education was an important indicator here: during the last 30 days, 63% of men with higher education searched for health information on the internet while in the case of nontertiary education, the indicator was only 56%. More than half of women with higher education (54%) sought health information in the last 30 days. For the rest, the respective figure was 50%.

Use of Health Information Sources. To the question "from which sources do you obtain most of the information on illnesses and health", the most frequently chosen answers were the following: "from a family doctor, outpatient clinics, hospitals, pharmacies" (73.5%), "from the internet" (57.3%), "print newspapers, magazines and books" (32.1%), "acquaintance, family" (27.7%), "TV and radio" (26.5%). "Library" and "social day care center" were the least popular options, at 3.2% and 2.4% respectively. The difference was statistically significant (p < .001, $\chi2$ (1) = 14.50), with 3.7% of women and only 0,5% of men choosing the "social center" option. It was noticeable that women were more active in all categories, as indicated by the t-test, which showed a statistically significant difference between the number of answers chosen by men and women: women chose statistically significantly more answers (M = 2.39, SD = 1.19) than men. (M = 2.04, SD = 1.13). p < .01, t (499) = −3.29).

The fact that the internet was the first so-called non-living source of information for both sexes gives a reason to study information behavior in the online environment more closely.

Preference for Online Health Information Sources. To the question – what are the main online sources you obtain health information from? - the option "arbitrary search results that Google displays first" was chosen in 47.2% of the cases. The option "designated e-health portals and websites on illnesses" (e.g., kliinik.ee, inimene.ee, web-based clinic, etc.) was mentioned in 39.9% of the responses, "online publications in the professional press, news portals and their health sections and health magazines" in 31.3% of the cases, and Wikipedia amounted to one fifth (20.2%). The remaining alternatives were chosen less frequently.

The choices of men and women were statistically significantly different only for the option: a) "special health and disease portals and websites", where 46.8% of women and only 31.3% of men chose this response (p < .01, $\chi 2$ (1) = 9.88), and "online publications of professional journalism, news portals and their health sections and health magazines" which was selected by 35.9% of women and only a quarter (25%) of men. The difference was statistically significant (p < .01, $\chi 2$ (1) = 5.43).

The prevalence of computer usage and the number of different internet sources were very weakly linked (rho = −.15, p < .01). The more diverse online sources the respondents reported, the more they were also interested in health-related applications (rho = −. 22, p < .001). The more topics the information was needed and the different sources the respondents referred to when searching for health information, the more different online sources they used (rho = .43, p < .001).

4.3 Vaccination Readiness

Contrary to the expectations, the results also indicated that men appeared to be more enthusiastic about getting vaccinated against Covid-19. 60,8% of men agreed to be vaccinated while the corresponding figure for women was 48.5%. The difference was statistically significant (p < .05, $\chi 2(2)$ = 7.54).

In the 65 + age group, for both sexes, the interest in vaccination was more active among respondents with higher education: 76% of men with higher education and 59% of men with lower level of education expressed such interest; for women the figures were 59% and 40% respectively.

It became apparent that the more often the need for health information arose (rho = .111) and the more often information was retrieved (rho = .137), the more ready the respondent was to be vaccinated. Higher attraction to digital applications seems to entail advanced readiness to vaccinate against Covid-19 (rho = .249). The willingness to vaccinate was also contingent on the respondent's income: the higher the income, the more he/she agreed to vaccinate (rho = −.116).

5 Discussion

The first hypothesis – men, especially the more educated and with higher income, report better access to computers and smart devices and are more willing to use digital solutions for health purposes and remote communication with medical personnel – was partially confirmed. Men indeed reported better access to computers and smart devices and were more willing to use digital apps and services for health purposes. In this regard the results of the study differed from earlier outcomes [53]. Perhaps the image of Estonia as a smart/digital nation also accounts for the fact that men are increasingly more interested in health information retrieved via digital channels.

However, the current study also revealed that women found it more important to communicate with a GP remotely during the Covid-19 crisis. Therefore, it can be concluded that women's and men's motivation to use ICT tools for health purposes proved to be somewhat different which was validated also by the Bidmon and Terlutter study [56]. This may be explained by the fact that men are fond of technology, but their desire to go to the doctor and communicate with him/her is lower. One possible explanation could be that although men enjoy technology, they are less enthusiastic about actually seeing a doctor or communicating with one.

The second hypothesis that men require less health information and are less likely to seek information on health and diseases was also partly true. There was no significant difference between genders in the frequency of feeling the perceived information need and in information seeking. In light of some previous studies conducted in the Nordic countries [4, 53] this finding was a little surprising. However, in the older age group ($\geq$65), female internet users claimed to search HI more frequently.

The third hypothesis that men and women prefer different information sources and men use less diverse information sources from a more limited range was also partly true. In terms of the sources where HI is mostly obtained from (e.g., other people, institutions such as libraries and social centers, traditional media and the internet), greater variability emerged for women. Ladies were apparently more active in all categories. With respect to online sources, although women opted for certain sources of HI (e.g., special health and disease portals and websites and online outlets of professional journalism) that men didn't, statistically significant differences between genders emerged only with respect to special health and disease portals/websites as well as online versions of professional journalism, which were both preferred by women. However, this does not mean that men preferred social or alternative media for the extraction of HI. Nevertheless, it is worrying that random search results displayed by Google first were fairly popular among men and women alike, suggesting modest levels of critical evaluation of the sources.

The fourth hypothesis that women are more enthusiastic about getting vaccinated against Covid-19 was overturned. Men, in fact, were more eager to get vaccinated, especially the older ones (65+). This result is noteworthy, because women are widely regarded as having better health behaviors and being more concerned about their health. The finding that older men are more active than women in terms of Covid-19 vaccination is consistent with the official statistics on vaccination.

As the questionnaire and study were both limited in their purview, a number of attributes (e.g., psychological characteristics of the respondents, past experience with ICT and information retrieval, trust in physicians, etc.) affecting a person's interest in electronic health information and behavior remained outside its scope, thus inviting further research to identify any such determinants.

6   Conclusions

This study focused on Estonian older adults' readiness to use ICTs for health purposes, HISB, and vaccination readiness for Covid-19. It demonstrated that despite the digital divide between generations, a large number of people aged 50 and over in Estonia are genuinely interested in using digital technology for health purposes.

Considering the rapidly ageing society which places added pressure also on its health-care system, it is indeed a rather positive outcome as digital technologies are expected to play an even greater role in acquiring and disseminating HI. It is common knowledge that a rapidly aging society puts the country's healthcare system under immense pressure; however, it is also comforting to learn that older people are willing to embrace future technologies for the acquisition and dissemination of HI. Use of the ICT tools by the elderly helps to ensure that they are better informed, and it also creates the necessary preconditions for coping with less serious health issues on one's own. Surely it provides easy access to the most relevant and up-to-date information i.e., it raises their awareness and hopefully enables them to tackle certain minor health problems without requiring any professional medical assistance.

The study largely contributes to the gender dimensions of HI research. It was found that gender differences in HISB were not particularly pronounced among 50+ people living in Estonia. The premise that men tend to be ignorant about their health was misguided. Perhaps the distinctive character of Estonia as a smart/digital country also accounts for the fact that men are increasingly more interested in HI retrieved via digital channels.

The positive disposition of men towards digital health devices enables us to surmise that digital information sources have every potential to improve their overall health behavior in the future. Subsequently, such indications should be given due consideration when developing various health services and apps as well as comprehensive health communication strategies.

Slightly different trends have emerged in Estonia compared to other similar surveys in the world, which could be explained by the peculiarities of Estonia as a top performer in the digitalization of its administration and public services.

Further research needs to examine which online services, digital content, websites, etc. the Estonian older population needs/would like to use. When trying to raise the digital competence level of its population, Estonia should give priority to the less educated older adults who work in positions where IT skills are not required and to those already retired or who have lost their jobs. It is most unfortunate that in our past attempts to equip people with much-needed digital competences we have (conveniently or inadvertently) neglected older adults, especially the ones with limited or absent ICT skills due to their lower professional qualifications or those already in retirement or unemployed. This fundamental shortcoming ought to be remedied in the immediate future.

References

1. Ihm, J., Hsieh, J.P.: The implications of information and communication technology use for the social well-being of older adults. Inf. Commun. Soc. 18(10), 1123–1138 (2021). https://doi.org/10.1080/1369118X.2015.1019912
2. Asla, T., Williamson, K., Mills, J.: The role of information in successful aging: the case for a research focus on the oldest old. Libr. Inf. Sci. Res. 28, 49–63 (2006). https://doi.org/10.1016/j.lisr.2005.11.005
3. Chu, L., Fung, H.H., Tse, D.C., Tsang, V.H., Zhang, H., Mai, C.: Obtaining information from different sources matters during the COVID-19 pandemic. Gerontologist 61(2), 187–195 (2021). https://doi.org/10.1093/geront/gnaa222. PMID: 33388758; PMCID: PMC7799117. https://pubmed.ncbi.nlm.nih.gov/33388758/
4. Eriksson-Backa, K., Enwald, E., Hirvonen, N., Huvila, I.: Health information seeking, beliefs about abilities, and health behaviour among Finnish seniors. J. Librariansh. Inf. Sci. 50(3), 284–295 (2018). https://doi.org/10.1177/0961000618769 971
5. Enwald, H., et al.: Health information behaviour, attitudes towards health information and motivating factors for encouraging physical activity among older people: differences by sex and age. In: Proceedings of ISIC: The Information Behaviour Conference, Zadar, Croatia, 20–23 September (2016). Part 2. http://informationr.net/ir/22-1/isic/isic1623.html
6. Choi, N.G., DiNitto, D.M., Marti, C.N., Choi, B.Y.: Telehealth use among older adults during COVID-19: associations with sociodemographic and health characteristics, technology device ownership, and technology learning. J. Appl. Gerontol. 5 (2021). https://doi.org/10.1177/073 34648211047347
7. Ekoh, P.C., George, E.O., Ezulike, C.D.: Digital and physical social exclusion of older people in rural nigeria in the time of COVID-19. J. Gerontol. Soc. Work 64(6), 629–642 (2021). https://doi.org/10.1080/01634372.2021.1907496. Epub 2021 May 27 PMID: 34042022
8. Frydman, J.L., Gelfman, L.P., Goldstein, N.E., Kelley, A.S., Ankuda, C.K.: The digital divide: do older adults with serious illness access telemedicine? J. Gen. Intern. Med. 37(4), 984–986 (2022)
9. Lambert, S.D., Loiselle, C.G.: Health information seeking behavior. Qual. Health Res. 17(8), 1006–1019 (2007). https://doi.org/10.1177/1049732307305199. PMID: 17928475
10. Kattel, R., Mergel, I.: Estonia's Digital Transformation. Mission Mystique and the Hiding Hand. Working Paper Series: IIPP WP (2018). https://doi.org/10.1093/oso/9780198843719.003.0008
11. European Social Survey. Round 9 (2018/2019) (2019). https://www.europeansocialsurvey.org/data/download.html?r=9
12. Unt, M., Kazjulja, M., Krönström, V.: Estonia. In: Ní Léime, Á., et al. (eds.) Extended Working Life Policies, pp. 241–249. Springer, Cham (2020). https://doi.org/10.1007/978-3-030-40985-2_17
13. The Active Ageing Index and its extension to the regional level (2014). https://webcache.googleusercontent.com/search?q=cache:HbywBEGAvPwJ:https://ec.europa.eu/social/BlobServlet%3FdocId%3D13544%26langId%3Den+&cd=3&hl=et&ct=clnk&gl=ee
14. Eurostat. At Risk of Poverty or Social Exclusion in the EU (2020). https://ec.europa.eu/eurostat/en/web/products-eurostat-news/-/edn-20211017-1. Accessed 11 Mar 2022
15. Statistics Estonia. At-Risk-of-Poverty Rate (2020). https://www.stat.ee/en/find-statistics/statistics-theme/well-being/social-exclusion-and-poverty/risk-poverty-rate. Accessed 11 Mar 2022
16. Future Health Care. The future healthcare in Estonia. Scenarios up to 2035. Ageing in the Digital Era (2021). UNECE Policy Brief on Ageing No. 26 July. https://unece.org/sites/default/files/2021-07/PB26-ECE-WG.1-38.pdf

17. Arthanat, S.: Promoting information communication technology adoption and acceptance for aging-in-place: a randomized controlled trial. J. Appl. Gerontol. **40**(5), 471–480 (2021). https://doi.org/10.1177/0733464819891045
18. Pourrazavi, S., Kouzekanani, K., Asghari Jafarabadi, M., Bazargan-Hejazi, S., Hashemiparast, M., Allahverdipour, H.: Correlates of older adults' e-health information-seeking behaviors. Gerontology **14**, 1–8 (2022). https://doi.org/10.1159/000521251. Epub ahead of print. PMID: 35034012
19. Hankewitz, S.: Estonian women among the most highly educated in Europe (2022). https://estonianworld.com/knowledge/estonian-women-among-the-most-highly-edu cated-in-europe/#:~:text=In%20Estonia%2C%20women%20are%20much,were%2047% 25%20and%2030%25
20. Eesti naised on endiselt Euroopa ühed kõrgemalt haritumad. [Estonian women are still among the most highly educated in Europe.] (2022). https://www.stat.ee/et/uudised/eesti-naised-endiselt-euroopa-uhed-korgemalt-haritumad?fbclid=IwAR2r0ONDstmsKrRzoF8iT_iZd32i MdnP-T2FZbNUov581szGO_Ymn6-bErU
21. Estonia. State of Health in the EU (2017). https://www.euro.who.int/__data/assets/pdf_file/ 0010/355978/Health-Profile-Estonia-Eng.pdf
22. Eurostat. Healthy life years at birth by sex. (2022). https://ec.europa.eu/eurostat/databr owser/view/tps00150/default/table?lang=en&fbclid=IwAR3_p1sJIGlaw90IFJW4gaZptN-mvzZOhWAeEa3nipo-9gMh68ogKTIkW98. Accessed 25 Jan 2022
23. Tervis, tervis arstiabi terviseseisund [Health, health medical care health condition]. https:// www.stat.ee/et/avasta-statistikat/valdkonnad/heaolu/tervis
24. Study: Estonians' health depends on gender, wage and education. ERR News (2020). https:// news.err.ee/1026573/study-estonians-health-depends-on-gender-wage-and-education
25. Pärli, M.: Mulluste liigsurmade taga on koroona, kuumalaine ja vananev rahvastik [Behind Last Year's Excess Deaths is a Corona, a Heat Wave and an Aging Population] (2022). https://www.err.ee/1608466241/mulluste-liigsurmade-taga-on-koroona-kuumalaine-ja-vananev-rahvastik
26. Terviseamet [Health Board]: Koroonaviiruse andmestik [Coronavirus Data] (2022). https:// www.terviseamet.ee/et/koroonaviirus/koroonakaart. Accessed 2 Mar 2022
27. Tervisemet [Health Board]: Covid-19 vaktsineerimise maakondade, vanuserühmade ja soolise jaotuse andmestik [Data on Counties, Age Groups and Gender Distribution of Covid-19 Vaccination] (2021)
28. Huisman, M., Joye, S., Biltereyst, D.: Searching for health: doctor google and the shifting dynamics of the middle-aged and older adult patient-physician relationship and interaction. J. Aging Health **32**(9), 998–1007 (2020). https://doi.org/10.1177/0898264319873809
29. Broekhus, M., van Velsen, L., ter Stal, S., Weldink J., Tabak, M.: Why my grandfather finds difficulty in using e-health: differences in usability evaluations between older age groups. In: Proceedings of the 5th International Conference on Information and Communication Technologies for Ageing Well and e-Health, 1 (ICT4AWE), Heraklion, Crete, Greece, pp. 48–57 (2019)
30. European Social Survey. Round 9 (2018/2019). https://www.europeansocialsurvey.org/data/ download.html?r=9
31. Eurostat. Individuals – frequency of internet use (2022). http://appsso.eurostat.ec.europa.eu/ nui/show.do?dataset=isoc_ci_ifp_fu&lang=en. Accessed 24 Jan 2022
32. ELSA. English Longitudinal Study of Ageing. Covid-19 Substudy (Wave 1). Digital inclusion and older people – how have things changed in a Covid-19 world? (2021). https://www.psl hub.org/learn/commissioning-service-provision-and-innovation-in-health-and-care/digital-health-and-care-service-provision/digital-inclusion-and-older-people-%E2%80%93-how-have-things-changed-in-a-covid-19-world-march-2021-r4342/

33. Shi, Y., Ma, D., Zhang, J., Chen, B.: In the digital age: a systematic literature review of the e-health literacy and influencing factors among Chinese older adults. Z Gesundh Wiss **4**(1), 9 (2021). https://doi.org/10.1007/s10389-021-01604-z. Epub ahead of print. PMID: 34104627; PMCID: PMC8175232

34. Goswami, A., Dutta, S.: Gender differences in technology usage—a literature review. Open J. Bus. Manag. **4**, 51–59 (2016). https://doi.org/10.4236/ojbm.2016.41006

35. Marston, H.R., Kroll, M., Fink, D., et al.: Technology use, adoption and behavior in older adults: results from the iStoppFalls project. Educ. Gerontol. **42**(6), 371–387 (2016). https://doi.org/10.1080/03601277.2015.1125178

36. Durndell, A., Haag, Z., Asenova, D., Laithwaite, H.: Computer self efficacy and gender: a cross cultural study of scotland and Romania. Personality Individ. Differ. **28**, 1037–1044 (2000). https://doi.org/10.1016/S0191-8869(99)00155-5

37. Qazi, A., et al.: Gender differences in information and communication technology use & skills: a systematic review and meta-analysis. Educ. Inf. Technol. **27**(3), 4225–4258 (2021). https://doi.org/10.1007/s10639-021-10775-x

38. Dixon, L.M., Brocklehurst, S., Sandilands, V., Bateson, M., Tolkamp, B.J., D'Eath, R.B.: Measuring motivation for appetitive behaviour: food-restricted broiler breeder chickens cross a water barrier to forage in an area of wood shavings without food. PLoS One **9** (2014)

39. Statistics Estonia. Statistika andmebaas: Sotsiaalelu. 16–74-aastased internetikasutajad elukoha ja kasutuseesmärgi järgi. (Statistical database: Social life. Internet users aged 16–74 by residence and purpose of use) (2021). http://pub.stat.ee/px-web. Accessed 5 Jan 2022

40. Menéndez Alvarez-Dardet, S., Lorence Lara, B., Perez-Padilla, J.: Older adults and ICT adoption: analysis of the use and attitudes toward computers in elderly Spanish people. Comput. Hum. Behav. **110** (2020). https://doi.org/10.1016/j.chb.2020.106377

41. Chaudhuri, S., Le, T., White, C., Thompson, H., Demiris, G.: Examining health information-seeking behaviors of older adults. Comput. Inf. Nurs. CIN **31**(11), 547–553 (2013). https://doi.org/10.1097/01.NCN.0000432131.92020.42

42. Pálsdóttir, A.: Health and lifestyle: icelanders' everyday life information behaviour. Informaatiotutkimus **25**(1) (2008). https://journal.fi/inf/article/view/2241

43. Allington, D., Duffy, B., Wessely, S., Dhavan, N., Rubin, J.: Health-protective behaviour, social media usage and conspiracy belief during the COVID-19 public health emergency. Psychol. Med. **51**(10), 1763–1769 (2021). https://doi.org/10.1017/S003329172000224X

44. Eriksson-Backa, K., Enwald, H., Hirvonen, N., Huvila, I.: Health information seeking, beliefs about abilities, and health behaviour among Finnish seniors. J. Librariansh. Inf. Sci. **50**(3), 284–295 (2018). https://journals.sagepub.com/doi/abs/. https://doi.org/10.1177/096100061 8769971

45. Choi, W.: Older adults' health information behavior in everyday life settings. Libr. Inf. Sci. Res. **41**(4) (2019). https://doi.org/10.1016/j.lisr.2019.100983

46. Sbaffi, L., Rowley, J.: Trust and credibility in web-based health information: a review and agenda for future research. J. Med. Internet Res. **19**(6), e218 (2017). https://doi.org/10.2196/jmir.7579

47. Kim, H., Xie, B.: Health literacy in the eHealth era: a systematic review of the literature. Patient Educ. Couns. **100**(6), 1073–1082 (2017). https://doi.org/10.1016/j.pec.2017.01.015. Epub 2017 Jan 28 PMID: 28174067

48. Bruine de Bruin, W., Bennett, D.: Relationships between initial COVID-19 risk perceptions and protective health behaviors: a national survey. Am. J. Prev. Med. **59**(2), 157–167 (2020). https://doi.org/10.1016/j.amepre.2020.05.001. Epub 2020 May 22. PMID: 32576418; PMCID: PMC7242956

49. Dryhurst, S., et al.: Risk perceptions of COVID-19 around the world. J. Risk Res. **23**(7–8), 994–1006 (2020). https://doi.org/10.1080/13669877.2020.1758193

50. Dai, H., Saccardo, S., Han, M.A., et al.: Behavioural nudges increase COVID-19 vaccinations. Nature **597**, 404–409 (2021). https://doi.org/10.1038/s41586-021-03843-2
51. Hu, G., Qiu, W.: From guidance to practice: Promoting risk communication and community engagement for prevention and control of coronavirus disease (COVID-19) outbreak in China. J. Evid. Based Med. **13**(2), 168–172 (2020). https://doi.org/10.1111/jebm.12387. Epub 2020 May 22. PMID: 32445287; PMCID: PMC7280730
52. Hallyburton, A., Evarts, L.A.: Gender and online health information seeking: a five survey meta-analysis. J. Consum. Health Internet **18**(2), 128–142 (2014)
53. Ek, S.: Gender differences in health information behaviour: a Finnish population-based survey. Health Promot. Int. **30**(3), 736–745 (2015). https://doi.org/10.1093/heapro/dat063
54. Sbaffi, L., Rowley, J.: Trust and credibility in web-based health information: a review and agenda for future research. J. Med. Internet Res. **19**(6), e218 (2017). https://www.jmir.org/2017/6/e218. https://doi.org/10.2196/jmir.7579
55. Nikoloudakis, I.A., et al.: Examining the correlates of online health information-seeking behavior among men compared with women. Am. J. Mens Health **12**(5), 1358–1367 (2018). https://doi.org/10.1177/1557988316650625. Epub 2016 May 18. PMID: 27193765; PMCID: PMC6142140
56. Bidmon, S., Terlutter, R.: Gender differences in searching for health information on the internet and the virtual patient-physician relationship in Germany: exploratory results on how men and women differ and why. J. Med. Internet Res. **17**(6), e156 8 (2015). https://doi.org/10.2196/jmir.4127

Telemedicine and Independent Living

Advancements on Technology Acceptance and Adoption by Older Adults in the Context of the Second Digital Divide

Cosmina Paul(✉) and Luiza Spiru

Ana Aslan International Foundation, Bucharest, Romania
cosmina.paul@anaaslanacademy.ro, lsaslan@brainaging.ro

Abstract. In the context of global ageing, the acceptance and adoption of the new technologies by older adults has become a focus point in society at large, as the actual and optimal usage of technology can improve independence and general well-being in the late life. This research sheds light on the importance of accounting for the psychological well-being as a key determinant in technology acceptance and adoption of the older adults. We employed two surveys. The first, in 2019, asked 125 older adults from the countries of Romania, Slovenia and Cyprus. The second, in 2021, asked the opinions of 32 older adults and their formal and informal caregivers from Romania and Cyprus. We have found that the older adults who are psychologically well accept new technologies as long as they bring new information relevant to them, while also give them a sense of social integration and entertainment. Those who are psychologically not well accept new technologies based on the social influence of the formal and informal care-givers. The first group adopt new technologies as long as they are easy to be used, but the second group adopt new technologies as long as they give them a sense of social integration and companionship, decrease their loneliness, and, not last, if they are easy to be used. We bring new evidence for how the psychological unwellness, and not the socio-demographic characteristics such as age, education or income, is the key factor for the unequal use of the online resources - the second digital divide.

Keywords: Older adults · Technology acceptance and adoption · Digital divide

1 Introduction

It is largely believed that the new and emerging technologies are meant to support and prolong older adults' independence and well-being, and so the topic of technology adoption is given increased attention at all levels: from decision-makers to technology developers and families. Nowadays, due to the development of the IT Revolution more and more people who enter retirement are familiar with various IT applications and even have already adopted many of these new technologies. Though, in spite of the increasing pervasiveness of internet technology at various societal levels, inequalities in the access of new and emerging technologies persist. This article will further refer to the term of new

L. A. Maciaszek et al. (Eds.): ICT4AWE 2021/2022, CCIS 1856, pp. 197–217, 2023.
https://doi.org/10.1007/978-3-031-37496-8_11

and emerging technologies with respect to the plethora of technologies developed so far which may be of high benefit to older adults, such as: telehealth, telecare, information and communication technologies, robotics, and gerontechnology, in line with similar studies which use the term of smart technologies [1–3].

Older adults are today more prepared to adapt to new and emerging technologies because of the technology familiarity and pre-retirement computer use and, thus, closing the first digital divide. Though, evidence show that older adults' technology acceptance, actual and optimal usage still lags behind expectations [4, 5], older adults being less willing to accept technologies, when compared with other groups [6–9]. Consequently, they do not benefit from the technological advancements and that contribute to their social exclusion.

An in-depth understanding of the conducive and limiting factors affecting new technology adoption by older adults becomes imperative in the context of global ageing of the population and the increase of societal pressure associated with that [10–12]. This understanding can be given by a employing a temporal perspective on the digital divide and a more effective analysis of its contextual factors or determinants.

Two decades ago, when the discussion on the existence of a digital divide and inequalities in access to and use of internet technologies arouse, it evolved around the impacts it has on life opportunities [13, 14]. Now it is understood as the first level digital divide, which is referring to the overall use of the internet, and is merely caused by socioeconomic inequalities. In time, internet skills and literacy came into focus and marked a second level digital divide [5].

The marginalization of the older adults in the internet usage due to the limited exposure, as well as their limited use of new and emerging technologies, has been also called the grey digital divide [15]. The grey digital divide is understood as a reverberation of the first digital divide, having its root causes in the group differences in gender, education and income but it is merely centered around the sub-optimal usage of new technologies by older adults and on the fact that technology bring poor improvements in the late life, compared to what has been expected.

The advanced age per se is not proved to be a factor, but the decline in cognitive abilities which comes with age has been found as a key variable [16]. When age-related impairments, such as the cognitive decline occurs, which obstruct new technology usage, the drop-out rate occurs. Gerontechnologies are developed for various impairments, as adaptive new technologies, tailored for the needs of the old older adults. For example, Kuerbis et al. [17] found that older adults between 50- and 70-years old use internet, and then the usage drastically decreases starting with 70+. A series of studies discusses the dissatisfaction older adults have with the new technologies conceived and designed for them, while emphasizing that the new technologies concepts and designs insufficiently addresses specific age-related impairments, such as visual, tactile, and cognitive impairments and age-related specificities such as the decreasing contact with outer world [17–19]. Though, it remains unclear if the generational effect or age per se may be blamed.

Though, nowadays, this first grey digital divide is shrinking, and the second grey digital divide is happening among the older adult population. It refers to the diminished access older adults have to available information, about their very limited use of new technologies, lacking knowledge and skills, training and interest to unlock the potential of new technology for their benefit. Research on the mobile phone usage by elderly adults shows [20–22] that older adults do not fully optimise technology, and not fully exploit the opportunity of communication and connectedness.

There are conflicting interpretations for the persistence or shrinking of this 'grey' divide in the future. Because older adults are the fastest growing group of online users [23, 24], some expect the divide to fade in the near future. Though, Pino et al., [25]; Kuerbis et al., [17]; Friemel, [5] argue that there is evidence that the divide will persist.

The common understanding was that those who aim at ageing in place are more likely to benefit from new technologies. That because it is largely assumed that new technologies give older adults health information and communication or just connectedness with the loved ones [1, 26]. Though, older adults might not perceive virtual communication and connectedness the same way the younger ones do and health information is much of relevance and interest to their caregivers.

Motivational indifference or the lack of relevance and deficient knowledge are at the core of technology rejection or limited use of technology, while cost is not anymore, a key factor [27, 28]. For example, the research carried by Loges and Jung [29] inquired into the centrality dimension of internet connectedness, specifically self-evaluation of the internet in the personal life, and found that too many older adults, internet is not central. Comparative to younger groups, older adults ascribe internet less centrality [30]. Many older adults believe modern technology is not relevant to them, or show little interest in the latest technology that might support them [31]. Loges and Jung [29] advise us to treat much more cautiously initiatives which encourage older adults to adopt new and emerging technologies as many initiatives as such can prove counterproductive. Nevertheless, the wide phrase used by older adults of 'being too old to learn certain technologies' which has been confirmed by research [32, 33], beside its reference to anxieties and familiarities towards tech [32, 34] may it also subtle implies the matter of relevance and irrelevance respectively of technologies on one's life.

If the first new digital divide is shrinking and the factors such as gender, education, income and costs have been overcome to a large extent, in the new context of the second digital divide, an interplay between psychological and social factors is emphasized in the research literature. For example, Huxhold et al. [35] show that gender and education differences in internet access were significantly less pronounced in 2014 in contrast to 2002, using longitudinal data from the German Ageing Survey (DEAS). For example, caring for a grandchild is significantly associated to internet consumption for an older adult [35, 36]. Arning and Ziefle [37] found that, comparative to youth and young adults, older adult users do not take into account the time and effectiveness of the new technologies but they put value on the results comparative to the adult consumers for whom time is a key ingredient when measuring the effectiveness of the new technologies. Moreover, the limited relevance of technology in one's late adulthood shall derive from what is called a natural tendency towards social withdrawal and increasing inward looking.

Conclusively, when discussing the second level digital divide, psychological and individualistic variables such as living arrangements, social and family connectedness prove to determine the acceptance of the new and emerging technologies and should be more emphasized in the new frameworks which aim at modeling the understanding of older adults' actual usage of technology.

2 Literature Review

2.1 The Models of Technology Acceptance by Older Adults in the Context of the First Digital Divide

This study aims to shed light on the intriguing phenomenon of technology adoption through emphasizing the high heterogeneity of older adults in needs, preferences and expectations, when compared to other younger groups. Older adults' relation with technology should not be seen through the lens of age, but through the interplay of more subtle inherent features of late adulthood in order to understand the conducive and limiting factors to technology acceptance. Age per se deceives research for that it may induce over-comparativeness to other younger groups, by emphasizing the have nots of the older adults rather than their needs, habits and preferences. The constant comparison with the younger generations may limit the understanding of the specific needs, wants and preferences of the older adults and refrain research from studying the diversity within the older adults' group.

For a deeper understanding of the factors affecting technology adoption or rejection by older adults, researchers and professionals started to refer to the now classic 'technology acceptance models' and to generate and tailor-made new ones based on specific technologies, i.e. internet, mobile phones and with reference to older adult population. Currently, a universal, accurate, highly effective and easy to apply model for technology acceptance and adoption by older adults is lacking, which impede on our understanding of the relationship between technology and late adulthood.

The models so far developed starting from the classic models are factoring in many variables and require sophisticated proficiency. That is merely because they were developed at the time of the first digital divide, when socio-demographic characteristics were still prevalent when explaining why some were using technology and other didn't. Though the adaptation of those classic models to the technology adoption of the older adults proves detrimental to our understanding, as the post-retirement contexts and technology pervasiveness in everyday life require now a more refine understanding of the topic. Some research argue that the classic models ignore or pay too little attention to key moderators for PU and PEOU [38–41]. The identification of the external variables which determine PU and PEOU has been the focus of research for the last two decades, as the meta-analysis of Lee et al. [21] shows. Yousafzai et al. [41] emphases that more the dozens of variables have been identified so far. These variables, when considered, were found to have a significant impact in TAM model [4, 7, 38, 42] claimed that the so many moderators of PU and PEOU lead to model development almost impossible. Due to that and more, following Zhang [43] recommendation to strengthen the conceptual models developed, we discuss here the psychological state of the older adult as a significant determinant for the acceptance and consequently the adoption and rejection of the new and emerging technologies.

The classic models of technology adoption also prove insufficient when trying to predict new technology adoption by older adults as they show some limitations both peculiar to the models themselves and other which arouse when applied to the older adults group. The models merely emphasize the product capacities instead of looking at the individual needs, preferences and expectation of the older adult consumers. The explanation is that these models have been constructed and developed having at their center youth and adult working population, whose social and psychological behaviour characteristics are much more homogeneous as well as their needs and expectations, when compared to the older adult group.

This is the case of the classic frameworks of Technology Acceptance Model (TAM) and Unified Theory of Acceptance and the Use of Technology (UTAUT) have been largely deployed for adult working population. At the core, they have been based on two variables: perceived usefulness (PU) and perceived ease of use (PEOU). The first has reverberated in relation to the job enhancements (Li et al. 2008; Venkatesch and Davis, 2000; 7; Venkatesh et al., 2012), while the second was defined as the extent to which a person believes that using the system will be free of effort [7].

Hence, these models show limited predictability [1] for the case of older adults because they fail to emphasize the relevance of individual factors rather than of the product experience. That was also confirmed by our previous field-research: older adults' habits, activities, interests and curiosities are the results of their life long experiences and, therefore, their adoption on new technologies will rather depend on individual factors or personal traits and less on the new technology products' attributes [47].

The models have at their core two key variables: perceived usefulness (PU) and perceived ease of use (PEOU). They are meant to predict the desirability to use the proposed technology, which is named as attitudes towards use (A), which lead to the acceptance of a technology. But the acceptance of a technology does not necessarily lead to its adoption, the actual usage. The second digital divide, the 'grey' divide is crucial to be accounted for when discussing the relation between technology and older adults who may make limited use of an accepted new technology. In the study conducted on the older adults' adoption of mobile phones, Gelderblom and Biljon [48] found that older adults neither accept nor reject mobile usage, but use them with limited functions. They identified age, mode of acquirement and the duration of ownership are predictors for full acceptance or rejection.

PU has a wide tested significance. Because the technology acceptance model has been constructed for employees, perceived usefulness (PU) was defined as 'the extent to which a person believes that using the system will enhance his or her job performance' [7] and the definition reverberated stressing or eluding 'the job' or the benefits obtained [44].

PEOU is defined as 'the extent to which a person believes that using the system will be free of effort' [7]. It has been hypothesized that the familiarization of people with new technology proposed make PEOU not to necessarily influence PU. Chung et al. [49] reveal that PEOU is not a significant indicator for PU, along Biljon and Renaud [50] who declared that PEOU affects the actual use of technology for the case of older adults, and it does not precede the intention to use. They found that poor ease of use especially and less than optimal confirmed usefulness hamper adoption [50].

The relationship between PEOU and PU has been strongly supported by research [51–53]. It is believed that an application should be ease to use in order for older adults to use it, though the perceived usefulness, the intention to use it, would precede the experimentation and exploration phase. To us that implies that perceived usefulness stays.

When referred to the 'perceived usefulness' (PU), critics pointed out that: a) a strong indication of the perceived usefulness does not necessarily lead to adoption, and so the models restrict to the 'Behavioural Intention to Use' without analyzing the 'Actual Usage' [54]; b) the perceived usefulness should be differently inquired into the post-retirement context, c) the higher heterogenity of the older adults when compared to the youth lead to factor in too many variables [55–57] and d) the age-related impairments add new limits to the easiness of the new technologies' usage.

When referred to the 'perceived ease of use' (PEOU), it has been hypothesized that the general familiarization with new technologies would make PEOU not to necessarily influence PU. Some researchers [43, 49] reveal that PEOU is not a significant indicator for PU. Biljon and Renaud [50] declared that PEOU affects the actual use of technology for the case of older adults, and it does not precede the intention to use. They found that poor ease of use especially and less than optimal confirmed usefulness hamper adoption [50].

2.2 The Need for New Models of Technology Adoption in the Context of the Second Digital Divide

Research shows that chronological age does not determine technology acceptance [47, 49, 58, 59]. That is because the physical and psychological state of health depends on how the individuals encounter various life-events [58, 60–62]. Hence, the decline which comes with ageing, largely varies: a person aged 60 shows a similar state of health as a person aged 70 or even 80. The functional capacity, which factors in the physical, psychological and social variables is intimately related with the technology adoption, but there is large variance within the age group in relation to the functional capacity.

For the last decades, there were various types of segmentations of the older adults' market which were employed by industry and marketing when developing and aiming at understanding of this market. The sociodemographic segmentation refers to objective characteristics such as age, income, education, living arrangements and others, the behavioural segmentation refers to activities and lifestyles, while the psychographic segmentation refers to the differences in values and attitudes [63]. Though, due to the large heterogeneity of older adults, segmentations such as sociodemographic, behavioural or psychographic proved insufficiently explanatory and, therefore, some use with the degree of dependency or frailty is used as a workable variable when older adults are defined into 3 groups: active, fragile and dependent in the French Silver Economy Strategy or with the 4 groups of gerontographics proposed by Moschis [58, 64]. On the same note of differentiating among the older adults based on their frailty or degree of independency, gerontographics segmentation indicates the well-being of older adults into categories which influence the relation with technology [47, 58].

To adjust the understanding of technology to the domain of older adults, researchers have sought to include variables relating to older adults' biophysical and psychosocial needs [65]. Peek [66] proposed therefore to include additional factors describing state-of-health, psychology, ability and specific challenge experienced by seniors. Along these studies, age stays just as a proxy variable.

Gerontographics has offered another framework to paint with a more refined brush the picture of old adulthood. Common understanding is supported by literature which emphasize that the formation of new memory connections is impaired with age [67–69], that it is the rate of learning which decline with age, especially because of the impaired vision, but not the ability to learn. Though, this is not a uniform process but it is a highly personalized process, so the age variable stays as a proxy.

In line with recent studies, gerontographics bring evidence for accounting for physical and psychological state of the older adults, rather than for demographic variables [58, 63, 70]. Data shows that the rate of depression drastically increases with age, as for the category of 74 and over, almost double compared to the group of those aged 65 to 74. It is not just that the rate of depression increases with age but it is also of relevance that for the case of males, the rate of depression almost triples. Isolation only worsen things and social integration is requested as the most urgent and pressing needs for this age-category [71, 72]. Hence, it is not age, but the psychological factor which needs to be accounted for.

Geronthographics proved to highly effective in predicting older adults' consumer behavior and reveals the individual differences in aging processes in late life. According to Moschis, the life experiences of the older adults' influence on the psychological factors, which ultimately, influence their needs, preferences and expectations. The gerontographics approach show that older adults manifest similar behaviour consumer activity as long as they had encountered similar circumstances, experiences and past events, based on the type of aging experience.

In a previous study [73] we have employed this type of segmentation of a continuum from independency towards dependency and from socially integrated towards socially isolated, working with the four groups of older adults, proposed by Moschis: healthy indulgers, frail recluses, ailing outgoers and healthy hermits. The four categories clearly show the target market of supportive and empowering technologies [74].

3   Research Methodology

The study was based on two surveys, among which the first was designed quantitatively and the second qualitatively. The first survey was conducted in Romania, Cyprus and Slovenia over the course of February and April, 2019 and the second survey was based on interviews with older adults from Romania and Cyprus in August and September 2020.

The first survey (Own survey, 2019) [73] had 125 participants, a convenient sample of members. In order to recruit participants, the administrators of day centers, nursing and retirement homes and older adults have been contacted. For the second survey, 32 interviews, 16 in each country were conducted in 2021

Members' physical and psychological wellbeing has been estimated through the Health Survey (SF12). The certified scale shows the physical and psychological state of the respondents. The "Verbal Fluency Test" (VFT), an instrument for cognitive assessment, was administrated in the case of the first survey and for the second survey, the exclusion criteria involved having intact the cognitive abilities.

The first survey included a total of 125 primary end-users who were grouped as following: 52 from Romania, 30 from Cyprus and 43 from Slovenia. For the case of Romania, there were 52 older adults pre-trial interviewed and the drop-out rate was of 20 seniors. The 125 respondents were 57–90 years old, and the average was 73, while the most frequent age was 70. Most respondents reported a general good state of health and an overwhelming majority declared that they feel blue and discouraged.

Those who were physically well but psychologically not well comprised about half of the sample (49% of respondents), and thus, an equal distribution of the psychologically well and those psychologically not well has been achieved. Half of them live in Slovenia and the other half was equally distributed across Romania and Cyprus.

The second survey (Own survey, 2021) has included a total number of 32 participants, among which 12 were older adults aged over 65, 10 were informal carers and 10 were formal carers providers. The older adults were aged 70+ years old and over, had no severe cognitive impairment but either physical or psychological limitations and voluntary participation in the research and giving their consent to participate.

The informed consent has been included for both studies and the focus of ethical concerns was the 1) anonymization, by which we made sure that the risk of somebody being identified in the data is negligible. 2) the minimization principle, according to which personal data which was collected was adequate, relevant and limited to what is necessary in relation to the purposes for which they will be processed.

'Cognitive Ability' has been assessed through the Verbal Fluency Test (VFT). Along the research evidence above presented, our research findings show that that age does not determine cognitive abilities. Our data show that chronological age is ineffectively associated with the cognitive abilities as the Pearson correlation is quite low (r = −224). That suggests that it is reasonable to think that as people age so there is a slowing down of mental and physical abilities but in a long space of time.

4 Results

4.1 Remarks on the Psychological Factor as Key Determinant in the Context of the Second Digital Divide

We grouped the older adults into those psychologically well and those psychologically not well and we have noticed radical differences between the two groups in the acceptance of new technologies.

We found that technological familiarity does not influence technology acceptance but technology adoption and that would lead to an optimal usage of the new technology. Though, our research findings clearly show that technology familiarity and other similar external factors such as age or education do not influence on the technology adoption.

Therefore, we have found that the current usage of technology does not depend on the starting age of using technology, as the ageing process changes the habits of usage of various technologies [73]. An explanation for that might be that those psychologically well, irrespective of their current physical state, encounter technology in their professional and social life prior to retirement. For those older adults, the life changes which occur after retirement decrease the necessity for technology adoption. On the contrary to that, those psychologically not well have a decreased interest in the newness of technology prior to retirement but, when their life after retirement radically brings more isolation and loneliness, their interest in technology increases as technology becomes the only source for meeting social and personal basic needs. We may also hypothesize that the predisposition of using technology is an early indicator or predictor of the psychological well-being of the type of the individual ageing process.

In our earlier analysis [73], which employed a gerontographics segmentation, we found that based on their psychological state, older adults have a different relation with technology. Those who are not psychologically well exhibit various usages of technology and have a clear predisposition for using new technologies. They are those who still use radio and landline phones and manifest a clear intention for using smart TV, computer and internet. Those who are psychologically well do not use anymore the old technologies and have a limited adoption of new technologies, while also preferring rather not to use the new technologies [47]. They started the relation with mobile phone, computer and internet at an earlier age on average, in the pre-retirement period but did not continue to endorse new technology after retirement.

Those psychologically well gave up to the usage of old technologies and followed the technological trends as long as the new technologies proved relevant in their life. The relevance merely refers to bringing new information to them, in the large sense, and, to some extent, entertainment. The older adults psychologically not well continue to keep and use to various degrees old technologies and manifest a large interest in new technologies. On average, this group has encountered the new technologies trends significantly later comparative to the other group, and often not much earlier their retirement. In the post-retirement period, the older adults psychologically not well have raised their interest in the new and emerging technologies, as these would serve their psychologically state derived from social isolation. The inquiry into the older adults' actual usage of the technology, be that old or new, show that there is no relationship between age per se, technology familiarity and actual technology usage along with other research evidence [73, 75].

External factors which were accounted for in the classic models of technology adoption and in the models which have been designed for understanding older adults' technology acceptance are not of relevance today. That is because we are referring to the second digital divide, which is not anymore, as it has been argued in the above section, a matter of sociodemographic factors which prevent technology adoption but a matter of individualistic preferences. Hence, the psychological state of the older adults plays a paramount role, as we will argue below. However, we should consider that we have reached this stage of overcoming socio-demographic characteristics because of the technological pervasiveness which led to technological familiarity prior retirement (Table 1).

Table 1. Technology acceptance based on the psychological state of the older adults

	Radio	Mobile phone	Internet	PC	E-mail	Smart tv	Smart watch
Psychologically well	Inconclusive	Adopted	Adopted	Adopted	Rather not	Rather not	Inconclusive
Psychologically unwell	Sub-optimal usage	Accepted	Adopted	Suboptimal usage	Accepted	Accepted	Accepted

Source: Adapted after Paul, C. Sterea, A., Mârzan, M. Economidou, A., Iztok, Garleanu, A. Why Do Seniors Accept or Reject New Technologies? (2019)

4.2 'Perceived Usefulness' and 'Social Influence' as Determinants of New Technology Acceptance Based on the Older Adults' Psychological Well-Being

We have found that the 'Perceived usefulness' (PU) is a determinant for the acceptance of a new technology by older adults psychologically well and the 'Social Influence' (SI) is a determinant for older adult psychologically not well in their acceptance of a new technology.

In the beginning, we have started by looking at the drop-out rates. In our research, the dropout rates occurred only for the older adults psychologically well, which indicate that the 'Perceived Usefulness' (PU) is key for the older adult group with a good psychological state. That indicates that the 'Perceived Usefulness' is considered only by those psychologically well, while those psychologically unwell are willing to enter the exploration and experimentation stage without questioning the usefulness of a new technology in the first instance.

We have observed significant differences in using the TV services, between the older adults psychologically well and those who are not. Evidence shows that none of those who are psychologically well use any of these TV services. Research findings clearly indicates that there is a high incidence of usage of TV Smart Application (Pearson R = .484) and also high correlations for the cases of TV Images (Pearson's R = .369) for older adults not psychologically well.

The below table is developed based on the previous carried analysis [73] (Table 2).

Table 2. The type of TV services used by older adults based on their psychological state.

	Radio	Teletext	Smart app	TV images	TV Video
Psychologically well	0%	0%	0%	0%	0%
Physically well and psychologically not-well	16,1%	16,1%	71,4%	51,8%	37,5%
Physically and psychologically not well	7,7%	20,5%	69,2%	56,4%	43,6%

Source: Paul, Cosmina, and Luiza Spiru. "From Age to Age: Key Gerontographics Contributions to Technology Adoption by Older Adults." (2021)

Social Influence (SI) stays for the degree to which an individual believes that what others feel if he or she should use a particular technology and it has been identified as a relevant factor in accepting technology [7, 21, 62, 76]. We have found that social influence matters only with respect to older adults who are psychologically unwell. We may advance the hypotheses that the research carried out in the 2000s reflect a time when SI could have had such an influence on the adoption of technologies such as Internet and smart phones, but that is not the case for non-revolutionary technologies. For example, in the case of mobile phone adoption, that is a revolution in communication and here, the pressure of the close others, be they relatives or peers, matter more than in the case of a specific technology which just meet the needs of the beneficiary.

4.3 The Determinants in Technology Adoption Based on the Psychological State of the Older Adult

We have found that for older adults psychologically well, the new information's relevance is key in technology acceptance, but for technology adoption, the easiness to use the technology would lead to its actual and optimal usage. In the case of older adults psychologically not well, the mentally ascribed meanings are the determinants for technology adoption, along the easiness to use.

The older adults psychologically well value new technologies to the extent to which new information and some enjoyments are brought. The new information and the entertainment are supposed to contribute significantly to their social integration. The older adults psychologically not well value technologies which also support them in reaching for new information and enjoyment but also decreasing loneliness, forming a ritual, giving a sense of companionship or entertainment. It worth to be noted that the older adults did psychologically not well did not care for the duplication of services, while that was of much relevance for those psychologically well. For example, having a new video-calling option or games through the means of a new device or service, alarm notifications, digital agenda, watching news and other as such, which are already offered through TV and smart-phones (Table 3).

In line with other research evidence, we emphasize that new technology is of limited relevance to the older adults psychologically well. They know very well their needs, preferences and expectations and refuse age-stigmatization, according to our own survey from 2021. The explanation for their limited relevance does not rely in the familiarity with technology, proficiency in technology usage, education or income but in the irrelevance and limited scope they see in the new technology. The relevance ascribed to technology in one's life is a dynamic process which change in time in close relation with the physical and psychological individual changes, according to the most participants from the survey from 2021.

More, both older adults either psychologically well or not, emphasized that video-calling, memory prompts, entertainment and other new technology services alike, do not bear for them the same value as offline socialization or the physical contact with the dear ones and, hence the limited ascribed meaning of the new technologies. However, those psychologically not well would adopt new technologies as long as they would contribute to their above ascribed mentally meanings even if to a lower extent.

Table 3. The mentally ascribed meanings of TV watching based on the psychological state of the older adults.

	Information	Entertainment	Decrease loneliness	C Companionship	Social integration	Ritual
Physically well and psychologically well	62.5%	37.5%	18.8%	31.3%	42.9%	36.0%
Physically not well but psychologically well	66.7%	66.7%	16.7%	33.4%	50.0%	–
Physically well but psychologically not well	80.3%	54.5%	83.6%	52.8%	57.7%	61.5%
Physically not well but psychologically well	72.9%	89.5%	76.5%	75.0%	60.6%	48.6%

Source: Paul, Cosmina, and Luiza Spiru. "From Age to Age: Key Gerontographics Contributions to Technology Adoption by Older Adults." (2021)

Thus, our research bring evidence that for the case of the older adults psychologically not well, the 'Perceived Usefulness' variable is not of relevance, as they prove to be heavily influenced by their informal entourage, more specifically by their relatives or informal carers.

Those psychologically not well ascribe to TV watching many mental associations, while those psychologically well do not. Information and social integration, along enjoyment are the two most important features associated to TV watching to those psychologically well, while those who are not psychologically well associate TV watching with: decreasing loneliness and companionship to a higher extent. The majority (62.5%) appreciate TV for 'information' and almost half of them (42.9%) appreciate TV for 'Social Integration'. The overwhelming majority of those in good health but without a social life associate TV watching with decreasing loneliness (83.6%) while also looking for information (80.3%), those who are bound due to poor health look first for enjoyment (89.5%) and decreasing loneliness (76.5%) and companionship (75%) as well.

Nevertheless, TV watching is associated with 'Social Integration', which matters for each category of older adults, though it increases in significance from those independent to those dependent, namely form those socially active who also have other means for social integration to those who lack that (42.9% to 60.6%) TV maybe being the only or one of a very few vehicles for their sense of belonging to society after retirement (Table 4).

Table 4. The information's relevance and the mentally ascribed meaning of TV watching based on the psychological state.

	Information	Enjoyment	Decrease loneliness	Companionship	Social integration	Ritual
Physically well and psychologically well	62.5%	37.5%	18.8%	31.3%	42.9%	36.0%
Physically not well but psychologically well	66.7%	66.7%	16.7%	33.4%	50.0%	–
Physically well but psychologically not well	80.3%	54.5%	83.6%	52.8%	57.7%	61.5%
Physically not well but psychologically well	72.9%	89.5%	76.5%	75.0%	60.6%	48.6%

Source: Paul, Cosmina, and Luiza Spiru. "From Age to Age: Key Gerontographics Contributions to Technology Adoption by Older Adults." (2021)

5 Discussion

The acceptance of a new technology precedes its adoption, and, even if a new technology is accepted, that would not necessarily lead to the actual usage and to the optimal usage. Hence, the first stage, when the technology is explored, is the stage of the acceptance or the rejection of the technology. Here, we have found that the psychological factor is the key determinant in the new technology acceptance process.

The importance of relevance of the new technologies in the life of the older adults psychologically well is paramount in their decision in accepting them. This is in line with other research findings, as the 'relevance' is shown to be the first and foremost factor in the acceptance and actual usage of new technologies [75]. For example, the older adults psychologically well adopted mobile phones, personal computers and internet often in their pre-retirement period but they did not continue necessary to use these new technologies after retirement. Older adults psychologically well did not manifest an interest in the duplication of some services or products in communication, information and others as such. For example, they did not find relevant in having the agenda or notifications electronically, pursing a video-call or having the news through various channels. Therefore, they need stronger incentives for using other PC or mobile phone applications as long as they have already acquired the needed information through other means, be they technological or not. Hence, having a hand-writing agenda, access to

210 C. Paul and L. Spiru

information on TV or video-calling through mobile phone, refrained many from the usage of PCs, e-mails, smart TVs and alike.

In a previous study [73] we aimed to build up a new model for technology adoption by older adults, with a better prediction power while also having an increased efficiency. Gerontographics segmentation gave us a more in-depth understanding of the relation between the older adults' technology habits and the predisposition towards the usage of new technologies or gerontechnologies.

Further, we show that in the case of older adults psychologically well, the 'Perceived Usefulness' of a new technology determines the acceptance or rejection of the technology, meaning here new information and the sense of social integration. The ascribed relevance is a dynamic process which change in time in close relation with the physical and psychological individual changes. For the case of those psychologically unwell, the influence of the formal and/or informal caregivers is decisive. For those psychologically well, once that the technology is accepted, the perceived ease of use will lead to the adoption or rejection of that technology, though that might preserve a limited usage of the technology in case, based on the relevance of that technology ascribed in one's life.

Research emphasizes that the use of technology has various meanings and the same technology does not serve the same purpose for everyone. For example, a mobile phone will be used by older adults psychologically well for getting information and feeling socially integrated, while those psychologically not well would expect mobile phones to decrease their loneliness, keep social relations and entertain them, thus using more games and mobile applications compared to those psychologically well. Moreover, people's relation with technology changes during the ageing process as retirement alters one's relation to the labor market and changes social contacts [77, 78]. For example, the assumption that older adults spent extensive amount of time in front of the TV and that lacks meaning for them, that there is no emotional and intellectual relationship established has been infirmed. Östlund's study [77] found that TV viewing fulfils the social needs of older adults, staying socially integrated, giving a rhythm and a structure to daily life, and answers to the needs of contemplation and reflection. Hence, older adults ascribe practical and symbolic meanings to technology, and integrate it into social relations and cultures as it contributes to the construction of a common experience of routines, of time and space and to their isolation or integration into society and family [78].

These findings emphasize relevant results for practitioners. If targeting older adults psychologically well, they need to have an older adults centered approach, as the older adults psychologically well would accept new technologies only as long as they would provide relevant new information to them and are not age-stigmatizing, but of universal usage.

If targeting older adults psychologically well, the developers should consider 1) to target the informal or formal care providers for advancing new technologies in the life of older adults psychologically not well, as their influence on the older adults in their technology acceptance is key; 2) to consider an adaptive nature of this technologies as the older adults psychologically not well have more physical and psychological impairments and that could prevent them from adoption. 3) To employ a user-centered approach, as the ascribed mental meaning of the technologies are complex for those psychologically not well and they need to meet these expectations: social integration, decreasing loneliness, increasing the sense of companionship, setting up a ritual and others.

Researchers and developers should further consider that even the first digital divide is shrinking in the sense that the access to online resources is more equal than before, the expectations from new technologies of the older adults psychologically well are totally different from the expectations of those psychologically not well. Thus, the technology familiarity prior retirement, or socio-demographic factors such as age, education, income, does not affect their relation with technology in the late life. Moreover, the familiarity with technology, the digitization, and external variables should be more carefully consider as they do not predict the usage of a new technology but only the ability and ease of use [63, 79–81].

6 Conclusion

In the context of the second digital divide, the relation of the older adults with technology and the barriers which have arose are differently experienced by those with dissimilar psychological well-being.

Our analysis indicates that older adults who are psychologically well see limited relevance in the new technologies and perceived the usefulness (PU) of the new technologies in terms of offering new information, social integration and, to some extent, entertainment. Thus, the acceptance of the new technologies strictly depends on the newness of the information received, meaning that that information can not be reached through other channels or means. The technology adoption, the actual usage of the new technology will depend on the ease of use (PEOU) (Fig. 1).

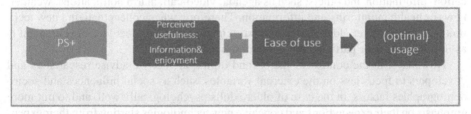

Fig. 1. Technology acceptance and adoption for older adults psychologically well.

In the case of the older adults psychologically not well, the acceptance of the new technologies depends on the social influence (SI) of their informal and/or formal caregivers. As long as the new technology offer them entertainment and has effect of decreasing loneliness and giving a sense of companionship and sets up a form of daily ritual, the technology will be adopted. The ease of use of the adopted technology determines its the optimal usage (Fig. 2).

We conclude that the new technologies should target those psychologically well differently from those psychologically not well, who will be actually targeted through their informal/formal carers.

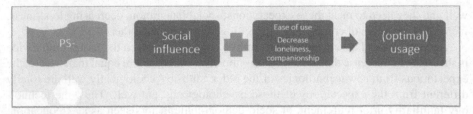

Fig. 2. Technology acceptance and adoption for older adults psychologically not well.

We have also shown that for the older adults, irrespective of their psychological state, the perceived ease of use (PEOU) does not determine technology acceptance but technology adoption. Acceptance of a not-easy to use technology leads to suboptimal usage of the new technology. Those psychologically not well are heavily socially influenced but also have specific expectations due to the mentally ascribed meanings they give to new technologies: decreasing loneliness, offering a sense of companionship, to ritualize their day and to increase their sense of being socially integrated.

This difference between 'perceived usefulness' and 'social influence' shows us that those who are psychologically not well are the target market for new technologies and gerontechnologies. They manifest a late interest in technology predisposition and usage, which is not shared by those who are psychologically well. Those who are psychologically well do not use anymore the old technologies and have a limited adoption of new technologies. They started the relation with mobile, computer and internet earlier on average but did not continue to endorse new technology after retirement.

We found that the first reason for the limited relevance of new technologies for older adults psychologically well is the redundancy or duplication of services in communication, information and others, such as agenda, video-call, alarm notifications, weather, news or health monitoring and information. Therefore, when conceptualizing new technologies which target older adults their participation in the project idea development is as important as their participation in the design of the project.

Nowadays, in the context of the second digital divide, we advise researchers and developers to focus less on the external variables, such as social influences and socio-demographics factors, in the case of older adults psychologically well, and to put more emphasis on their expectations and conceive new technologies starting from their expectations. In the case of older adults psychologically not well, from the onset of the new technologies' development, the expectations of their formal/informal carers should be considered and the testing should analyse the degree to which the new technologies answer to the mentally ascribed meanings of the targeted people.

7 Limitations of this Study

There are two main limitations of this study: the cultural and digital inclusion factors. Romania and Cyprus are lagging behind in terms of digital inclusion. The share of the elderly who use internet at least once a week in Cyprus is 26% and in Romania is 13%, while the EU average is 45%. Both Cyprus and Romania find themselves much under the European Union average. Romania is among the top five countries that have the highest rates of non-users in the EU [82]. We need also to account for cultural variations as the countries of our focus are collectivist cultures where group cohesiveness is still expressed through the extended family where members offer help and loyalty, strengthening the familialism paradigm. Greece and Romania are more of masculine societies, where men are caring for the families [83].

Acknowledgements. This work was performed in the frame of the EU project iCan. Inclusive online platform for Senior Adults (AAL-2019-6-182) project funded by the AAL Programme – April 2019), co-funded by the European Commission and the National Funding Authorities of Cyprus, Spain and Romania.

References

1. Golant, S.M.: A theoretical model to explain the smart technology adoption behaviors of elder consumers (Elderadopt). J. Aging Stud. **42**, 56–73 (2017)
2. Davenport, T.H., Barth, P., Bean, R.: How 'big data' is different, pp. 22–24 (2012)
3. Kaye (2017)
4. Wildenbos, G.A.: Mobile health for older adult patients: using an aging barriers framework to classify usability problems. Int. J. Med. Inform. **124**, 68–77 (2019)
5. Friemel, T.N.: The digital divide has grown old: determinants of a digital divide among seniors. New Media Soc. **18**(2), 313–331 (2016)
6. Morris, M.G., Venkatesh, V.: Age differences in technology adoption decisions: implications for a changing work force. Pers. Psychol. **53**(2), 375–403 (2000)
7. Venkatesh, M., et al.: User acceptance of information technology: toward a unified view. MIS Q. **27**(3), 425–478 (2003). https://doi.org/10.2307/30036540
8. Czaja, S., Schulz, R.: Innovations in technology and aging introduction. Generations **30**(2), 6–8 (2006)
9. Yao, Y., Murphy, L.: Remote electronic voting systems: an exploration of voters' perceptions and intention to use. Eur. J. Inf. Syst. **16**(2), 106–120 (2007)
10. Bae, H., Jo, S.H., Lee, E.: Why do older consumers avoid innovative products and services? J. Serv. Mark. **35**(1), 41–53 (2020). https://doi.org/10.1108/JSM-10-2019-0408
11. Vasiliadis, H.M., Dionne, P.A., Préville, M., Gentil, L., Berbiche, D., Latimer, E.: The excess healthcare costs associated with depression and anxiety in elderly living in the community. Am. J. Geriatr. Psychiatry **21**(6), 536–548 (2013)
12. Hazra, N.C., Gulliford, M.C., Rudisill, C.: 'Fair innings' in the face of ageing and demographic change. Health Econ. Policy Law **13**(2), 209–217 (2018)
13. Gibson, G., et al.: The everyday use of assistive technology by people with dementia and their family carers: a qualitative study. BMC Geriatr. **15**(1), 1–10 (2015). https://doi.org/10.1186/s12877-015-0091-3
14. Warren, S.J., Lee, J., Najmi, A.: The impact of technology and theory on instructional design since 2000. In: Spector, J.M., Merrill, M.D., Elen, J., Bishop, M.J. (eds.) Handbook of Research on Educational Communications and Technology, pp. 89–99. Springer, New York (2014). https://doi.org/10.1007/978-1-4614-3185-5_8
15. Morris, M.E., Adair, B., Miller, K., Ozanne, E., Hansen, R., Pearce, A.J.: Smart-home technologies to assist older people to live well at home. J. Aging Sci. **1**(1), 1–9 (2013)
16. Singer, J., Rexhaj, B., Baddeley, J.: Older, wiser, and happier? Comparing older adults' and college students' self-defining memories. Memory **15**(8), 886–898 (2007)

17. Kuerbis, A., Mulliken, A., Muench, F., Moore, A.A., Gardner, D.: Older adults and mobile technology: Factors that enhance and inhibit utilization in the context of behavioral health (2017)
18. Mitzner, T.L., et al.: Technology adoption by older adults: findings from the PRISM trial. Gerontologist 59(1), 34–44 (2019). https://doi.org/10.1093/geront/gny113
19. Hedman, A., Kottorp, A., Almkvist, O., Nygård, L.: Challenge levels of everyday technologies as perceived over five years by older adults with mild cognitive impairment. Int. Psychogeriatr. 30(10), 1447–1454 (2018). https://doi.org/10.1017/S1041610218000285
20. Chen, K., Chan, A.H.S.: Gerontechnology acceptance by elderly Hong Kong Chinese: a senior technology acceptance model (STAM). Ergonomics 57(5), 635–652 (2013)
21. Lee, M.M., Carpenter, B., Meyers, L.S.: Representations of older adults in television advertisements. J. Aging Stud. 21(1), 23–30 (2007)
22. Ziefle, M., Bay, S.: How older adults meet complexity: aging effects on the usability of different mobile phones. Behav. Inf. Technol. 24(5), 375–389 (2005)
23. Smith, J.L., Hollinger-Smith, L.: Savoring, resilience, and psychological well-being in older adults. Aging Ment. Health 19(3), 192–200 (2015)
24. Anderson, M., Perrin, A.: Tech adoption climbs among older adults. Pew Res. Center 17 (2017)
25. Pino, M., Boulay, M., Jouen, F., Rigaud, A.S.: Are we ready for robots that care for us?" Attitudes and opinions of older adults toward socially assistive robots. Front. Aging Neurosci. 7, 141 (2015)
26. Orlov, L.M.: Technology survey: older adults, age 59–85+. Aging in Place Technology Watch, Mason (2016). https://www.ageinplacetech.com/files/aip/Linkage202016:20
27. Peacock, S.E., Künemund, H.: Senior citizens and Internet technology. Eur. J. Ageing 4(4), 191–200 (2007)
28. Juznic, P., et al.: Who says that old dogs cannot learn new tricks? A survey of internet/web usage among seniors. New Libr. World (2006)
29. Loges, W.E., Jung, J.-Y.: Exploring the digital divide: internet connectedness and age. Commun. Res. 28(4), 536–562 (2001)
30. Abbey, R., Hyde, S.: No country for older people? Age and the digital divide. J. Inf. Commun. Ethics Soc. 7(4), 225–242 (2009). https://doi.org/10.1108/14779960911004480
31. Mohadis, H.M., Ali, N.M., Smeaton, A.F.: Designing a persuasive physical activity application for older workers: understanding end-user perceptions. Behav. Inf. Technol. 35(12), 1102–1114 (2016)
32. Barnard, Y., Bradley, M.D., Hodgson, F., Lloyd, A.D.: Learning to use new technologies by older adults: perceived difficulties, experimentation behaviour and usability. Comput. Hum. Behav. 29(4), 1715–1724 (2013). https://doi.org/10.1016/j.chb.2013.02.006
33. Wilson, C.: No one is too old to learn: neuroandragogy: a theoretical perspective on adult brain functions and adult learning. iUniverse (2006)
34. Tsai, T.H., Lin, W.Y., Chang, Y.S., Chang, P.C., Lee, M.Y.: Technology anxiety and resistance to change behavioral study of a wearable cardiac warming system using an extended TAM for older adults. PLoS ONE 15(1), e0227270 (2020)
35. Huxhold, O., Fiori, K.L., Webster, N.J., Antonucci, T.C.: The strength of weaker ties: an underexplored resource for maintaining emotional well-being in later life. J. Gerontol.: Ser. B 75(7), 1433–1442 (2020)
36. Evans, J.: Mapping the vulnerability of older persons to disasters. Int. J. Older People Nurs. 5(1), 63–70 (2010)
37. Arning, K., Ziefle, M.: "Get that camera out of my house!" conjoint measurement of preferences for video-based healthcare monitoring systems in private and public places. In: Geissbühler, A., Demongeot, J., Mokhtari, M., Abdulrazak, B., Aloulou, H. (eds.) ICOST 2015.

LNCS, vol. 9102, pp. 152–164. Springer, Cham (2015). https://doi.org/10.1007/978-3-319-19312-0_13

38. Bagozzi, R.P.: The legacy of the technology acceptance model and a proposal for a paradigm shift. J. Assoc. Inf. Syst. **8**(4), 3 (2007)
39. Benbasat, I., Barki, H.: Quo vadis TAM? J. Assoc. Inf. Syst. **8**(4), 7 (2007)
40. Sun, Y., et al.: Stress and depression among Chinese new urban older adults: a moderated mediation model. Soc. Behav. Pers.: Int. J. **48**(9), 1–10 (2020). https://doi.org/10.2224/sbp.9446
41. Yousafzai, S.Y.: A literature review of theoretical models of Internet banking adoption at the individual level. J. Financ. Serv. Mark. **17**(3), 215–226 (2012). https://doi.org/10.1057/fsm.2012.19
42. Gefen, D., Straub, D.W.: Gender differences in the perception and use of e-mail: an extension to the technology acceptance model. MIS Q. **21**(4), 389–400 (1997). https://doi.org/10.2307/249720
43. Zhang, S., et al.: A predictive model for assistive technology adoption for people with dementia. IEEE J. Biomed. Health Inform. **18**(1), 375–383 (2014). https://doi.org/10.1109/JBHI.2013.2267549
44. Lee, I., Choi, B., Kim, J., Hong, S.J.: Culture-technology fit: effects of cultural characteristics on the post-adoption beliefs of mobile Internet users. Int. J. Electron. Commer. **11**(4), 11–51 (2007)
45. Venkatesh, V., Davis, F.D.: A theoretical extension of the technology acceptance model: four longitudinal field studies. Manag. Sci. **46**(2), 186–204 (2000)
46. Venkatesh, V., Thong, J.Y.L., Xu, X.: Consumer acceptance and use of information technology: extending the unified theory of acceptance and use of technology. MIS Q. **36**, 157–178 (2012)
47. Paul, C., et al.: Why do seniors accept or reject new technologies? In: The Fourth International Conference on Neuroscience and Cognitive Brain Information, BRAIN INFO 2019 (2019). http://www.thinkmind.org/download_full.php?instance=BRAININFO+2019
48. Gelderblom, H., van Dyk, T., van Biljon, J.: Mobile phone adoption: do existing models adequately capture the actual usage of older adults? In: Proceedings of the 2010 Annual Research Conference of the South African Institute of Computer Scientists and Information Technologists (2010)
49. Chung-Yan, G.A.: The nonlinear effects of job complexity and autonomy on job satisfaction, turnover, and psychological well-being. J. Occup. Health Psychol. **15**(3), 237–251 (2010). https://doi.org/10.1037/a0019823
50. Renaud, K., Van Biljon, J.: Predicting technology acceptance and adoption by the elderly: a qualitative study. In: Proceedings of the 2008 Annual Research Conference of the South African Institute of Computer Scientists and Information Technologists on IT Research in Developing Countries: Riding the Wave of Technology (2008)
51. Adams, D.A., Ryan Nelson, R., Todd, P.A.: Perceived usefulness, ease of use, and usage of information technology: a replication. MIS Q. **16**(2), 227–247 (1992). https://doi.org/10.2307/249577
52. Chen, L., Gillenson, L., Sherrell, L.: Enticing online consumers: an extended technology acceptance perspective. Inf. Manag. **39**(8), 709–719 (2002). https://doi.org/10.1016/S0378-7206(01)00127-6
53. Gefen, D., Karahanna, E., Straub, D.W.: Trust and TAM in online shopping: an integrated model. MIS Q. **27**(1), 51–90 (2003). https://doi.org/10.2307/30036519
54. Bouwhuis, S., et al.: Distinguishing groups and exploring health differences among multiple job holders aged 45 years and older. Int. Arch. Occup. Environ. Health **92**(1), 67–79 (2018). https://doi.org/10.1007/s00420-018-1351-2

55. Hunsaker, A., Nguyen, M.H., Fuchs, J., Djukaric, T., Hugentobler, L., Hargittai, E.: He explained it to me and I also did it myself: how older adults get support with their technology uses. Socius 5, 2378023119887866 (2019)

56. Stone, J.A., et al.: A preliminary examination of over-the-counter medication misuse rates in older adults. Res. Soc. Adm. Pharm. 13(1), 187–192 (2017). https://doi.org/10.1016/j.sapharm.2016.01.004

57. Quan-Haase, A., et al.: Dividing the grey divide: deconstructing myths about older adults' online activities, skills, and attitudes. Am. Behav. Sci. 62(9), 1207–1228 (2018)

58. Moschis, G.P.: Consumer Behavior over the Life Course: Research Frontiers and New Directions. Springer, Cham (2019). https://doi.org/10.1007/978-3-030-05008-5

59. Steenstra, I.A., et al.: Predicting time on prolonged benefits for injured workers with acute back pain. J. Occup. Rehabil. 25(2), 267–278 (2015)

60. McCloskey, R., Jarrett, P., Stewart, C., Keeping-Burke, L.: Recruitment and retention challenges in a technology-based study with older adults discharged from a geriatric rehabilitation unit. Rehabil. Nurs. 40(4), 249–259 (2015)

61. Czaja, S.J., Lee, C.C.: Information technology and older adults. In: Human-Computer Interaction, pp. 35–50. CRC Press (2009)

62. Mallenius, S., Rossi, M., Tuunainen, V.K.: Factors affecting the adoption and use of mobile devices and services by elderly people–results from a pilot study. In: 6th Annual Global Mobility Roundtable, vol. 31, p. 12 (2007)

63. Nimrod, G.: Older audiences in the digital media environment. Inf. Commun. Soc. 20(2), 233–249 (2017)

64. Moschis, G.P., Lee, E., Mathur, A.: Targeting the mature market: opportunities and challenges. J. Consum. Mark. 14(4), 282–293 (1997). https://doi.org/10.1108/07363769710188536

65. van der Valk, M.J.M., et al.: Long-term outcomes of clinical complete responders after neoadjuvant treatment for rectal cancer in the International Watch & Wait Database (IWWD): an international multicentre registry study. Lancet 391(10139), 2537–2545 (2018)

66. Peek, S.T.M.: Understanding technology acceptance by older adults who are aging in place: a dynamic perspective. Dissertation Tilburg University (2017)

67. Burke, D.M., Mackay, D.G.: Memory, language, and ageing. Philos. Trans. R. Soc. Lond. Ser. B: Biol. Sci. 352(1363), 1845–1856 (1997). https://doi.org/10.1098/rstb.1997.0170

68. Keoleian, V., Polcin, D., Galloway, G.P.: Text messaging for addiction: a review. J. Psychoactive Drugs 47(2), 158–176 (2015)

69. Gaddam, A., et al.: Design & development of IoT based rehabilitation outdoor landscape for gait phase recognition. In: 2019 13th International Conference on Sensing Technology (ICST). IEEE (2019)

70. Sthienrapapayut, T., Moschis, G.P., Mathur, A.: Using gerontographics to explain consumer behaviour in later life: evidence from a Thai study. J. Consum. Mark. 35(3), 317–327 (2018). https://doi.org/10.1108/JCM-02-2017-2083

71. Zhang, Y., et al.: Exploration of users' perspectives and needs and design of a type 1 diabetes management Mobile app: mixed-methods study. JMIR mHealth uHealth 6(9), e11400 (2018). https://doi.org/10.2196/11400

72. Valladares-Rodriguez, S., et al.: Design process and preliminary psychometric study of a video game to detect cognitive impairment in senior adults. PeerJ 5, e3508 (2017). https://doi.org/10.7717/peerj.3508

73. Paul, C., Spiru, L.: From age to age: key gerontographics contributions to technology adoption by older adults. In: International Conference on Information and Communication Technologies for Ageing Well and e-Health, ICT4AWE 2021 (2021)

74. Vichitvanichphong, S., Talaei-Khoei, A., Kerr, D.: Elderly's perception about the value of assistive technologies for their daily living: impacting factors and theoretical support. In: Proceedings of the 50th Hawaii International Conference on System Sciences (2017)

75. Krzystanek, M., et al.: A telemedicine platform to improve clinical parameters in paranoid schizophrenia patients: results of a one-year randomized study. Schizophrenia Res. **204**, 389–396 (2019). https://doi.org/10.1016/j.schres.2018.08.016
76. Or, C.K.L., Karsh, B.-T.: A systematic review of patient acceptance of consumer health information technology. J. Am. Med. Inform. Assoc. **16**(4), 550–560 (2009). https://doi.org/10.1197/jamia.M2888
77. Östlund, B.: Watching television in later life: a deeper understanding of TV viewing in the homes of old people and in geriatric care contexts. Scand. J. Caring Sci. **24**(2), 233–243 (2010)
78. Silverstone, R., Hirsch, E., Morley, D.: Information and communication technologies and the moral economy of the household. In: Consuming Technologies: Media and Information in Domestic Spaces, pp. 15–31 (1992)
79. Schomakers, E.-M., Ziefle, M.: Privacy perceptions in ambient assisted living In: ICT4AWE (2019)
80. Agyapong, V.I.O., Ahern, S., McLoughlin, D.M., Farren, C.K.: Supportive text messaging for depression and comorbid alcohol use disorder: single-blind randomised trial. J. Affect. Disorders **141**(2–3), 168–176 (2012). https://doi.org/10.1016/j.jad.2012.02.040
81. Hall, C.M., Bierman, K.L.: Technology-assisted interventions for parents of young children: emerging practices, current research, and future directions. Early Childhood Res. Q. **33**, 21–32 (2015)
82. Stojanovska, M., et al.: Mixed reality anatomy using Microsoft HoloLens and cadaveric dissection: a comparative effectiveness study. Med. Sci. Educ. **30**(1), 173–178 (2019). https://doi.org/10.1007/s40670-019-00834-x
83. Insights, Country Comparison-Hofstede. "Home-Hofstede Insights." Copyright©, we can get a good overview of the deep drivers of the Czech culture relative to other world cultures (2020). Dostupné z: https://www.hofstedeinsights.com/country-comparison/czech-republic

Technological Model Based on Blockchain Technology for Genetic Information Protection in the Health Sector

Julio Arroyo-Mariños, Karla Mejia-Valle, and Willy Ugarte(✉)

Universidad Peruana de Ciencias Aplicadas, Lima, Peru
{u201424125,u20161a572}@upc.edu.pe, willy.ugarte@upc.pe

Abstract. In the health industry, the transparency of product data registration in the supply chain is a critical aspect in determining the source of genetic data. Various upcoming technologies, such as blockchain, can help with this challenge. Blockchain is a shared and immutable database that makes recording transactions and tracking assets in a commercial network easier. Currently, genetic information is regarded as a vital asset in the health sector, as more precise diagnostic samples in medical genomics enable improved treatments for patients suffering from a variety of disorders. Since actions connected to the storage or management of data might have several areas of vulnerability, this paper describes the development of a technological model employing Blockchain as technology to assure the protection of genetic information in the private health sector. Furthermore, unauthorized activities such as registration and access control in the exchange of genetic information have been carried out, primarily through entities that manage the eligibility of users with genomics information and grant access to specific data sets, demonstrating a lack of harmonization in access policies between the owners of genetic information and the health entities that manage it. A proof-of-concept was carried out to evaluate the model's capabilities and ensure that a larger-scale deployment could be carried out. Experts agreed with our proposal, and consumers would be prepared to employ proof of concept to assure traceability and security of their data, according to the evaluation.

Keywords: Genetic information · Blockchain · Patient · Healthcare

1 Introduction

Nowadays, medicine takes the patient's genetic information into account as a variable is already a reality. In clinical practice, genetic testing yields results that are used to confirm or improve the diagnosis of genetic illnesses, determine treatment, or measure the risk of relapse in diseases including cancer and its derivatives, hepatitis, and others.

In Peru, the administration of genetic information in health entities is not well developed; as a result, the Nation Institure of Neoplastic Diseases (INEN) presents a comparison of prior years, highlighting that the average waiting time for a consultation is 60 min. In addition, from 2013 to 2018, the average number of genetic information consultations was 450 per year[1].

---

[1] Chief Resolution (In Spanish) N 490-2019-J - https://bit.ly/2RQ0k5X.

L. A. Maciaszek et al. (Eds.): ICT4AWE 2021/2022, CCIS 1856, pp. 218–233, 2023.
https://doi.org/10.1007/978-3-031-37496-8_12

New emerging technologies, such as blockchain, are being used in various industrial sectors, such as agriculture [10], [9], food [20], clothing [12], and so on, to provide cost savings, veracity, and availability of information in real-time for the operations performed. Blockchain is a distributed technology in which each node of the network retains a copy of the transactions, ensuring that the data is always available [16]. Blockchains would contribute to our proposal as a result of this progress, with the benefits of transaction and record openness as well as information integrity [11].

In light of this, the rapid advancement of technical development has resulted in a significant and profound development of human genomic information in the field of health. Various genetic analysis approaches, as well as the biological implementations required for the interpretation of detected changes, have also been used [25].

The digitization of the genome is a good illustration of this, as it was prompted by the necessity to save genetic data digitally. Doctors can use this to speed up the diagnosis and treatment of patients. However, just as with personal information, it is critical to protect a person's genetic information for privacy reasons, and they also pose a significant challenge in terms of transporting and storing personal genetic information in a simple, secure, and anonymous manner because people do not want their data to be manipulated[2]. Many national and international programs and initiatives for its implementation and utilization place a strong emphasis on encouraging open and responsible exchange of genomics data.

Nonetheless, due to the constraints faced by these central mechanisms and the non-automated nature of traditional data access and exchange to establish central mechanisms in data access management [25], there are some challenges based on the adoption of centralized approaches to data storage, exchange, and access. Because data storage and management operations that incorporate genetic information have several sources of vulnerability, genomic data security threats are highlighted. Even if there are procedures for protecting patient data in health facilities, they are frequently the target of computer assaults even with the regional laws regulations.

For example, a Ponemon survey in 2016 found that 90% of health care institutions and partner corporations have experienced a data breach, with 64% reporting a violation including the disclosure of patient medical records [28]. In the context of genetic data, new technologies have recently arisen with the goal of enhancing data access, patient empowerment, and interoperability. For example, the use of Cloud Computing technology for genetic data storage and sharing, which allows for flexible scalability of genetic data and simplicity of use for users [29].

However, unauthorized activities such as registration and access control in the exchange of genetic information have been carried out, primarily through entities that manage the eligibility of users with genomic information and grant access to specific datasets, demonstrating a lack of harmonization in access policies between the owners of genetic information and the health entities that manage it.

Adopting an "authorized" structure using Blockchain technology, where transparency in these transactions will be enabled by a framework based on Blockchain technology, which limits access to a patient's data and allows the owner of that genomic information to maintain and manage it. Although everyone on the system has access to

---

[2] Emerging Tech 2015: Digital Genome - https://bit.ly/3ePkBDm.

the metadata that the datasets describe, this does not mean that everyone can read the data stored in Blockchain. This is because Blockchain is based on pseudo anonymity and public key infrastructure (PKI), which allows Blockchain content to be encrypted in a way that is difficult to decrypt.

Here, we present significant extensions of our recent paper [3] on the proposal of a technological model for storing genetic information with blockchain. First, we detail the method framework based on blockchain theory. Second, we describe the architecture that benefits from it. Third, the key element of the framework, the architecture is described which is a cornerstone of our method. Finally, we present an empirical study which includes different datasets and comparisons. This enables us to draw some lessons on the strengths and weaknesses of each method.

Implementing such technology could allow for the discovery of existing datasets while also protecting people's privacy by limiting access to just those who have been authorised. With Blockchain technology, we propose a technological approach for managing genetic information security. Our contributions are as follows:

- We define a technological model that enables actions such as receiving the correct information, in the right format, for the right person, at the right time, and in the right place.
- The components employed assure openness and data integrity because the chain's participants are known, and there is no risk of information manipulation or theft.
- For data processing with minimum resource consumption, we employ the Ethereum Framework.

This paper is organized as follows. Section 2 discusses Related Works. Section 3 describes the relevant concepts and definitions related to this document and the details of our contribution. Section 4 shows the analysis of the results obtained. Finally, Sect. 5 shows the conclusions and perspectives.

2 Related Works

In [13], the authors offer a light system for safeguarding the privacy of medical records, which is made up of the generation and storage of medical data. In contrast, our idea, includes the process of information distribution.

In [19], the authors propose a registration and authentication-based security storage paradigm for medical data. Our solution, on the other hand, offers the owner of the information and the process of disseminating that information access control.

In [18], the authors propose a Blockchain-based Zenome system design, with three roles outlined in their system: Person, Data Consumer, and Service Provider. However, because the literature discusses different levels of privacy for such information, our idea incorporates other access to the person's information, which is granted directly to the other roles in our situation.

In [23], the authors propose a Blockchain-based medical data sharing system that incorporates procedures such as healthcare and data exchange. Our approach, on the other hand, encompasses both the recording and distribution of information.

Shanna et al. [2], on the other hand, present the construction of a four-layer traceability system architecture for the capture of information on products: infrastructure layer, integration and network layer, and application layer. They also provide information on the traceability system's economic viability. Our approach, on the other hand, uses blockchain technology to isolate assets during the tracing process.

Qijun et al. [20], for example, present a food traceability system based on blockchain and EPCIS technologies. The installation of smart contracts that can detect data manipulation is the most important component of this paradigm, which also incorporates the use of ON-Chain and Off-Chain. In the garment sector, Kristoffer et al. [12] established the criteria for evaluating the degree of availability when implementing blockchain technology in the supply chain. The degree of knowledge, confidence, security, and social context were all listed as criteria. Each of these criteria reflects a different component of end-user behavior and enables for examination of new technology uptake.

Choi [9], on the other hand, discusses his operations management (OM) research focused on supply chain operations utilizing BTS systems for diamond verification and certification. Furthermore, he claims that new trends in technology for determining a product's origin, whether based on supply chain traceability or simply tracking systems, may be used to the retail sector of selling and buying diamonds. The author also explains how blockchain may offer value to the supply chain by focusing on security, implementation, data consistency, and other elements. Finally, models of supply chain architectures were discovered employing blockchain technology as the primary component.

Similarly, Antonios et al. [21] present a full examination of blockchain and how it fits into the supply chain sector through their methods. By highlighting various aspects of blockchain that affect the supply chain (e.g., scalability, performance, consensus method, privacy considerations, testing, and cost), the potential influence of blockchain on supply chain disruption within the industry can be demonstrated.

Most of these studies cover data logging and storage but not distribution or access control, or vice versa, if they attack distribution or access control but not data recording and storage. Most of these studies cover data logging and storage but not distribution or access control, or vice versa, if they attack distribution or access control but not data recording and storage.

As a result, with our approach, we hope to consider both the generation and distribution of genetic information on a global scale.

3   Blockchain for Genetic Information in Health Sector

3.1   Preliminary Concepts

This section explains the concepts that will be used in the construction of the model that will be offered for the security of genetic information in the private health sector utilizing Blockchain technology.

Definition 1 (Blockchain [27]). *Blockchain is defined as a distributed and immutable digital ledger that provides data transparency and user privacy.*

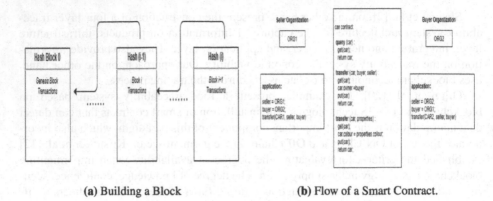

(a) Building a Block   (b) Flow of a Smart Contract.

Fig. 1. Blockchain Structure [3].

This concept is based on cryptography and peer-to-peer (P2P) networks, in which data from a given structure is sorted into blocks and arranged into a data chain in chronological order in a chain structure, establishing a blockchain [8].

Similarly, there is no central authority, and the digital ledger is accessible to all peers. While this notion was originally associated with financial transactions, technical advancements and their huge benefits have made this technology a component of a variety of industries where record security is critical [27].

Example 1. Each block is created by generating the genesis block, often known as block "0", and the transactions that go with it. As shown in Fig. 1a, each block in this structure includes a unique identifier called a hash, which is generated each time the contents of the block are modified, with the preceding block's header becoming the hash of the following block. Because any update to the data in each block necessitates updating hash values throughout the chain, this block interconnect provides the blockchain with security, making it difficult to modify or hack information [27].

Definition 2 (Encryption [4]). *At Blockchain, encryption is responsible for ensuring the integrity of the information and the anonymity of the owner of that information using algorithms.*

A hash function is used in conjunction with this technology to allow fresh data to be added to the block. Specifically, any modifications to the ledger, such as the addition of a new transaction, must be recalculated [4].

The use of digital signatures ensures that the transaction was received by the intended recipient and that the sender is not a forger [4].

Definition 3 (Smart Contract [24]). *In Blockchain, Smart Contracts are a set of instructions that have special storage for information related to the developing application.*

This store contains a record, which is copied and transmitted to all nodes in the network [30]. This, for example, enables the usage of notifications in health apps to be automated, resulting in improved device integration [7].

It also enables for the study of medical data, allowing for the activation of alarms for certain unexpected activities [15].

Example 2. As shown in Fig. 1b, two Org1 and Org2 organizations are observed, which define a Smart Contract for consulting, transferring and updating cars[3].

Some of main components of a blockchain platform are:

- **Hyperledger Fabric:** A blockchain framework that is open-source. This platform's design is highly scalable and adaptable, allowing it to be used in a variety of use cases across diverse industries [1].
- **Kubernetes:** A platform for managing workloads and services that is open-source. It provides container-focused management environments by assembling a set of components and tools that allow for rapid, scalable, and customized application deployment [5].
- **Microservices:** Microservices can be used as a software architecture to create cloud-based applications that are extremely scalable. These architectures are made up of smaller services that are deployed independently of one another [26].

Definition 4 (Blockchain in the Health Sector [22]). *The health sector has data security and privacy requirements due to the existence of legal standards in the protection of patient information established by governments.*

Malicious assaults that threaten the integrity of such information as a result of the usage of the internet in the sharing of patient data [17] are now a source of worry.

As a result, Blockchain technology envisions requirements in the health industry such as medical and genomic data exchange and transfer, as well as authentication and interoperability [22].

3.2 Method

Now, as illustrated in Fig. 2, we outline our proposal for a Blockchain-based technology model for the preservation of genetic information.

Roles. The following roles have been identified for the design of the technical model:

- *Generator Agent* with the following activities:
  - **Generation:** The Generator Agent is in charge of recording the genetic information of the patient who granted him the registration permit, so that the data recorded in the blockchain may be kept and traced later.
  - **Authorization/Validation:** The Generator Agent has permission to add the patient's genetic information.
- *Consumer Agent* with the following activities:
  - **Distribution:** The Consumer Agent is able to look up the patient's genetic information in the system.

---

[3] Smart Contracts and Chaincode - https://bit.ly/3kvgwG2.

- **Authorization/Validation:** The Patient's Genetic Information can be consulted and visualized by the Consumer Agent.
- *Patient* with the following activities:
  - **Generation:** The patient gives the Generator Agent permission to register them so that the generator can upload their genetic data.
  - **Authorization/Validation:** To control their genetic data, the patient grants the appropriate permissions as a Generator Agent or Consumer Agent.
  - **Distribution:** The patient gives the Consumer Agent permission to confer with them so that he or she can use their genetic data.

Our solution's architecture, which will support the aforementioned applications. Now we'll go over the key elements of the suggested architecture:

1. **CouchDB**: Representation of the CouchDB database instance which supports powerful queries when the data values of the chaincode instances as JSON format. Besides, it is a data store of JSON documents rather than a store of pure key values, thus allowing document content indexing.
2. **Smart Contracts - Chaincodes**: These are programs developed in node.js instantiated in a channel, which runs in Docker containers. Additionally, they will allow the management of the information about the accounting general ledger. Likewise, all the business logic is inside the chaincodes represented as assets which will be used to trace the information. Similarly, chaincodes have a data model that was determined based on the analysis of the logging process.
3. **API Gateway**: This component represents an intermediary system to protect and manage the exposed APIs. It has as main characteristics, the speed limit, oAuth, and CORS.

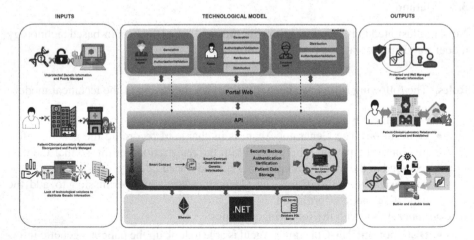

Fig. 2. Proposed Technology Model [3].

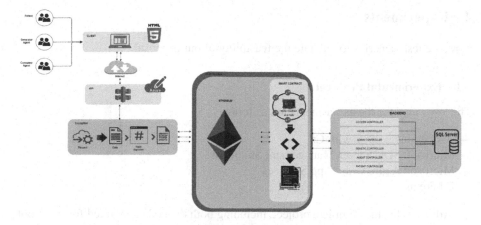

Fig. 3. Web Portal Architecture [3].

Web Site. The model will feature a web portal representation to demonstrate the registration of the patient's genetic information and the regulation of accesses to that information by the same actor. HTML5 for the client view, ASP.Net for the back end, SQL Server as the database management, and the Microsoft Azure Cloud platform were used to create this application.

The Genetic Information Generation Smart Contract was developed using the Ethereum Framework, and each time such information is recorded, a transaction is made that provides the block ID, the transaction creation date, and the cryptographic hash generated.

The architecture of the gateway in Fig. 3 demonstrates this with user administration, traceability, certificate management, and report display modules were implemented in this application:

- The first module allows you to manage your network's registered users, including adding participants and assigning them roles, as well as removing them if necessary.
- The second module allows you to see the assets that have been registered in the blockchain network in three stages.
- The third module allows you to see and update the status of authorization certificates.
- The fourth and final module allows you to see the reports that the mobile app generates.

Blockchain Platform. The Blockchain platform works as the technology with the ability to record transactions made in the web application and transfer them to a network of nodes where this network is worth the transaction for transactions made in the development of the model.

Furthermore, each transaction has a cryptographic hash to confirm claims made against the blockchain's recorded and controlled assets, which in this case is genetic information.

4   Experiments

Now, we test scenarios to validate the feasibility of our proposal.

4.1   Experimental Protocol

The tools used for the experiments are as follows:

- Visual Studio 2017 with C#
- Microsoft SQL Server Management Studio 18
- Microsoft Azure with "App Services"
- Ethereum

Additionally, the complete project, including both the code generated for the proof-of-concept that confirms the model's functionality and the data stored in the database, is freely accessible at the following link: https://bit.ly/37HAcDk

In addition, using the Zoom platform, virtual presentations were prepared for the validation of the proof of concept, in which the project idea was described to the experts chosen. Following the presentations, surveys were sent out in order to get input from professionals and users.

For this, we divided surveys into several categories based on expert groups, such as Blockchain Expert and Laboratory Expert, as well as the user.

1. **Blockchain Expert Survey:** The 13 questions in the Blockchain Expert survey were designed to get input on your Blockchain experience as well as your thoughts on our proposal. In addition, two Blockchain experts have been chosen.
2. **Laboratory Expert Survey:** The Laboratory Expert's survey will consist of 14 questions with the goal of receiving feedback on the Model's functional level as well as comments on our proposal. In addition, two laboratory experts are chosen.
3. **User Survey:** A survey was conducted on the user, who represents the patient in our model.
   We have a sample of 40 people who are between the ages of 20 and 30 years old for the sake of our proposal.
   All of these sample users live in Lima Metropolitana and have undergone genetic testing at least once.
   "What amount of priority do you think should be given to the security of your genetic information?" are some of the questions they will be asked and "How willing are

Table 1. Expert Survey Data [3].

	Validation Date	Expert	Recording Link	Survey Link	Answers
Blockchain	06/10/2020	Expert 1	https://bit.ly/3kVQFYr	https://bit.ly/31uVArq	https://bit.ly/3mqyoCV
	07/10/2020	Expert 2	https://bit.ly/34sRTEL	https://bit.ly/31uVArq	https://bit.ly/3mqyoCV
Laboratory	06/10/2020	Expert 1	https://bit.ly/3dYeYCs	https://bit.ly/3dOrwMv	https://bit.ly/3kTXeuB
	09/10/2020	Expert 2	https://bit.ly/37CukLH	https://bit.ly/3dOrwMv	https://bit.ly/3kTXeuB

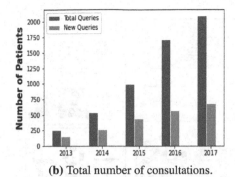

(b) Total number of consultations.

Medical Genetics Consultation	Average Time (minutes)
Patient Admission	5
Medical Consultation	5
Exams	40
Genetic Pretest Counseling	10
Total	60

(b) Average genetic consultation time.

Fig. 4. Relationship between old consultation system per year and new consultation system of the Medical Genetics Office [3] (See Footnote 1).

you to share your genetic information with others?". There are nine questions in this survey, and the user survey URL is avaiable at https://bit.ly/2TRl5iA.

The URLs to the Survey given to Blockchain and Laboratory experts, the links to the recordings created, the dates of the sessions, and the platform on which the presentation was made are all listed in Table 1.

Similarly, INEN collected statistical data, as shown in Fig. 4b, which shows the average genetic consultation time, which is expected to be 60 min and includes patient identification, genetic testing registration, and diagnosis.

In addition, Fig. 4a shows a statistic collected by INEN describing the increase in genetic information consultation transactions from 2013 to 2018 achieving an average of 450 consultations per year and identifying a gap between supply and demand.

4.2 Experimental Results

For validating our proposal, two test scenarios were considered, which will prove transparency in the genetic information managements.

Scenario 1. On the one hand, experts agree that transparently protecting genetic information and using Blockchain as a technology to secure the administration and assurance of this asset is the right choice. They also agree that the patient owns and controls his or her genetic information.

However, they suggested that more encryption procedures be added to the model in order to gain stronger guarantee of genetic information and to define the model's components, which can be reused for the building of future architectures and solutions because it is a model.

Laboratory scientists, on the other hand, said they support the proposed project since it makes it easier to register and retrieve genetic data while also securing it with Blockchain technology.

They also discovered that the need identified by the vulnerabilities that frequently occur within health systems is correct, that the model's design is simple and easy to

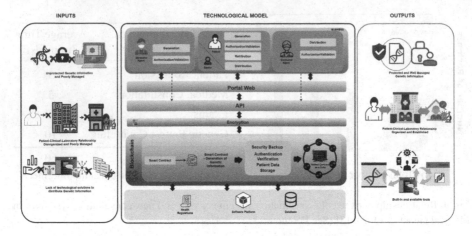

Fig. 5. Final Proposal for the Technology Model [3].

understand, that the roles managed are sufficient, and that they prefer a web environment for proof of concept for management issues in health facilities.

Whereas they emphasized that the patient may not always be able to manage their information because, depending on the clinical condition that he is experiencing, he may require the assistance of a doctor for management, and that genetic information can be classified as paternity studies, autoimmune diseases, and degenerative diseases, among other things.

Based on the comments and recommendations provided by the experts, the following components were added in Fig. 5:

- The encryption layer, which adds additional encryption processes to provide greater security.
- A "Health Regulations" component, which aims to detail that the Legal Rules regarding the use of patient information are considered.
- A "Doctor" role, which assume the patient's activities according to the patient's clinical picture.

From the survey responses:

- Figure 6a shows that 58% rate as "Very High" the level of importance to be considered with the security of their genetic information.
- Figure 6b also shows that 45% of all respondents define "Unlikely" in sharing their genetic information with others.
- And this is supported by Fig. 6c, as the percentage of respondents who do not feel confident that their genetic information is on the internet reaches 63% of the total.
- However, by using our proof of concept, 60% would be willing to share your information, this can be viewed in Fig. 6d.

Similarly, we have the metric of the average time of genetic consultations which with our proposal we seek to reduce the time of this metric, for which a comparison was made with the current time and the average time offered by the proposal.

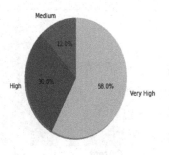

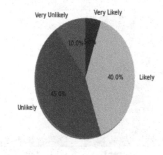

(a) Security importance level of genetic information

(b) Level of sharing of genetic information with
other people

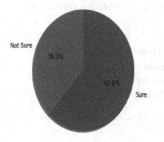

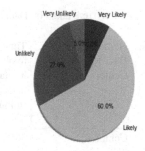

(c) Perception of having genetic information
over the Internet

(d) Level of willingness to share genetic information with our proof of concept

Fig. 6. Perception results [3].

- As seen in Fig. 7a, the current average time is 60 min, while our proposal's average time is 5 min, reducing the current average time by 92%.
- Nevertheless, another metric that is handled is that of the number of genetic queries. As shown in Fig. 7b, the current number of consultations is 450, while our proposal is 700, which is increased by 56%.

Scenario 2. Nowadays, due to the multiple participants within the macro process of information management, it is difficult to obtain information regarding the current state of the assets for those who are involved in the genetic information in health sector.

In this scenario, a data set will be generated to simulate a transparent process from the transaction registration into the blockchain network to allow the traceability of the assets involved within the authorization document. The names of the participants were censored and replaced by fake ones to ensure the confidentiality of the data. Table 2 shows an extract of 13 genetic informations distribution center and the time in calendar days to know the status of the OP.

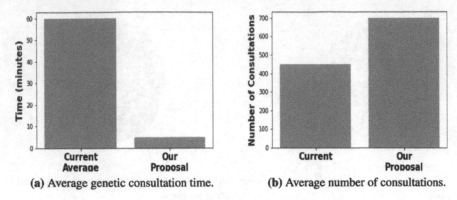

(a) Average genetic consultation time.   (b) Average number of consultations.

Fig. 7. Comparison of Current Situation with Our Proposal [3].

Table 2. Time taken by Data Recolection Centers to obtain information.

Name of the Data Recolection Center	Time to obtain its status manually (minutes)	Time to obtain its status manually (seconds)	Time to obtain its status with our solution (seconds)
Center 1	505	30,300	15.06
Center 2	141	8,460	21.62
Center 3	141	8,460	24.66
Center 4	94	5,640	24.15
Center 5	434	26,040	22.95
Center 6	23	1,380	18.03
Center 7	212	12,720	19.00
Center 8	739	44,340	14.15
Center 9	140	8,400	14.02
Center 10	285	17,100	13.50
Center 11	486	29,160	15.38
Center 12	38	2,280	11.86
Center 13	710	42,600	16.75
Average	303	18,180	17.78

1. **Business Process:** The supervision process consists of monitoring and control the status and the assets involved in the document. This process is carried out in a physical way in which the supervising entity receives and verifies the information manually.
2. **Validation Steps:** The following are the validation steps:

- *Generation with Attached Assets:* Registration with attached information with our proposal.
- *Traceability:* Search for the data set traced through the proposed technology solution using the Apache JMeter performance measurement tool.
3. **Metrics:** For this scenario, we are only going to use one metric: **Average time in obtaining the status**. Since we aim to prove the effectiveness of our approach.

Once the experimental protocol and validation metrics were defined, unit tests of the web application's traceability module were performed with each of the generated cases corresponding to those presented in Table 2. After the execution of each iteration with the Apache JMeter tool, an average time of 17.78 s was achieved in obtaining the status. Table 2 shows the results obtained by consulting and the average time to obtain their status.

5   Conclusions

To summarize, we have demonstrated that Blockchain technology is useful and efficient because, whereas a typical genetic consultation takes 60 min, our technology allows us to complete it in 5 min, saving up to 92% of the time.

Furthermore, it allows us to increase the number of genetic information queries, as the current average is 450, but with the use of this technology, a total of 700 is expected, an increase of 56%, and users are much more willing to share their genetic information if they have a platform that ensures the traceability and protection of their data.

According to our findings, implementing a technology solution such as the one presented in the health sector would provide significant benefits to the participants and allow them to assure asset data security. Evenmore, additional experiments could be carried out to illustrate asset traceability during logging management percent using real data in a proof of concept to acquire more accurate findings.

However, it would be interesting to be able to work with geolocalisation [6, 14], which would allow for the classification of a patient's genetic information in order to deliver a better diagnosis based on their location, or the usage of a chatbot to detect user interaction.

References

1. Andola, N., Raghav, Gogoi, M., Venkatesan, S., Verma, S.: Vulnerabilities on hyperledger fabric. Pervasive Mob. Comput. **59**, 101050 (2019)
2. Appelhanz, S., Osburg, V.S., Toporowski, W., Schumann, M.: Traceability system for capturing, processing and providing consumer-relevant information about wood products: system solution and its economic feasibility. J. Clean. Prod. **110**, 132–148 (2016)
3. Arroyo-Mariños, J.C., Mejia-Valle, K.M., Ugarte, W.: Technological model for the protection of genetic information using blockchain technology in the private health sector. In: ICT4AWE (2021)
4. Benil, T., Jasper, J.: Cloud based security on outsourcing using blockchain in e-health systems. Comput. Netw. **178**, 107344 (2020)

5. Bernstein, D.: Containers and cloud: From LXC to docker to kubernetes. IEEE Cloud Comput. **1**(3), 81–84 (2014)
6. Cheikhrouhou, O., Koubâa, A.: Blockloc: secure localization in the internet of things using blockchain. In: IWCMC, pp. 629–634. IEEE (2019)
7. Chen, Y., Ding, S., Xu, Z., Zheng, H., Yang, S.: Blockchain-based medical records secure storage and medical service framework. J. Medical Syst. **43**(1), 1–9 (2019)
8. Cheng, X., Chen, F., Xie, D., Sun, H., Huang, C.: Design of a secure medical data sharing scheme based on blockchain. J. Medical Syst. **44**(2), 52 (2020)
9. Choi, T.M.: Blockchain-technology-supported platforms for diamond authentication and certification in luxury supply chains. Transp. Res. Part E: Log. Transp. Review **128**, 17–29 (2019)
10. FAO: E-agriculture in action: Blockchain for agriculture opportunities and challenges. Food and Agriculture Organization of the United Nations and the International Telecommunication Union (2019)
11. Figorilli, S., et al.: A blockchain implementation prototype for the electronic open source traceability of wood along the whole supply chain. Sensors **18**(9), 3133 (2018)
12. Francisco, K., Swanson, D.: The supply chain has no clothes: technology adoption of blockchain for supply chain transparency. Logistics **2**(1), 2 (2018)
13. Fu, J., Wang, N., Cai, Y.: Privacy-preserving in healthcare blockchain systems based on lightweight message sharing. Sensors **20**(7), 1898 (2020)
14. Goyat, R., Kumar, G., Alazab, M., Saha, R., Thomas, R., Rai, M.K.: A secure localization scheme based on trust assessment for WSNs using blockchain technology. Future Gener. Comput. Syst. **125**, 221–231 (2021)
15. Griggs, K.N., Ossipova, O., Kohlios, C.P., Baccarini, A.N., Howson, E.A., Hayajneh, T.: Healthcare blockchain system using smart contracts for secure automated remote patient monitoring. J. Medical Syst. **42**(7), 1–7 (2018)
16. Gupta, M.: Blockchain For Dummies. IBM Limited Ed, 3rd edn. (2018)
17. Khezr, S., Moniruzzaman, M., Yassine, A., Benlamri, R.: Blockchain technology in healthcare: a comprehensive review and directions for future research. Appl. Sci. **9**(9), 1736 (2019)
18. Kulemin, N.: The zenome project : whitepaper blockchain-based genomic ecosystem (2017)
19. Kuo, T., Kim, J., Gabriel, R.A.: Privacy-preserving model learning on a blockchain network-of-networks. J. Am. Med. Inform. Assoc. **27**(3), 343–354 (2020)
20. Lin, Q., Wang, H., Pei, X., Wang, J.: Food safety traceability system based on blockchain and EPCIS. IEEE Access **7**, 20698–20707 (2019)
21. Litke, A., Anagnostopoulos, D., Varvarigou, T.: Blockchains for supply chain management: architectural elements and challenges towards a global scale deployment. Logistics **3**(1), 5 (2019)
22. McGhin, T., Choo, K.R., Liu, C.Z., He, D.: Blockchain in healthcare applications: research challenges and opportunities. J. Netw. Comput. Appl. **135**, 62–75 (2019)
23. Murugan, A., Chechare, T., Muruganantham, B., Kumar, S.: Healthcare information exchange using blockchain technology. Int. J. Electr. Comput. Eng. (IJECE), **10**, 421 (2020)
24. Ozercan, H.I., Ileri, A.M., Ayday, E., Alkan, C.: Realizing the potential of blockchain technologies in genomics. Genome Res. **28**, 9 (2018)
25. Shabani, M.: Blockchain-based platforms for genomic data sharing: a de-centralized approach in response to the governance problems? J. Am. Med. Inform. Assoc. **26**(1), 76–80 (2019)
26. Taherizadeh, S., Grobelnik, M.: Key influencing factors of the kubernetes auto-scaler for computing-intensive microservice-native cloud-based applications. Adv. Eng. Softw. **140**, 102734 (2020)
27. Tripathi, G., Ahad, M.A., Paiva, S.: S2HS- a blockchain based approach for smart healthcare system. Healthcare **8**(1), 100391 (2020)

28. Ujibashi, Y., Kawaba, M., Harada, L.: Proposal of a database type and aggregation function for accelerating medical genomics study on RDBMS. In: EDBT. OpenProceedings.org (2016)
29. Yang, J.: Cloud computing for storing and analyzing petabytes of genomic data. J. Ind. Inf. Integr. **15**, 50–57 (2019)
30. Zhang, P., White, J., Schmidt, D.C., Lenz, G., Rosenbloom, S.T.: FHIRChain: applying blockchain to securely and scalably share clinical data. Comput. Struct. Biotech. J. **16**, 267–278 (2018)

Designing Pervasive Games Oriented Towards the Elderly: A Case Study

Raquel Lacuesta[1] (ID), Jesús Gallardo[1] ([⊠]) (ID), Silvia Hernández[2] (ID), and Álvaro Pérez[1]

[1] Department of Computing and Systems Engineering, University of Zaragoza, Teruel, Spain
{lacuesta,jesus.gallardo}@unizar.es
[2] Pre-departmental Unit of Fine Arts, University of Zaragoza, Teruel, Spain
silviahm@unizar.es

Abstract. Elderly people is a segment of population that is quickly increasing during the last years. In the digital society where we live, it is not bearable that this segment of population remains out of the advances in information and communication technologies. In fact, such advances have the potential to improve aspects such as memory or physical condition. This is the case of computer games, and, specifically, of pervasive games. They are a new genre of games in which some of the traditional boundaries of computer games get exceeded. Therefore, in this chapter we explain the design process of a pervasive game oriented towards the elderly and some assessment activities to validate it. The game implies the elderly moving in the real world searching some targets that have to be scanned with a mobile device with the game running. When this happens, the game unlocks a memory, which is a piece of information about a past event, a person or a place. Players store the memories unlocked in an album that can be accessed at any time. Testing of the game in a real environment has started, with some interesting feedback collected.

Keywords: Pervasive games · Elderly people · Augmented reality

1 Introduction

We are currently experiencing an increase in the segment of population that we may name as elderly people, which is the one of people over 65 years old. This is why it is important to take advantage of their learning capacity to engage them in initiatives that enable their personal development [1]. In Spain, the use of computer games leads the ranking of digital entertainment, as it supposes more than half of the total time spent. It is worth mentioning that computer games are no longer only played by children and young people, but they are being used by almost every age range. This is due, among other facts, to the fact that computer games are being used for other purposes than those of entertainment, such as socialization, education and others.

AEVI (Spanish Association of Video Games) states that 47% of the total turnover of computer games worldwide comes from mobile games, being observed that they are experiencing a great growth year after year (12.8% more than in 2017) [2]. This is not

L. A. Maciaszek et al. (Eds.): ICT4AWE 2021/2022, CCIS 1856, pp. 234–255, 2023.
https://doi.org/10.1007/978-3-031-37496-8_13

a surprise and confirms that smartphones are nowadays the main platform for playing computer games.

Also, having elderly people involved in Information and Communication Technologies is quite important for removing the digital divide. Digital divide can suppose exclusion and dependency for those who are not integrated into the information society. And, again, computer games play an important role. Allaire et al. [3] carried out a study among 140 people of average age 77,5 years, and concluded that those who regularly or occasionally played computer games showed better values in the socio-emotional field than those who had never played such games.

When developing software for the elderly, and computer games are not an exception, some specific requirements have to be met. Specifically, as the elderly are now being introduced to computer games, the proper motivation has to be found for them to finally play the game. In this sense, the adoption of a user-centered approach for the design and implementation of the game is an interesting start point that may help to fulfill this issue, as this kind of approach involves users from the beginning of the process and considers their peculiarities.

Computer games have evolved throughout history, following the advances in technology that have occurred. In recent years, a new paradigm has emerged, as it is the one of pervasive games. Montola [4] states that pervasive games are a genre of play that breaks the traditional boundaries of the game, defined in terms of spatial, temporal and social dimensions. These games, which gained popularity when Pokémon Go was launched, are characterized by the pervasive expansions in the axes of time, space and social interaction, which are not present in traditional games. Usually, pervasive games make use of novel technologies, such as virtual/augmented reality or geolocation. This way, game experiences go further than in a traditional computer game that is framed within the aforementioned game boundaries.

With all the above mentioned into consideration, we have designed and developed a pervasive game oriented towards elderly people, with the aim of improving their quality of life, both physically and at a cognitive level. The physical improvement comes as players will have to move around their environment to progress in the game, whereas the cognitive one is linked to the fact that the game is about unlocking memories. The game consists of searching some photos that, when found, cause the appearance of a virtual object through augmented reality. Touching that object will unlock a memory that can be reviewed and afterwards is stored on an album. This game is pervasive on a spatial level, as it can be and potentially played in any location, on a temporary level, as it can be played at any time, and also on a social level, as people who play can interact in the meantime with other people who are not players in order to progress. A first description of the game can be found on [5]. In that paper is also described a first validation of the game, in which a TAM-based questionnaire was used to test the technological acceptance of the game, and, specifically, its perceived usefulness of the game and its perceived ease of use. In this chapter, we carry out a more exhaustive description of the game, of its development process, and of the selection of the elements chosen for the engagement of the elderly when playing the game. Also, we describe briefly how the game has been used by elderly people and which feedback we have already collected. Lastly, in this chapter we also introduce a full assessment of the accessibility of the game.

The rest of the chapter is organized as follows. Section 2 introduces the concept of pervasive games. Section 3 includes some examples of computer games for the elderly. Section 4 is about specific requirements of computer games for the elderly. In Sect. 5 we talk about usability and accessibility for the elderly. Section 6 is where we introduce our game and talk in detail about it. This sections includes the description of the gamification elements and their assessment. Section 7 is the one with the conclusions of the chapter and future lines of work. Lastly, we have included an appendix with the assessment of the accessibility of the game.

2 Pervasive Games

The growth of the field of pervasive games has been strong recently, as some studies have proved [6]. In [7] it can be found a review with several developments of pervasive games in fields such as health, education, tourism, entertainment and others. A possible definition of pervasive games from the point of view of user experience is the following: "A pervasive game offers the player an enriched game experience through an evolution of game dynamics, expanding the game space according to the context in which it is played. In this way the limits of the game world are broken, making reality part of it, and the elements present in that reality can have an influence on the game" [8]. The same work identifies some of the main concepts included in this kind of games, which are mobile devices, pervasive context, social interaction, time, space, multi-reality and crossmedia. All those components are integrated by means of a pervasive narrative.

Pervasive games, consequently, can develop one or several dimensions of the ones that are present in them. As we mentioned in the introduction, usually there are three dimensions that may be overcome when developing a pervasive game, that are the temporal, spatial and social. Temporal pervasiveness is usually achieved when playing the game is not restricted to a specific game session. Spatial pervasiveness implies that the game is not restricted to be played at a specific place. And social pervasiveness happens when not only the players can have an influence on the game, but also other people that are not considered players. Also, another kind of pervasiveness can be considered in these games, which is the pervasiveness of the dynamics. This would happen when the dynamics and rules of the game are not static, but can be altered during the game for any reason. All these dimensions of pervasiveness can be present in pervasive game at different levels, so it can be necessary to know at which degree does a given game cover each one of those dimensions.

3 Computer Games for the Elderly

In recent years, there is a lot of activity in the development of games for elderly people. In addition, the authors of these works have drawn interesting conclusions as to what should be taken into account when developing video games for adults. Several relevant works in this area will be mentioned below. In [9], the authors conducted a study on aspects that lead elderly people to play games for the mobile phone. The study consisted of developing a catalogue of games, so that the preferred genres of elderly people were identified. From there, the authors developed a game called Traveling the World, with several mini-games of the genres preferred by the elders. Through this work, the authors identified several elements of motivation relevant to the elderly people, such as, for example: the interaction of the player always has an associated result, the difficulty increases gradually, the mechanics are simple, information about the benefits of playing, or aspects of usability, such as color contrast or large, clear images.

Another interesting example of a game, which has certain similarities with the one we will present later, is the one described in [10]. This game, also designed for mobile phones, combines a classic game of looking for identical cards with the search for specific physical locations. In this way, we could say that there is also something pervasive about it. It is a game that can be collaborative, and thus enhance the social aspect. After the evaluation of the game, called Walk2Win, the authors drew certain recommendations, such as: this type of games should reach as wide an audience as possible (even if certain elders participate passively), rules should be minimized, it is interesting to introduce elements of familiar games, gender distinctions should be eliminated, and the environment should be customizable.

Another type of games is the one in which, using devices such as Microsoft Kinect or other similar, the elderly people are sought to perform some type of exercise, either within the scope of a rehabilitation plan or simply to keep them active. An example would be described in [11]. In that case, the authors used Nintendo Wii to develop a game called SilverPromenade that simulated virtual rides while posing certain mini-games to older people. From the experience, the authors drew three useful conclusions for developers of this type of game: the capabilities of the target audience should be carefully explored, the right choice of metaphors is fundamental to making it easy to enter the game, and games should be designed to suit a wide range of players and situations.

Lastly, we are going to mention another example of activity for adults which shares with the game that we will introduce some points such as the use of virtual or augmented reality and the aim of stimulating players' memory. This is the Virtual Maze Task [12]. This activity is not presented by their authors as a game, but it includes some aspects that we may understand as gamification elements, as users have to learn routes in a maze. In this work, authors studied the difference in performing this activity with an immersion approach or with physical activity, regarding satisfaction, interaction and other aspects.

4   Requirements of Games for the Elderly

According to the study "Video Game use habits in Spain of people over 35 years of age" by Parra, David et al. [13], around 24% of people over 65 years use computer games. Nevertheless, only 7.9% of those over 65 are regular gamers. Some aspects that are increasing the predisposition and interest of elderly to its use are: the incorporation of aspects of games, such as gamification or serious games, in areas such as education, health and quality of life improvement; and the introduction of new themes, types of games or ways of playing. Also, new generations of elderly people are closer to technology. This will increase the use of computer games for this group of people.

Design adaptation and personalization of computer games must be considered in the design requirements both at a physical and at a cognitive level, considering the different modes of interaction, limitations and capabilities of users. Some goals that are pursued in its design may be playful or serious such as improve active aging, treatment and following of illnesses, improvement of isolation and social insertion.

The use of games for the elderly can be focused on different levels. In the first place we could use gamification elements. With gamification elements we will use game mechanisms to drive engagement in non-game business scenarios. Also we intend to change behaviors in the target audience. Some elements used in this area are the use of points, resources collections, avatars, badges, level of complexity, progressions, leaderboard and quests. When the intention is the use of game tools for more serious uses like education and health, we could design and develop serious games. They are built in the same style of entertainment games, but are intended for more serious objectives, such as learning. Some elements used are relatively more complex game dynamics, avatars, instant rewards and levels of challenges. Simulation is used usually for skill transfer to the real world. We transfer from the reality word to the simulation scenarios real world experience, using well defined rules, processes and structures. Real-life outcomes are based on metrics and levels of difficulty and complexity. Lastly, if our intention is to blend the virtual game play with the physical game providing a 360 degrees gaming experience, we design a trans-reality game. This type of game could involve elements of gamification, serious games and simulations. In this scenario we have real and/or fictional experiences. One challenge in this scenario is to define the interface between real and virtual world components. In this case, some elements used are alternate reality, mixed reality and location augmented games. Also we can find different levels of difficulty and complexity. This last paradigm will allow the user to be in contact with reality while they perform the gambling activity.

Requirements in the design of interactive systems for elderly people need to include cognitive and physical requirements. Also other elements, such as social issues must be considered.

At a cognitive level, we need to consider impairments related to reduced short-term memory, difficulty of concentrating and distraction factors. At that level, some main recommendations to follow are: use of simple instructions and navigation, with clear explanations; use of adapted, interesting and varied themes with different levels of difficulty and different game modalities; possibility of repeating the game after each failure; absence of negative motivational messages; and use of intuitive screens. Some serious goals of game tools could be to improve the user's learning and stimulation, or to improve orientation, perception, and mental agility.

Regarding game themes, current preferences focus on questions, puzzles, logic, sports and strategy activities. Games must present adequate realistic images, as well as attractive color and sound. If we focus on the use of game tools for serious aspects, we have examples that work for the control of health and improvement of the quality of life.

At a physical level, we will consider senses aspects and physical abilities. Some aspects to analyze include impairments related with contrast sensitivity, color perception and hearing. Also, impairments related to reduced dexterity and fine control should be analyzed. These limitations could make difficult the reading and hearing of audios. Also, physical aspects could impede the use of a mouse and click small targets. Some requirements to be considered in the design will be the use of large letters and drawings, which are easy to read and view, the use of accessible on and off buttons, the possibility of playing without moving, and that users should not need to press too many buttons at the same time to play. It is also important that the interface, the controls and the screen are easy to use and intuitive, and that the device can be carried.

At a social level, it is required that more than one person can play. The intervention aspects will focus on working in the areas of socialization, empathy, values and emotional control, taking into account motivation and the need of sense of belonging to a group. Another requirement in the selection of the topic will be the gender analysis of the end user.

At all levels, requirements of customization to specific profiles and users' preferences must be included, since the group of elderly people includes significant differences among users.

5 Usability and Accessibility for the Elderly

In the design of gaming activities, usability principles (ISO 9241-11) must be followed, taking into account specific users, specific objectives, levels of effectiveness, efficiency and satisfaction, and the context of use. Principles of universal accessibility must be analyzed in the design of the interactive systems. The goals are to design systems that are understandable and usable by all people in conditions of safety and comfort and in the most autonomous and natural way possible. The motivation and analysis of satisfaction in the use of applications or video games will be essential in the analysis process.

The WAI-AGE project by the W3C Web Accessibility Initiative[1] was focused on the analysis of the needs of older web users. The established guidelines focus on generating perceptible, operable, understandable and robust content. Thus, the main aspects to consider are those related to perceptible information and user interface, operable navigation and user interface, understandable user interface and information, and robust content and reliable interpretation. For each principle, a series of recommendations and examples of techniques to be considered in the design of these interfaces are presented.

The established principles should establish a balance between user experience, principles of strategy and challenge, and usability/accessibility for the elderly, assessing the difficulty dimension associated with the "levels of difficulty" and not with "levels of ease of use". Players are generally more favorable to games with less usability and some game difficulty. Other aspects to assess will be the learning rate and the intrinsic motivation to play. In any case, required skills must be established.

6 Presentation of a Pervasive Game for the Elderly

In this section, we are going to detail the process of design and development of our pervasive game oriented towards elderly people. The game is named EncuéntraTe, and it makes use of augmented reality technology. Game action implies players moving in a given environment searching for memories to be unlocked.

---

[1] https://www.w3.org/WAI/WAI-AGE/.

6.1 Requirements

The idea behind this project was to develop a pervasive game for helping to improve life quality in the elderly, working on aspects such as getting their mind exercised, boosting their social abilities or keeping them active. We counted with the support of a residential complex for elderly people for the design and development of the game. This complex has apartments for non-dependent people, a residential center for dependent people and a senior day center. From the very beginning of the development process, we followed a user-centered design approach so that the final idea of the game was generated jointly by the development team, the staff in the residential complex and a group of residents. Therefore, two meetings in which the idea of the game was produced were organized. The first meeting was attended by members of the development team and members of the staff of the complex. In this meeting, the idea of the game was generated. This idea consisted of locating certain elements placed in the complex and unlocking memories when doing that. The memories also had to get stored in an album and they had to make the game to advance. The elements of the game that allow the memories to get unlocked would appear by means of augmented reality.

Later on, a second meeting was organized. It was a focus group in which some residents of the complex participated, together with staff members and members of the development team. This meeting served for validating the approach of the game, and for creating a list of categories in which the memories could get classified. The categories chosen were sports, music and cinema, culture, personalities, and history. Also, a decision was taken in the sense that, when choosing the memories, a special interest would be given to memories from the region of Aragon. This is the region where the residents live.

The user-centered analysis stage not only included the first meeting and the focus group. Also, an observation process of the elderly in the residential complex was carried out. From this observation we conclude that a great disparity of profiles coexists in the complex. Thus, residents that are dependent to a higher or lower degree live together with some other residents with a high level of autonomy.

After this analysis, the goals defined for the design of the app were the following:

- To develop a pervasive mobile game adapted for its use by elderly people.
- That the game uses augmented reality for integrating it with the environment in which it will be played (i.e., the residential complex).
- To elaborate an album of memories with which the user gets identified. Those memories will get unlocked when playing the game.
- To develop the game experience in a way in which players get encouraged to keep exploring their environment in search of more memories to unlock.

Specific Requirements for the Elderly. Regarding the requirements established in the previous analysis, the following are requirements for elderly people considered at both physical and cognitive level.

The first requirement is the use of simple instructions and navigation. We need to use short sentences and user language with clear explanations about those instructions with more difficulty of understanding.

The themes will be adapted to end users, to their experiences, motivation and interest. Therefore, the topics selected must be close to users. In this case, after a first analysis we selected old memories. Also, we tried to use a game strategy easy to follow, accessing real images in a real scenario.

The idea has been to stimulate physical movement and cognitive thinking using an easy way of playing. This implies to adapt the content with clear letters, to make it easy to read and easy to understand, and to provide the possibility of hearing the content with adaptable sound. The difficulty of memory understanding does not have to increase along the different levels. The game must be played with autonomy by users. The device can be carried, as it is a mobile device.

The choice of memories was a key element in the development of this research. The objective was to create a collection of memories that would be recognizable to the elderly in the residence, would help them remember moments of their youth and would be familiar to them so that they could work on their memory as well as having fun obtaining them.

In the game, we do not include different game modalities. However, it is possible to adapt the location of real images to real areas or rooms. People with reduced mobility could have access to the content with images closer to them in their place of stay. In that way they could play without having to move around the place.

We will never use negative motivational messages; instead, we will use positive reinforcement when playing. The game will not have a limit for tries and players will be able to repeat the game as much as they need to. Also, they will be able access the content every time they want to, to better understand the content, by using the album. It will not be necessary for users to remember any aspect of the game.

Screens will be designed simple and intuitive, with short and clear text and with no technical language. Attractive colors will be chosen. A graphic designer is in charge of doing the screen templates.

Images in the walls are real images with beautiful images of Teruel province (the city where the residence is located). Also memories are interesting facts or places information designed with attractive color and sound. Audio can be adapted to different hearing difficulties.

The game does not need to click small targets. All the icons and buttons will be designed with long size. Users do not need to press many buttons at the same time.

At a social level, it is requested that more than one person can play. Assistant workers focus on the area of socialization, where several residents play at the same time and then they do meetings to comment on memories found. They create in that way the sense of belonging to a group. In other ways, competition can be done by users, but finally they can help each other.

In this case we have not considered gender analysis of users. In the future, we plan to establish requirements of customization that have not been included in this research. Users will be able to establish preferences and different profiles will be included, since the group of elderly people includes significant differences among users.

6.2 Design and Implementation

Now, we are going to detail the design of our pervasive game. The first element we are going to talk about is the architecture of the app. The game works over the Android operating system, the most used in mobile devices. The environment chosen for the development of the game was Unity, an engine for multi-platform computer games that is widely used by the community of computer game developers. Google Firebase has been chosen as a platform for the support of programming thanks to its APIs, which make it easier to handle features such as authentication. Lastly, with regards to augmented reality (RA), Vuforia has been chosen as RA platform. Vuforia's SDK allows tracking a great diversity of both 3D and 2D objects using almost any camera integrated in a mobile device. This leads to a great level of compatibility with most actual devices. In Fig. 1 it can be seen a schema of the architecture of the app.

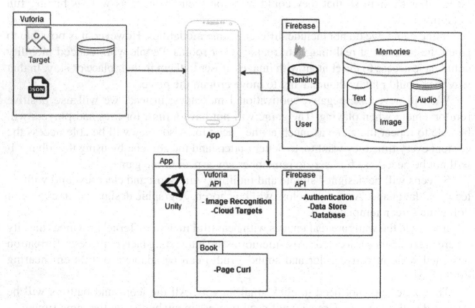

Fig. 1. Architecture of the system [5].

Game action consists of the player locating certain images in the real world so that, when the mobile device focuses on them, a RA virtual object appears on the screen. These images are photographs that are stored in the app database. The RA object is a button that belongs to a certain category, from the ones that the game includes. When this button is touched by the player, a memory from that category gets unlocked. Therefore, a screen with the information about that memory appears. This screen includes an image, a brief description of the memory and some controls for listening to the narration of the description. Some memories have a video instead of an image. After this screen is exited, a positive support will be shown to the player, so that he/she gets encouraged to keep on playing. Also, if after this progress the player has achieved a certain number of memories in this category, a medal will be awarded to him/her. Moreover, he/she will be asked about his/her opinion on the memory unlocked. This is made with a thumbs up/thumbs down system. All memories that have already been unlocked are stored in the album, which is available through a button in the main game screen. Also, a ranking screen is implemented and the player can go to it by means of another button in the same screen.

Next, we are going to show some screenshots of the game so that its user interface and visual appearance get presented. Firstly, in Fig. 2 we show the main game screen. In it, three static buttons appear. The button in the upper part of the screen allows the player to go to the screen in which the awards achieved when unlocking memories are shown. The two buttons in the lower zone of the screen are for going to the ranking screen and to the album with all the memories already unlocked, respectively. Regarding the central button, it is a RA virtual object that has appeared when focusing the mobile device on an image that the game identifies as a target. In this specific case, this virtual button will unlock a memory of the sports category.

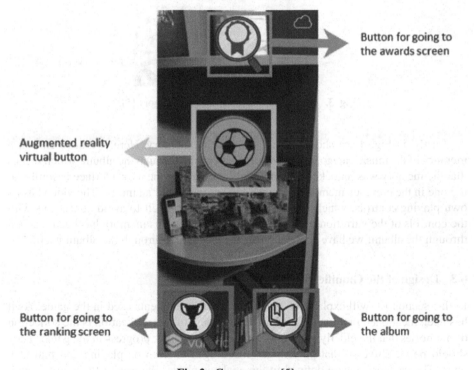

Fig. 2. Game screen [5].

As a second example, in Fig. 3 we depict an example of a screen of a memory. Specifically, it is a memory of the personalities category. This memory has been shown directly after being unlocked by the player. It can be seen how the interface includes an image about the memory (here, a person's photo), a description, and controls for handling the narration of the description. This way, the description can be read, listened, or both, depending on the player's preference.

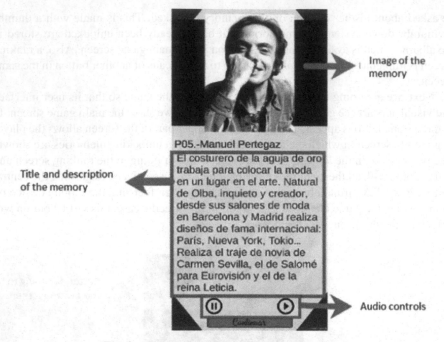

Fig. 3. Memory of the *personalities* category [5].

Lastly, in Fig. 4 we show another example of memory. Here, we have chosen a memory of the music category, and we have accessed it through the album, which means that the memory was unlocked time ago. It is shown how the user interface is similar to the one in the previous memory, but with a video instead of an image. The video has its own playing controls, which are shown over the video itself to avoid confusions with the controls of the narration of the description. Also, as this memory has been reached through the album, we have some controls for navigating through the album itself.

6.3 Design of the Gamification System

In this section we will explain the main gamification elements used in the game. As it has been mentioned previously, a critical component of the application is the collection of memories that the elderly people will unlock during their progress in the game. They should be attractive so that players get encouraged to keep on playing and find new ones. The categories were defined in the analysis phase. We used a focus group with potential players to decide what topics were more attractive for potential users. The goal was to create a collection of memories recognizable for the residents, which help them to remember moments of their life and to learn curiosities of their environment. Thus, memories from the 50s until our days were chosen. Then, the development team selected specific memories. Another gamification element selected was the use of points. The goal with this element would be to motivate users and establish a way of giving users feedback about their progression. The sense of progression usually helps to motivate continued

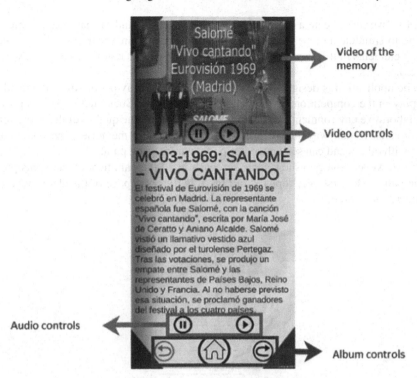

Fig. 4. Memory of the *music* category [5].

effort. Badges and achievements act as visual symbols to give rewards and signals of accomplishments of users, therefore was another gamification element included in our design. These badges are shown with positive reinforcement sentences. In that way users are able to see their progress and receive medals in a category. For this last point, we create an algorithm that compares the number of memories unlocked in a category with the number of memories pending to be unlocked in this category. Subsequently, based on this percentage, the player is awarded a medal with 50% of unlocked memories being bronze, 75% silver and 100% gold (levels of challenges - element included also in serious games.).

We use leaderboards and rankings to display points and positions of individuals in the competition in order users can visualize their stand relative to the competition. With the use of albums users will be able to browse the memories obtained and enjoy its content. The album acts as progress bar, helping users to know how far along they've come and how much resources they have collected and also as a multimedia element to enjoy content. Also, we design a video explaining the way of playing. With this element we try to incentivize and help users with the learning process.

Moreover, we create a scenario where real elements and virtual ones are blended. Trying to simulate a game where users interact with real in a real place, but including virtual elements in this word through the use of augmented reality (goal of trans-reality games).

The application is designed as a social network, as only people from the residence can play in the competition, so they all know each other. Social networks can promote a collaborative environment, improving cooperation and the quality of the game for the participants. In that way, they can help each other to get memories, can comment on them with others and can see how other people are getting points.

Next, we are going to show some screenshots of the gamification elements present in the game. The first one, depicted in Fig. 5, is the front page of the album where the memories get stored.

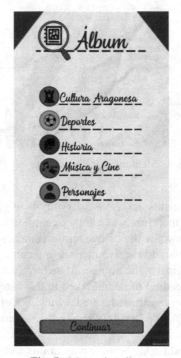

Fig. 5. Memories album.

The next one is an example of how badges are presented to users when they are achieved. This is shown in Fig. 6.

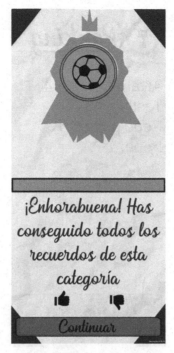

Fig. 6. Badge achievement.

Lastly, in Fig. 7 we can see an example of ranking. Data is just for testing purposes.

In order to perform a first assessment of the gamification elements in the game, it was used by some elderly people from the residential complex where the user-centered design activities were carried out at the beginning of the project. After two weeks playing the game, we carried out an interview with two elderly people who had been playing. Some interesting feedback was collected, being the following the most relevant pieces of information collected:

- Rewards are too hard to collect, and the point system is not easy to understand.
- The game was not played in a competitive way, so the ranking was not useful for them.
- Cooperative search of memories was being carried out, followed by the players talking about what they had found.
- Positive reinforcements are well received.

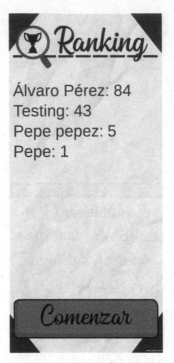

Fig. 7. Ranking of the game.

7 Conclusions and Future Work

In this chapter we have described "EncuéntraTe", which is a pervasive mobile game aimed at elderly people. The game has been developed for its use in centers for elderly people. The game consists of searching some *targets* in the real world so that the game unlocks some memories that can stimulate the players' memory. The game has an achievement and ranking system to encourage the player to keep playing. Thus, we have designed and implemented a novel game that uses current technologies and consider specific requirements that are needed in the development of games for the elderly. This way, the game puts together the ideas of pervasive games with the aim of stimulating the elders' memory and having them performing physical activity.

We have included two assessment activities in the chapter. In the first one, referred to the elements for encouraging the use of the game, some elderly people who have played the game have provided us with valuable feedback that will help use to improve the game. In the second one, which is detailed in the appendix of the chapter, we have tested how the accessibility of the game is the demanded when a game is oriented toward the elderly.

As future work, we will improve the game following the feedback provided by the players that have played the game. In particular, we will consider including captions in the videos, the possibility of changing the size of icons, text and graphics, alternative texts in images, and controls adapted to the player's sensitivity. Also, more complete studies with a larger number of users will be carried out so that the assessment of the game gets more complete. Finally, we will also consider the possibility of the game getting adapted to the player, so that the memories that he/she unlocks depend on the feedback provided in previous memories.

Acknowledgments. Work partly funded by the Spanish Science and Innovation Ministry, the National Research Agency (AEI) and the EU (FEDER) through the contract RTI2018-096986-B-C31, by Fundación Bancaria Ibercaja through the contract JIUZ-2020-TEC-04, and by the Aragonese Government (Group T60_20R).

Appendix

Accessibility Assessment

In order to validate the application, we have analyzed the accessibility aspects considered according to WCAG 2.0 "Applies to Older People".

Perceivable Information and User Interface. This section explains how many of the Web Content Accessibility Guidelines (WCAG) 2.0 guidelines and success criteria specifically meet the needs of older web users. Although not all the WCAG 2.0 success criteria are applied here, we use WAI recommends meeting at least all WCAG 2.0 Level A and AA success criteria.

This section is organized under the four principles of web accessibility from WCAG 2.0: perceivable, operable, understandable, and robust. Success criteria are listed thematically, to help readability. Sometimes they are drawn from different guidelines to address a particular aspect.

Text Size
Large text has been applied due to decreased vision, including text in form fields and other controls. According to WCAG 2.0 success criteria:

- *Resize text* (AA): Text can be resized in the application without assistive technology up to 200 per cent without loss of content or functionality. We've applied techniques:

  - Using relative font-sizes such as percent (C12) or ems (C14) and ensuring text containers resize (C28).
  - Avoiding the use of text in raster images.

Text Style and Text Layout
The following aspects regarding the style of the text and its visual presentation have been taken into account. Since they influence the difficulty or ease of reading for people, especially older people with vision problems.

- *Visual Presentation* (AAA) some of the requirements on text style, text justification, line spacing, line length, and horizontal scrolling. We've applied techniques:

  - Avoiding fully-aligned text (C19)

– Using readable fonts
– Using upper and lower case according to the spelling conventions of the text language
– Avoiding chunks of italic text
– Avoiding overuse of different styles on individual pages and in sites

Color and Contrast

We apply various specifications for the use of color, paying special attention to those aspects that older people find it difficult to recognize, such as contrast and others:

- *Use of Color* (A) Color is not the only means of transmitting information, we normally apply it together with other indicators such as signs or text to identify buttons or the various sections of the app. Applied technique:

  – G14: Ensuring that information conveyed by color differences is also available in text

- *Contrast* (Minimum) (AA) as required a contrast ratio of at least 4.5:1 is applied for the visual presentation of text and images

  – Using a light pastel background rather than a white background behind black text to create sufficient but not extreme contrast
  – G18: Ensuring that a contrast ratio of at least 4.5:1 exists between text (and images of text) and background behind the text

- *Contrast* (Enhanced) (AAA) as required a higher contrast ratio of at least 7:1 for the visual presentation of text and images

  – G17: Ensuring that a contrast ratio of at least 7:1 exists between text (and images of text) and background behind the text

– Using a light pastel background rather than a white background behind black text to create sufficient but not extreme contrast

Multimedia
Because the hearing or vision of many older people decreases, we have applied the following requirements:

- *Extended Audio Description* (Prerecorded video) (AAA) Applying the technique:

  – G158: Providing an alternative for time-based media for audio-only content

1. *Low or No Background Audio* (Prerecorded) (AAA). Applying the technique:
   1. No Background: The audio does not contain background sounds.

Text-to-Speech (Speech Synthesis)
We do not apply speech synthesis.

CAPTCHA
Captcha systems offer reading difficulties. Older people with low vision may not be able to distinguish characters in a CAPTCHA, especially since CAPTCHAs often have low contrast and do not increase in size when users have larger text. As a measure of success:

1. *Non-text Content* (A) includes a requirement for alternative CAPTCHAs. we decided not to apply forms with CAPTCHA, as is contemplated in the technique:
   1. Not requiring CAPTCHAs for authorized users

   Operable User Interface and Navigation

Links
As many older people need the links to be particularly clear and identifiable due to impaired vision and cognition, we apply the following requirements:

1. *Link Purpose* (In Context) (A) the purpose of a link can be determined from the link text alone, or from the link text together with its surrounding context. We apply the technique:
   1. G91: Providing link text that describes the purpose of a link
   2. Limiting the number of links per page
   3. Making links visually distinct

2. *Focus Visible* (AA) requires a visible keyboard focus indicator that shows what component on the web page has focus. We apply the technique:
   1. Highlighting a link or control when the mouse hovers over it, or when it receives keyboard focus

Navigation and Location
Many older people require particularly clear navigation due to decreased cognitive abilities. The adaptations that we have taken into the app are the following:

1. *Page Titled* (A): "web pages have titles that describe topic or purpose". We apply the techniques:
   1. G128: Indicating current location within navigation bars
   2. Providing a link to the home page or main page

Mouse Use
It is difficult for some older people to use a mouse due to declining vision or dexterity. This section is in relation to aspects that we have already described previously. We apply the following success requirements:

1. *Focus Visible* (AA) says that focus indicators should be visible. As we said previously we use the technique:
   1. Highlighting a link or control when the mouse hovers over it
2. *Resize Text* (AA) says that text should be resizable up to 200 percent. We apply the technique:
   1. Using real text with relative font size (C12, C14) and avoiding the use of text in raster images as larger text is easy to click.

Keyboard Use and Tabbing
The content cannot be operated with a keyboard interface, as it is an app developed for a mobile phone. This precept does not apply.

Distractions
Some older people are particularly distracted by any movement and sound on web pages. So we have included controls in the audio and video elements following the success requirements:

1. *Pause, Stop, Hide* (A): "a mechanism for the user to pause, stop, or hide" moving or blinking content. We apply the technique:
   1. G4: Allowing the content to be paused and restarted from where it was paused
2. *Audio Control* (A): "a mechanism is available to pause or stop the audio". We apply the techniques:
   1. G4: Allowing the content to be paused and restarted from where it was paused
   2. G171: Sound playing only on demand.

Understandable Language
Many older people find it particularly difficult to understand complex sentences, unusual

words, and technical jargon. For this reason, the sections have been drafted as clearly as possible:

1. *Reading Level* (AAA) requires providing a version that "does not require reading ability more advanced than the lower secondary education level". We apply the technique:
   1. Using the clearest and simplest language appropriate for the content

Consistent Navigation and Labeling

For people who are new to the web, and older people with some types of cognitive decline, consistent navigation and presentation is particularly important.

1. *Consistent Navigation* (AA) requires that navigation is presented in the same relative order across a website. We apply the technique:
   1. G61: Presenting repeated components in the same relative order each time they appear
2. *Consistent Identification* (AA) requires that components with similar functionality are identified consistently. We apply the technique:
   1. G197: Using labels, names, and text alternatives consistently for content that has the same functionality

Pop-Ups and New Windows

Some older people experiencing cognitive decline can be confused or distracted by pop-ups, new windows, or new tabs.

This is how we have eliminated pop-ups that open without user request. As success requirements:

1. *On Focus* (A) says "when any component receives focus, it does not initiate a change of context"
2. *Change on Request* (AAA) says "changes of context are initiated only by user request or a mechanism is available to turn off such changes"
   1. G107: Using "activate" rather than "focus" as a trigger for changes of context

Page Refresh and Updates

Some older people with declining vision or cognition can miss content that automatically updates or refreshes in a page.

1. *On Focus* (A) says "when any component receives focus, it does not initiate a change of context". We apply the techniques:
   1. G80: Providing a submit button to initiate a change of context
   2. G107: Using "activate" rather than "focus" as a trigger for changes of context
2. *On Input* (A) says that changing a setting does not automatically change the context unless the user has been advised beforehand
3. *Change on Request* (AAA) says "changes of context are initiated only by user request or a mechanism is available to turn off such changes"
   1. G76: Providing a mechanism to request an update of the content instead of updating automatically. We apply the techniques:

2. SCR19: Using an *onchange* event on a select element without causing a change of context

Instructions and Input Assistance
It is difficult for some older people to understand the requirements of forms and transactions. Thus, to make the application more accessible, we have developed the following elements:

1. *Labels or Instructions* (A) says "labels or instructions are provided when content requires user input" we apply the technique:
   1. G184: Providing text instructions at the beginning of a form or set of fields that describes the necessary input
2. *Consistent Identification* (AA) says "components that have the same functionality within a set of Web pages are identified consistently" we use the technique:
   1. G197: Using labels, names, and text alternatives consistently for content that has the same functionality

Error Prevention and Recovery
It is difficult for some older people to use forms and complete transactions due to declining cognitive abilities.

1. *Error Prevention* (All) (AAA) says that users can check and correct any information they submit. So that we use the technique:
   1. G98: Providing the ability for the user to review and correct answers before submitting

Robust Content and Reliable Interpretation

Older Equipment/Software
Some older people will use older systems that may not be as capable or fault tolerant as current versions.

1. Parsing (A) requires that markup is used correctly according to specification:
   1. G134: Validating Web pages
   2. G192: Fully conforming to specifications

Taking all the aforementioned into account, we understand that our application fulfills in a satisfactory way most accessibility requirements, so it is suitable for its use by elderly people.

References

1. Morillas, A.S., Martínez, G.: La influencia de las nuevas tecnologías: videojuegos, redes sociales e internet, en los consumidores seniors en España. In: I Congreso Internacional de Comunicación y Sociedad Digital. Logroño, Spain (2013)
2. AEVI (Asociación Española de Videojuegos): La Industria del videojuego en España. Anuario 2018. LLYC (2019)

3. Allaire, J., McLaughlin, A., Trujillo, A., Whitlock, L.A., LaPorte, L., Gandy, M.: Successful aging through digital games: socioemotional differences between older adult gamers and non-gamers. Comput. Hum. Behav. **29**, 1302–1306 (2013)
4. Montola, M.: Exploring the edge of the magic circle: defining pervasive games. In: Proceedings of DAC, vol. 1966, pp. 16–19 (2005)
5. Pérez, A., Gallardo, J., Lacuesta, R., Hernández, S.: A pervasive game for elderly people with augmented reality: description and first validation. In: ICT4AWE 2021, 7th International Conference on Information and Communication Technologies for Ageing Well and e-Health (2021)
6. Kasapakis, V., Gavalas, D.: Blending history and fiction in a pervasive game prototype. In: 13th International Conference on Mobile and Ubiquitous Multimedia, pp. 116–122 (2014)
7. Arango-López, J., Collazos, C.A., Gutiérrez Vela, F.L., Castillo, L.F.: A systematic review of geolocated pervasive games: a perspective from game development methodologies, software metrics and linked open data. In: Marcus, A., Wang, W. (eds.) DUXU 2017. LNCS, vol. 10289, pp. 335–346. Springer, Cham (2017). https://doi.org/10.1007/978-3-319-58637-3_27
8. Arango-López, J., Gallardo, J., Gutiérrez-Vela, F.L., Cerezo, E., Amengual, E., Valera, R.: Pervasive games: giving a meaning based on the player experience. In Interacción 2017 (2017)
9. Cota, T.T., Ishitani, L., Vieira Jr, N.: Mobile game design for the elderly: a study with focus on the motivation to play. Comput. Hum. Behav. **51**, 96–105 (2015)
10. Mubin, O., Shahid, S., Al Mahmud, A.: Walk 2 win: towards designing a mobile game for elderly's social engagement. In: People and Computers XXII Culture, Creativity, Interaction (HCI) (2008)
11. Gerling, K., Schulte, F., Masuch, M.: Designing and evaluating digital games for frail elderly persons. In: ACE 2011, Lisbon, Portugal (2011)
12. Cárdenas-Delgado, S., Méndez-López, M., Juan, M.C., Pérez-Hernández, E., Lluch, J., Vivó, R.: Using a virtual maze task to assess spatial short-term memory in adults. In: International Conference on Computer Graphics Theory and Applications, vol. 2, pp. 46–57. SCITEPRESS (2017)
13. Parra, D., García de Diego, A., Pérez, J.: Habits of use of videogames in Spain between older than 35 years. Revista Latina de Comunicación Social **64**, 694–707 (2009)

A Technological Solution to Supervise CoViD-19 Symptoms in Senior Patients in Lima

Sara Haro-Hoyo, Edgard Inga-Quillas, and Willy Ugarte(✉)

Universidad Peruana de Ciencias Aplicadas, Lima, Peru
{u201317016,u20141A776}@upc.edu.pe, willy.ugarte@upc.edu.pe

Abstract. The article's objective is to outline the application of a technological solution based on wearable technology that provides for the best possible monitoring of elderly patients with CoViD19. This is a pressing issue right now because the epidemic has caused numerous problems for senior patients. For example, because older persons are more susceptible to CoViD19, they must limit social contact or adhere to stricter lockdown protocols. In order to do this, a thorough assessment of the relevant scientific literature in the phases of planning, development, and analysis was conducted. The use of technology models in real time, the monitoring of CoViD19 symptoms, and the usage of IoT for geriatric patient monitoring are all topics covered in this paper. Our findings demonstrate the viability of our strategy.

Keywords: CoViD19 · Technological solution · IoT · Monitoring · Patients

1 Introduction

On January 30, 2020, the World Health Organization (WHO) reported the existence of a total of 7,818 people infected with CoViD19 worldwide, most of them from China.

According to the Pan American Health Organization (PAHO), the WHO declared China as very high risk and the other countries as high. Likewise, the WHO published the Strategic Preparedness and Response Plan of the international community, to help states with poor health systems to protect themselves from the new virus.

More than 2.9 million people worldwide have died from the new SARS-CoV-2 coronavirus and about 134.1 million infected. It is worth mentioning that the country most affected by 2021 is the United States with more than 31 million infections and 560,000 deaths; Brazil follows, with over 13.2 million diagnosed and with 345,000 deaths; and India exceeds 13 million infected and 167,000 deaths.

According to the latest report from the Ministry of Health of Peru (MINSA), as of September 2021, 199,727 deaths were registered in our country, where the most affected province was Metropolitan Lima with 81,389 deaths, with a 9.23% fatality rate of the virus. With these indicators, many countries are in a state of health emergency due to this pandemic, hence the need to find technological solutions based on innovation within the field of medicine.

Hence, this article aims to contribute with a proposal for improvement in the process of monitoring patients with symptoms of this disease, as well as in the recovery

L. A. Maciaszek et al. (Eds.): ICT4AWE 2021/2022, CCIS 1856, pp. 256–272, 2023.
https://doi.org/10.1007/978-3-031-37496-8_14

process of the patient infected with this virus. A precedent is the study of Remote health monitoring of elderly through wearable sensors [1], which focused on the design and implementation of an intelligent health monitoring system that can observe the elderly remotely, see Fig. 1.

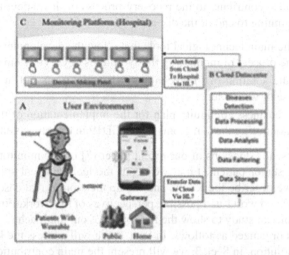

Fig. 1. High-level overview of SW-SHMS system architecture [1].

For the development of this research, a compilation of various articles indexed in journals categorized in quartiles within Scopus and Web of Science was made, in the period 2019 to 2021. As well as testimonies through interviews of the 4 main actors: patient, caregiver, doctor, and laboratory.

The objective of this article is to present a technological solution based on 2 mobile applications:

– "CoViDSalud_Paciente" and
– "CoViDSalud_Atención"

In addition, this system allows to collect data that is sent to the corresponding medical units to assess the patient's situation. At the end of the validation, an improvement was observed regarding the nutritional status of the person, cognitive functions and the execution of daily activities of the participants [1]. By identifying this type of solution, it has been validated what to know about the health status and impairment of a patient's cognitive functions makes it easier for the doctor to generate accurate recommendations regarding the advancement of the patient's disease.

Seeking to optimally monitor the symptoms of CoViD-19 in elderly patients in Metropolitan Lima, offering an excellent service. Therefore, the main matrix of the technological solution is to have a mobile application that can be linked to a "wearable" device; to obtain constant control and monitoring of the patient. This application presents a friendly interface; in other words, it is easy to use for the target audience, who are older people, who present specific and distinctive needs, as well as significant demands regarding the use of ICTs.

The development of this APP contributes as a data control and monitoring tool that can refer to a possible CoViD19 alert; o provide support in the process of a patient who has already been diagnosed and that these can serve as an accurate reference for the doctor and thus also contribute to the recovery process of the patient throughout their process from beginning to end of the disease.

- We analyze the main technological tools that allow the development of the solution to optimize the process of monitoring the symptoms of CoViD19 in elderly patients.
- We validate the solution of the technological model proposed in elderly patients through the use of wearable.
- We propose a business continuity plan for the implementation of the technological solution for monitoring the symptoms of CoViD19 in elderly patients.

Here, we present extensions of our recent paper [7] on the monitoring the CoViD-19 symptoms in senior patient. First, we detail the technological solution wih more detail. Second, we describe the results and the application to real cases. Furthermore, we discuss the related works and possible perspectives of this work. Finally, we present an extensive empirical study to show the feasibility of our approach.

This paper is organized as follows. In Sect. 2, we will address the key concepts for developing our solution, in Sect. 3, we will present the main contributions of the study. In Sect. 4, we will describe the differences and comparisons with other works about technological solutions for health care. Subsequently, in Sect. 5 we will present the validation of the technological model functionalities in a simulated scenario. Finally, in Sect. 6 we will specify our main conclusions and results of the finished application.

2   Context

In this section, the main concepts involved in our research will be developed.

We propose that, for each concept, there is a definition and a respective example based on a review of the literature on depressive disorder and facial and voice recognition.

Definition 1 (Use of IoT Technologies [4, 12, 14, 16, 17]**).** *The concept of IoT refers to a digital interconnection of everyday objects with the internet. It is the internet connection more with objects than with people.*

According to Forbes, with the appearance of CoViD19, at the beginning of 2020, thermometers began to be used, which were connected by a 5G network, such as smart rings and/or bracelets that had the function of collecting data from patients such as the blood oxygen level and heart rate [10], see Fig. 2.

Example 1. In [16], the research, presents a system based on IoT that provides us with a program where the patient can perform his totally personalized rehabilitation and is reviewed by a professional to monitor the performance and efficiency of workouts from any device. This work used a ReMoVES architecture which has 4 layers as shown in Fig. 2:

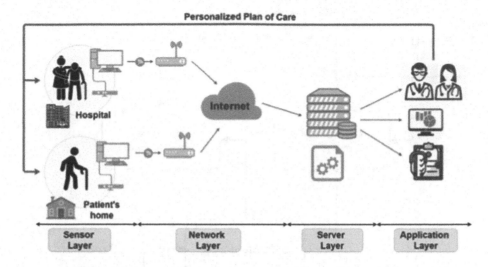

Fig. 2. Remote Monitoring Validation Engineering System (ReMoVES) Architecture [16].

2.1 Wearable Sensors

Advanced technology to "carry", mobility is its main characteristic and the IoT the basis of its approach, since sensors allow data to be constantly collected and transmitted to different devices, accessories, and garments.

While it might seem like most wearables are worn on the wrist, there are devices designed to be worn almost anywhere on the body. For this reason, in addition to bracelets, wearables can be found in rings, necklaces, headbands and even shoe inserts with advanced functions [13].

According to Filho [12], an analysis of the various previous studies for the spread of CoViD19 based on IoT technologies, cloud computing and mobile applications can be carried out. Which are already being used to process patient data regarding health monitoring and obtain an immediate response as soon as the patient needs it. See Fig. 3.

2.2 Depression

According to the Pan American Health Organization (2021), the epidemiological update caused by SARS-CoV 2 has had different variants that affect public health. In October 2020, a new variant was detected in India called B.1.617, which is under investigation. Also, other variants of great interest for public health have emerged, such as variant P.1, lineage B.1.1.28 on January 9, 2021, in Japan, which was detected in travelers coming from Brazil.

According to the virologist Kamil, one of the mutations of this new variant is like those identified in the countries of Brazil and South Africa and he considers it to be less infectious compared to the variant in the United Kingdom[1].

---

[1] Epidemiological Update - PAHO.

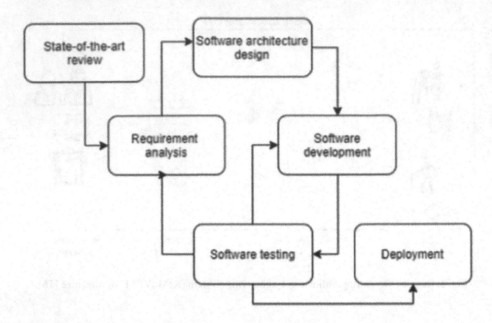

Fig. 3. Methodology to develop PAR [12].

According to [14], the authors propose the use of monitoring of 15 symptoms of infected patients in an-ANN-based system to manage patient data, to improve the classification of CoViD19 infected patients. The model used in this research is the multi-layer perceptron network (MLP) which is considered a type of ANN those researchers often use frequently, see Fig. 4.

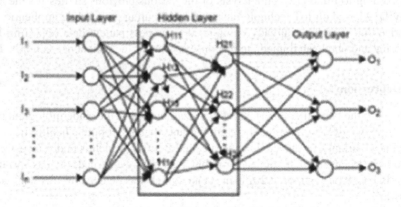

Fig. 4. Multilayer perceptron architecture network [14].

3   Main Contribution

Prior to the development and proposal, a benchmarking analysis was carried out as the methodology to extract the data, using Gartner[2], which has a wide field regarding the evaluation of tools from different areas.

On this occasion, this methodology was adapted to generate a quantitative report that serves to qualify the tools in question.

3.1   Phases

The project development approach was based on five phases, which are detailed below:

- In the first phase, the scope of the project was defined together with the Product Owner. Likewise, an in-depth investigation was generated regarding the initially agreed requirements. With these premises, the Project Charter documentation begins.
- For the second phase, an analysis was carried out regarding the technologies that would be involved for the proposed solution.
- In the third phase, the technological model was designed, validated by the Product Owner.
- During the fourth phase, the development of the proposed solution (product) that was delivered to the Product Owner was carried out. Additionally, the corresponding validations were generated based on the initial requirements.
- Finally, in the fifth phase, the results of the project (final product) were presented.

3.2   Execution

Two mobile applications will be developed for the Android operating system as part of the technological solution, which will bear the name of "CoViDSalud_Paciente" whose main purpose will be to optimize the monitoring of main symptoms of elderly patients to rule out or accompany the CoViD19, using a wearable device via Bluetooth connection.

And it will work together with another application called "CoViDSalud_Atención", whose main purpose will be to contribute to the management of doctors, caregivers and laboratories, to be able to provide medical assistance to patients, by appointment in an efficient manner.

This technological solution will contribute with the monitoring of the main symptoms to prevent the patient from getting worse his state of health, as well as keep a record in the reports of symptoms that keep the patient stable and collaborate with the tranquility of this (see Fig. 5).

This research is aimed at elderly patients, that is, 60 years and older, since according to WHO research statistics (2020), they are the society with the greatest vulnerability and/or risk against CoViD19. This part of the population has a weaker immune system

---

[2] Benchmark Analytics.

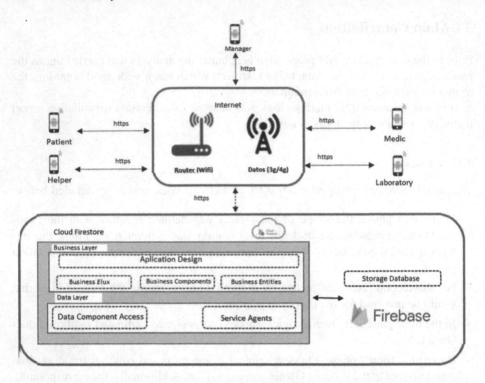

Fig. 5. Physical Architecture Diagram [7].

and, in most cases, they have one or more chronic diseases, such as diabetes, hypertension, cardiovascular and pulmonary conditions (COPD), so their ability to respond to infections is less.

The objective of this architecture, see Fig. 6, is to be able to identify the requirements that have an impact on the software structure and reduce the risks associated with its construction.

The architecture must support future changes in software, hardware and functionality demanded by customers (which occur very often).

Similarly, it is the responsibility of the software architect to analyze the impact of his design decisions and establish a compromise between the different quality requirements, as well as between the compromises necessary to satisfy the users, the software, and the business objectives, and which are functional and quality requirements, hence it is vital to determine the type of software to be developed, see Fig. 7.

Presentation Layer. It is the part of the system with which the user interacts. Your screens, forms are all user interfaces (UI) that are part of the presentation layer User interfaces can make use of components or user process controllers (UIC) to communicate with the back end and navigate or process the user interface.

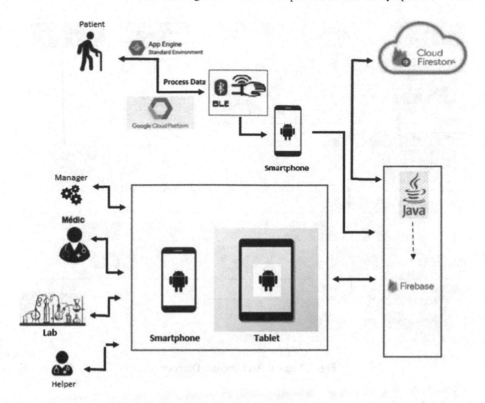

Fig. 6. Integrated Architecture Diagram [7].

Service Layer. The services layer in the architecture allows the functionality of the system to be exposed to client and external applications. It is also the key to achieving cross-platform and interoperable solutions. Service components expose the functionality of the components through contracts, which are the interfaces where service providers and service consumers agree and must be immutable.

Business Logic Layer. It contains all the processing logic to make the application possible. The Component is where you put this processing logic where each one can be coded in independent methods.

Data Layer. The data layer is where we save our components as CRUD operations, which handle the insertion (Create), the selection (Read), the modification (Update) and the elimination (Delete) of data, see Table 1. In this presentation we show the different modules with their respective responsibilities.

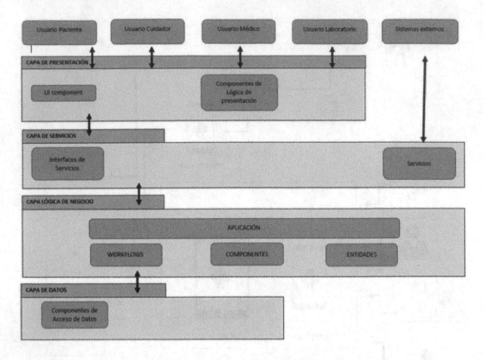

Fig. 7. Logical Architecture Diagram.

3.3 Elaboration

In the construction phase, the web and mobile application was developed using the programming language C# and Kotlin respectively. As a database support using the non-relational database, Mongo DB.

The wearable used for capturing vital signs (blood pressure and oxygenation) and sleep status was Smartband S5. The cloud platform used for web application deployment was Microsoft Azure.

During this stage, the applications that compose part of the technological solution were developed: mobile and web.

On the one hand, the coding of the mobile application included the libraries android-smartband-sdk-sxrblejy2aidl-release.aar and android-smartband-sdk-sxrblejy2library-release.aar to establish the connection with the wearable Smartband S5. Likewise, this library allowed obtaining data related to vital signs (arterial pressure and blood oxygenation) and sleep status. Additionally, stimulation games aimed at the following cognitive functions were included: memory, concentration and calculation. The data related to vital signs, sleep status and scores in the cognitive stimulation games were stored in the MongoDB Atlas database and the visualization functionality was integrated through reports with the support of the AAChartCore-Kotlin library.

On the other hand, the code of the web application includes the development of functionalities for displaying reports related to the patient's health status with support of the Chart JS library. Likewise, the functionality of recording recommendations for each patient was incorporated.

Table 1. Modules and responsibilities.

Module	Responsibility
User interface (UI)	Forms are all user interfaces (UI) that are part of the presentation layer
Presentation logic components	Process a request, generating response content, and formatting the page for the client
Contracts (Service interfaces)	Allows data transfer, it applies specific actions (POST, GET, PUT and DELETE) on resources
Services	Provide additional services that the application requires
App	Expose the business logic
Workflows	Organize the flow that carries out the execution of the business process
Components (edit)	Component that performs business tasks
Entities	Component that represents custom business classes
Data access components to Data	Components that deal with the database tables

4   Related Works

For the development of the proposed technological solution, 2 mobile applications were implemented that are linked to a "wearable" device to obtain constant control and monitoring of the patient with CoViD19. For this, an analysis of the state of the art was carried out, selecting its most relevant scientific articles:

In the paper [11], the author achieved the optimization in the information reporting processes of the main symptoms of CoViD19, so that it serves as part of the process of studies considered in possible diagnoses. What differs from our paper is that we will consider four measurement indicators, temperature, heart rate, sleep status and blood saturation.

In the same way, in the paper [12], the authors manage to demonstrate the need for an intelligent diagnosis and monitoring of infected patients to reduce hospital care, since they are the most vulnerable people, and this could have great consequences. The objective of this research is to present a platform designed for constant monitoring of patients in critical condition, using portable sensors to monitor patients infected with coronavirus. What sets us apart from this paper is that we not only rely on monitoring, but we also provide virtual medical assistance to those who use our application.

Another study that follows the same line of research is the paper [14], which delves into the 2 studies already mentioned, since it explains the importance of the use of AI in the health sector, mainly, in medical systems, which can be very useful to automate and remotely quantify CoViD19 patients and improve recognition of infected patients in the early stages of contagion. What differentiates us from this paper is that they are based on the first stages of contagion, however, we already work with patients infected with CoViD-19, providing them with continuous monitoring, medical and laboratory assistance from day one.

Furthermore, in [2], the authors present another assisted technology that helps people affected by dementia, such as the MSI-MDD digital platform. In addition, this article presents another assisted technology that allows helping people affected by dementia, such as the MSI-MDD digital platform.

Nevertheless, it is also evidenced that the authors of [15], through a mobile application evaluate and improve the emotional state of caregivers, allowing to optimize the stimulation process for the caregiver, applying medical metrics. On the other hand, it is also evidenced that the authors, through a mobile application evaluate and improve the emotional state of caregivers, allowing optimization of the stimulation process for the caregiver, applying medical metrics.

Finally, in [5], the authors showed that web-based video services can be used on tablets, allowing to improve mood in people living with dementia and improve perceptions of caregivers about the daily interaction that older adults may have with their caregivers, showing that video services based on the web can be used on tablets, allowing to improve mood in people living with dementia and improve perceptions of caregivers about the daily interaction that older adults may have with their caregivers.

Hence, when we are faced with the inexplicable situation of a pandemic that has not yet been overcome, the motivation of the researchers of the paper [8] is observed, to propose extensive analyzes and evaluations on the technological solutions that can help in the fight against the expansion of CoViD-19, and thus continue to inspire other researchers to continue making their contributions to mitigate the damages of the pandemic. What differentiates us from this paper is that we already apply a solution to CoViD-19 patients monitoring the main symptoms and there will also be a caregiver who will also follow the steps of a respective patient.

However, one of the most vulnerable groups and that suffered high mortality rates were the elderly, therefore, in paper [6], it refers to the importance of constant monitoring with the elderly, since they are more vulnerable due to the possible congenital diseases, or those already developed by age. Therefore, and according to the positions, it is vitally important to interconnect with the integrated systems developed to combat CoViD19. Compared to this paper, our solution implements an alert system to our elderly patients that is sent both to the patient, caregiver, and GP.

5 Experiments

In this section we are going to treat an experimental study to show the feasibility of our project, in each of the following paragraphs the experimental protocol, the results measuring the efficiency of the proposal and a short discussion will be detailed.

5.1 Experimental Protocol

For the development of our solution, an IDE called Android Studio 3.6 was used, where the Java and Kotlin language were used for the entire Front-end part.

Firebase cloud-based platform for the back end, HMS Core (Huawei Mobile Services) for wearable and mobile device connectivity. However, for those users who do not have mobiles with an Android operating system, an emulator called Blue Stacks 5 with an instance in Android 9.0 was used to run the tests of our application.

In the same way, to run the programs used, a computer with 10th generation Core i7, 16 GB of RAM and a 10 GB reserved storage for the application was used. Likewise, to carry out the respective tests, a Samsung Galaxy Note 20 Ultra cell phone with Android 11.0 operating system was used, accompanied by a Huawei Band 6 Smart Band with Bluetooth connection.

Then install the Huawei Health Kit and create an account that will be associated with the wearable. When opening the app, it will ask to connect with Huawei services, for this Huawei HMS Core will be downloaded. Immediately after downloading it, you will enter the application and you will be prompted to enter your Huawei account email and password.

Finally, it will ask for the permissions to read your data, it should be noted that all the data it reads is saved in Firebase. Our code and our data are publicly available at the following links, for the main apk: https://github.com/retto710/CoViDSaludAppAndroid and for the patient apk: https://github.com/retto710/CoViDSaludPaciente.

5.2 Results

This section will show the solution developed from the proposed architecture.

In addition, to validate the developed solution, the test to which it was subjected, and the results obtained from it in different elderly patients with different morbidities are shown. Our final IoT-enabled prototype is designed with a Huawei Band 6 wearable and a mobile device where the measurements of the main symptoms will be displayed. The accuracy of heart rate and oxygen saturation measurement are compared using two handheld devices: CONTEC-CMS50D and AFK-YK009. As shown in scenario 1, see Table 2, measurements with the Band 6 device are more effective, see also Fig. 8a for variations.

On the other hand, the temperature measured by the device is compared with the Thermometer mercury thermometer. It can be seen in Table 2 that the results shown for 5 patients with different ages by the proposed IOT-enabled wearable device are almost close to the values obtained by the smart band and the thermometer.

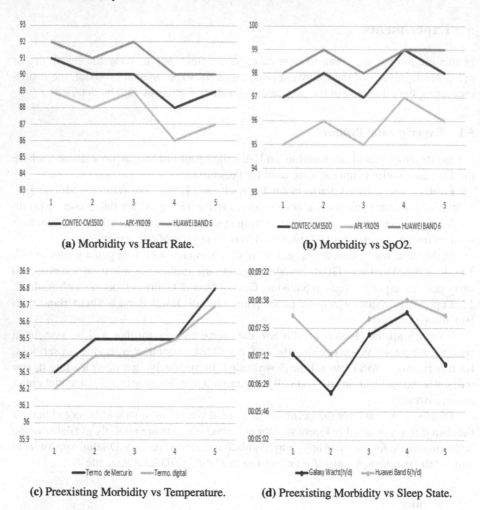

(a) Morbidity vs Heart Rate.

(b) Morbidity vs SpO2.

(c) Preexisting Morbidity vs Temperature.

(d) Preexisting Morbidity vs Sleep State.

Fig. 8. Comparison of results [7].

Finally, for the sleep state, a comparison was made between two wearable devices: Galaxy Watch and Huawei Band 6, in which the following results are shown (see Table 2).

The validation approach has focused on analyzing the results obtained in the pre-validation and post-validation survey that was performed as the final step of the desirability stage, allowing to obtain the values related to costs during Alzheimer's disease and the time associated with the tasks of monitoring the disease.

Supporting Physical Exercise Activities: we identified that this task (see Fig. 9) was previously performed between 11 to 20 min (20% of the time) and around 21 to 60 min (80% of the time) (see Fig. 9a), however, it can now be all performed in 30 min in average (see Fig. 9b). The reduction to perform this activity, like the previous activity,

Table 2. Scenarios [7].

Patient	1	2	3	4	5
Preexisting Morbidity	Alzheimer's	Irritable colon, Gastritis	Type 2 diabetes	Low back pain	Migraine
Age	89	89	67	65	61
Heartrate (bpm)					
CONTEC-CMS50D	91	90	90	88	89
AFK-YK009	89	88	89	86	87
HUAWEI BAND 6	92	91	92	90	90
SpO2 (%)					
CONTEC-CMS50D	97	98	97	99	98
AFK-YK009	95	96	95	97	96
HUAWEI BAND 6	98	99	98	99	99
Temperature (°C)					
Thermometer Mercury	36.3	36.5	36.5	36.5	36.8
Thermometer Digital	36.2	36.4	36.4	36.5	36.7
DreamState					
Galaxy Wacth (h/d)	7:15	6:15	7:46	8:20	7:00
HUAWEI BAND 6	8:15	7:15	8:10	8:40	8:15

was achieved by the use of the mobile application, which includes recommendations for physical exercises, which is suggested by the patient's doctor. For this reason, the search time for physical exercises decreases, according to the values indicated above.

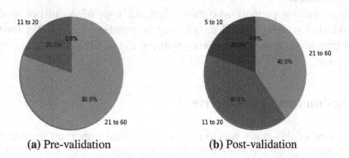

(a) Pre-validation   (b) Post-validation

Fig. 9. Supporting Physical Exercise Activities (in minutes).

Communication with an Specialist in case of complication: we identified that this task (see Fig. 10) was previously performed between 11 to 20 min (60% of the time) and around 21 to 60 min (40% of the time) (see Fig. 10a), however, it can now be all performed in 22 min in average (see Fig. 10b). The reduction to perform this activity, like the last two mentioned before, was achieved by the use of the mobile application, which includes a section on "Generate alert" for the doctor, in case the ranges of the variation of the patient's vital signs are outside the limits established by the doctor and by the information that the he maintains on the website of the patient's results. For this reason, the time taken to explain to the doctor how the patient's health behavior has been in a given period is reduced because the doctor has all the variation generated day by day.

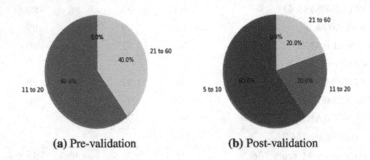

(a) Pre-validation   (b) Post-validation

Fig. 10. Communication with an Specialist in case of complication (in minutes).

5.3 Discussion

In Fig. 8, the main results are depicted for the main indicators of a person health, and its improvement with our solution.

We describe the implementation and impact of a CoViD-19 senior monitoring solution, in which we found that the RPM program was associated with significantly lower risk from our endpoint and the percentage of hospitalized or readmission patients hospitable has decreased.

In addition, among patients who have used our app, 67% did not produce alerts for symptoms that require manual monitoring, suggesting that PROM for CoViD-19 patients can provide extensive monitoring without the need to directly contact a physician for a review.

6 Conclusions and Perspectives

The primary goal of this study was to examine the most important technical resources in relation to the various forms of follow-ups for patients with CoViD-19 during the early stages of infection.

The data collection for health monitoring, and laboratory-based results interpretation are all addressed in the our work.

The use of IoT technology and a wearable to collect data on blood oxygenation, heart rate, and sleep state allowed researchers to track the development of the primary symptoms of CoViD-19 patients and validate the solution of the technological model. The experimental findings of the suggested approach employing Huawei's smart band 6 device demonstrate improved precision and quicker response times in many functions of our application.

As a result, this initiative serves as a pilot study, a model for future technological advancements in the Peruvian healthcare system, and a call to action for private enterprises to participate in I+D+I, or research, development, and innovation. Additionally, using genetic data to look for historical patient data [3] or monitoring symptoms [9] for additional disorders.

References

1. Al-khafajiy, M., et al.: Remote health monitoring of elderly through wearable sensors. Multimed. Tools Appl. **78**(17), 24681–24706 (2019). https://doi.org/10.1007/s11042-018-7134-7
2. Alexandru, A., Ianculescu, M.: Enabling assistive technologies to shape the future of the intensive senior-centred care: a case study approach. Stud. Inform. Control. **26**(3), 343–352 (2017)
3. Arroyo-Mariños, J.C., Mejia-Valle, K.M., Ugarte, W.: Technological model for the protection of genetic information using blockchain technology in the private health sector. In: ICT4AWE (2021)
4. Blas, H.S.S., Mendes, A.S., Encinas, F.G., Silva, L.A., González, G.V.: A multi-agent system for data fusion techniques applied to the internet of things enabling physical rehabilitation monitoring. Appl. Sci. **11**(1), 331 (2021)
5. Gilson, A., Dodds, D., Kaur, A., Potteiger, M., Ford, J.: Using computer tablets to improve moods for older adults with dementia and interactions with their caregivers (preprint). JMIR Form. Res. **3**(3), e14530 (2019)
6. Gordon, W.J., et al.: Remote patient monitoring program for hospital discharged COVID-19 patients. Appl. Clin. Inform. **11**(5), 792–801 (2020)
7. Haro-Hoyo, S., Inga-Quillas, E., Ugarte, W.: Technological solution to optimize the monitoring of COVID-19 symptoms in seniors patients in lima. In: ICT4AWE, pp. 17–25 (2022)
8. He, W., Zhang, Z.J., Li, W.: Information technology solutions, challenges, and suggestions for tackling the COVID-19 pandemic. Int. J. Inf. Manag. **57**, 102287 (2021)
9. Jorge-Lévano, K., Cuya-Chumbile, V., Ugarte, W.: Technological solution to optimize the Alzheimer's disease monitoring process, in metropolitan lima, using the internet of things. In: ICT4AWE (2021)
10. Milenkovic, M.: Internet of Things: Concepts and System Design. Springer, Switzerland (2020). https://doi.org/10.1007/978-3-030-41346-0
11. Mohammadzadeh, N., Gholamzadeh, M., Saeedi, S., Rezayi, S.: The application of wearable smart sensors for monitoring the vital signs of patients in epidemics: a systematic literature review. J. Ambient Intell. Humaniz. Comput. **14**(5), 6027–6041 (2020)
12. de Morais Barroca Filho, I., Aquino, G., Malaquias, R.S., Girão, G., Melo, S.R.M.: An IoT-based healthcare platform for patients in ICU beds during the COVID-19 outbreak. IEEE Access **9**, 27262–27277 (2021)
13. Motti, V.G.: Wearable Interaction. Human-Computer Interaction Series. Springer, Cham (2020). https://doi.org/10.1007/978-3-030-27111-4
14. Rathee, G., et al.: ANN assisted-IoT enabled COVID-19 patient monitoring. IEEE Access **9**, 42483–42492 (2021)

15. Sikder, A.T., Yang, F.C., Schafer, R., Dowling, G.A., Traeger, L.N., Jain, F.A.: Mentalizing imagery therapy mobile app to enhance the mood of family dementia caregivers: feasibility and limited efficacy testing. JMIR Aging **2**(1), e12850 (2019)
16. Trombini, M., Ferraro, F., Morando, M., Regesta, G., Dellepiane, S.G.: A solution for the remote care of frail elderly individuals via exergames. Sensors **21**(8), 2719 (2021)
17. Vedaei, S.S., et al.: COVID-SAFE: an IoT-based system for automated health monitoring and surveillance in post-pandemic life. IEEE Access **8**, 188538–188551 (2020)

What Helps to Help? Exploring Influencing Human-, Technology-, and Context-Related Factors on the Adoption Process of Telemedical Applications in Nursing Homes

Julia Offermann[1]([✉]) [iD], Wiktoria Wilkowska[1] [iD], Anne Kathrin Schaar[1] [iD], Jörg Christian Brokmann[2] [iD], and Martina Ziefle[1] [iD]

[1] Human-Computer Interaction Center, RWTH Aachen University, Campus-Boulevard 57, 52074 Aachen, Germany
{offermann,wilkowska,schaar,ziefle}@comm.rwth-aachen.de
[2] Emergency Department, University Hospital RWTH Aachen, Pauwelsstraße 30, 52074 Aachen, Germany
jbrokmann@ukaachen.de

Abstract. Currently, the shortage of personnel and the increasing proportions of older individuals in need of care pose enormous challenges to care facilities. Some of the resulting hospitalizations in nursing home are not medically necessary for geriatric patients and can even cause a deterioration of their health. Using telemedical consultations in nursing homes represents one approach aiming at the reduction of unnecessary hospitalizations of geriatric patients and support of care personnel in acute and uncertain situations. Hence, the patients' as well as the care personnel's perspectives and their acceptance are essential for a successful implementation of these telemedical consultations. This paper presents qualitative and quantitative results of acceptance patterns in using telemedical consultations from a social communication science perspective within the Optimal@NRW project. An initial qualitative interview study with residents and care personnel of different nursing homes (N = 28) identified attitudes, perceived advantages, and concerns as well as requirements regarding the usage of telemedical consultations. These results provided the basis for further quantifications and for the comparison of acceptance parameters of using telemedical consultations in nursing homes across the entire duration of the project. In a second step, we present the results of a first quantitative study (N = 145) that quantified and validated the previously identified qualitative parameters. Insights of the current empirical approach should be considered within the conceptualization and implementation of telemedical services in nursing homes to fulfill the needs of the respective users, in particular geriatric patients and their care personnel.

Keywords: Telemedical consultations · Technology acceptance · Nursing homes · Geriatric patients · Empirical research · Qualitative and quantitative analyses

L. A. Maciaszek et al. (Eds.): ICT4AWE 2021/2022, CCIS 1856, pp. 273–295, 2023.
https://doi.org/10.1007/978-3-031-37496-8_15

1 Background

First, the theoretical and empirical background is presented, starting with the motivation to use telemedical applications, followed by the current state on telemedical applications as well as insights regarding empirical technology acceptance research. Based on that, the underlying research project is introduced. Focusing on a social communication science perspective, the two-step empirical approach of this study, its specific research aims, and the underlying research questions are described.

1.1 Motivation

Previous research identified that 20% of nursing home residents are hospitalized once a year, and from these hospitalizations 40% turn out to be premature or even unnecessary [1, 2]. Apart from stressful emotional components, hospital admissions can even cause harm to this vulnerable group of patients, causing for instance deteriorations of health due to delirium. Moreover, when a resident of a nursing facility is taken to an emergency room for an acute medical situation that could have been treated by a general practitioner, the resident joins the ranks of other patients whose reasons for visiting the emergency room can often be more urgent and critical. Long waiting times in an unfamiliar environment, such as stays in the emergency room or in hospitals in general, often trigger delirium – in particular related to patients with dementia. It is not unusual for nursing home residents to spend weeks recovering from the rigors of a short stay in an emergency room. In cases where delirium occurs, for example, it is even likely that a higher level of dependency will persists due to the underlying frailty [3]. So far, the primary reasons of these so called "ambulatory-care sensitive conditions" are not finally clarified. As this effect can be observed especially outside the regular consultation hours of general practitioners and combined with an increasing workload of the care personnel in the facilities (i.e., shortage of care providers during night shifts), suboptimal outpatient medical care of nursing home residents often seems to be responsible for this situation.

Precisely at this point, the Optimal@NRW project aims at support and relief for the residents and staff of nursing facilities offering telemedical acute care 24/7. The idea is to provide technology for telemedical consultations as well as an early warning system implemented in 25 participating senior care facilities. The overall goal of the project lies in preventing nursing residents from unnecessary hospital admissions. Thereby, the usage of an early warning system aims at the preventive counteracting of a potential health deterioration, running regular non-invasive measurements of vital parameters. Beyond the technical infrastructure itself, the aim is to link the data of the patients with the nursing home documentation system via interfaces. This way, every physician who is not familiar with the patient's disease history has access to the relevant preliminary medical information and, in turn, is able to document on the acute telemedical setting and therapy in a way that is visible to other therapists and the general practitioner. Here, it needs to be emphasized that this approach does not aim at a substitution of personal doctor-patient interaction by telemedicine, but it rather aims at supplementing standard medical care, in particular related to situations in which hospital admissions are the only option left. Moreover, positive economic side effects can be assumed by a reduction in hospitalizations and ambulance transports.

1.2 Telemedical Applications

Developments in the field of innovative digital applications offer the opportunity to address the main challenges in healthcare, i.e., high numbers of older individuals with long-term care needs, shortages of medical personnel, and a lack of financial resources [4, 5]. Combining the advantages and the potential of Internet as well as sensor-based innovations and ambient technologies enable the conceptualization and design of specific monitoring concepts being applied in hospitals, private settings, and nursing institutions. In recent years, the value of information and communication technologies (ICT) as well as their socioeconomic benefits in healthcare were highly acknowledged [6]. According to this, also efforts in the design and development of eHealth and telemedical applications have been immensely accelerated: in the field of telemedicine, applications addressing doctor-patient communication but also applications for the communication between medical professionals, i.e., tele-intensive care [7] or tele-emergency care [8, 9], have been focused. Supporting current developments in research and industry, diverse telemedicine and eHealth approaches are funded in terms of national and international research projects. The EU-project PAAL (Privacy-Aware and Acceptable Lifelogging services for older and frail people) represents one international example that aimed at the development and combination of diverse video-, sensor-, and speech-based systems supporting older and frail people in their everyday lives [10]. Another project AIDA focused on medical care of residents in nursing homes and aimed at a preparation of nursing facilities for using telemedicine to ensure adequate care for geriatric patients [11].

So far, the potential and purposes of such research projects are promising. However, a concrete transfer of the project phases into the standard care of the national health insurance funds is still difficult and has not yet occurred. Beyond financial difficulties, especially the acceptance of all involved stakeholders (i.e., patients/nursing home residents, their treating physicians, and their care personnel) poses an important prerequisite for a successful and sustainable rollout of innovative technical concepts such as telemedical consultations being applied in nursing homes.

1.3 Technology Perception and Acceptance Research

In accordance with the increasing technical advances in the development of innovative digital applications, approaches referring to technology acceptance research have rapidly grown in the last decades. Initially, and differentiating between acceptance subjects, objects, and contexts [12], technology acceptance has been researched based on established acceptance models like TAM [13] and further model developments and adaptions such as UTAUT [14]. These models were reduced to the adoption of ICT in the working context and identified in particular two relevant parameters as good predictors for the behavioral intention to use a specific technical application: the perceived ease of use and perceived usefulness. Till today, these models are frequently applied and usually adapted to different contexts (for an overview see [15]).

Beyond these well-established models and especially in early project or technology development phases, acceptance research is often challenged by the fact that it relates to areas that have not been researched before: here, it is required that the status quo is identified first. At the beginning of the project, when interaction with technical applications has not yet started and only theoretical deliberations were made, adequate explorative approaches are needed, especially in such sensitive context as nursing home environments. In a first step, qualitative and scenario-based approaches are one suitable measure to gain insights into the respective stakeholders' associations and to identify existing mental models, perceived (dis)advantages, needs, wishes, and the requirements of using specific applications in a specific context.

1.4   Project Context: Optimal@NRW

Although telemedicine approaches are promising to tackle the described healthcare challenges, there are no solutions so far that either realized a concrete transfer of the approaches to standard care of the national health insurance nor have been rolled out large-scale. Connecting to the efforts of the AIDA project [11], central tasks for future research lie in the implementation and standardization of telemedical processes, the proof of medical evidence, analyzing ways of cost coverage by the health insurance companies as well as the investigation of acceptance of the involved stakeholders. All these steps are relevant and necessary in order to enable a sustainable and widespread use of telemedical care in nursing homes. The project Optimal@NRW realizes these tasks, representing a new intersectoral approach to provide acute care and support for geriatric patients based on the integration of telemedical consultation systems in 25 nursing homes within the region of Aachen in Germany. In particular, the major aim of the project lies in the avoidance and reduction of inadequate hospital admissions in ambulatory care-sensitive hospital cases [2] as well as improved medical care in nursing homes. Thereby, a central emergency number acts as a virtual hub for the care of geriatric patients. Here, it is the idea of the project that the participating nursing homes firstly contact the doctor's call center in case of medical problems or acute situations. Then, the call center is responsible for an initial medical assessment, and has to decide about the case's urgency and following treatments. When the general practitioner is not available, or if the call from the nursing home is received outside the opening hours of the general practitioner, the physicians of the resident health service are contacted to provide a visit. If timely contact cannot be guaranteed (neither by the general practitioner nor the resident health service), telemedical consultations by the tele-physicians can be carried out at any time.

Besides medical research and evaluation of the efficacy of the implemented structure and processes, the project is also accompanied by a social communication science perspective and respective research approaches. In more detail, user-related acceptance is investigated focusing on the perceptions, requirements, and wishes of the relevant stakeholders – in particular, the residents of nursing homes and their care personnel. Due to the fact that in nursing homes especially the actions and opinions of the care personnel determine whether new structures and process are applied in the professional everyday life, it is precisely the perspective of this specific user group that has to be considered, analyzed, and understood throughout and within the entire project. This way, central perceived barriers, concerns, and requirements especially of these relevant stakeholders can be timely identified. This early identification enables in turn iterative technical and/or medical adaptions of the telemedical infrastructure and processes.

Overall, three phases of the project have to be distinguished: pre-implementation, implementation, and post-implementation. During the pre- and post-implementation phases relevant parameters, processes, and structures can be identified directly at the beginning of the project, and offer the opportunity for comparisons of perceptions and acceptance patterns with regard to the usage of the telemedical infrastructure over the whole project period. In each of the three phases, technology acceptance and perception are investigated, applying multi-faceted empirical approaches consisting of qualitative interview and quantitative survey studies. In addition, the implementation phase enables to evaluate interactions with the telemedical infrastructure in the participating nursing homes, thus in real and not in scenario-based or laboratory settings. The entire project, including the individual studies of the different project partners, was reviewed and approved by the Ethics Committee at the RWTH Aachen Faculty of Medicine.

This paper presents first results from an initial qualitative interview study, identifying the wishes, needs, concerns, and requirements of the two most relevant user groups, the geriatric patients and their care personnel, prior to the real use of the telemedical consultations. In a second step, results of a first subsequent quantitative study with professional caregivers are presented to provide first insights regarding a quantification and validation of the previously identified acceptance-relevant parameters.

2 Empirical Concept

From the perspective of social communication science, the project aims at the understanding and identification of acceptance-relevant parameters of the telemedical consultations in nursing homes.

The present study describes the results of interviews with geriatric patients and care personnel from different nursing homes within the pre-implementation phase in a first step. Hence, the identification of opinions, attitudes, requirements, and wishes is focused prior to first interactions with the telemedical infrastructure. The qualitative approach as a first step was necessary to enable subsequent quantifications and weightings of the identified acceptance parameters. In a second step, the identified parameters were quantified and validated in an online survey. Beyond that, the investigation in the initial phase of the project provides a baseline for the comparisons of acceptance and the identification of impacting parameters in later project phases. The underlying research questions for this qualitative study were the following:

- RQ1a: How do geriatric patients and care personnel in nursing homes generally perceive telemedical consultations in emergency situations?
- RQ2a: Which benefits related to telemedical consultations in emergency situations do geriatric patients and care personnel perceive in nursing homes?
- RQ3a: Which barriers and concerns related to telemedical consultations in emergency situations do geriatric patients and care personnel perceive in nursing homes?
- RQ4a: Which requirements related to telemedical consultations in emergency situations are relevant for geriatric patients and care personnel in nursing homes?

Using the results of the initial interview study, a survey was conceptualized focusing on all identified acceptance-relevant parameters, addressing the professional caregivers of the participating nursing homes aiming for a quantification and validation of the previously identified parameters. Based on the mentioned two-step empirical concept, the specific underlying research questions for the subsequent quantitative study were the following:

- RQ1b: How do geriatric patients and care personnel evaluate their intention to use telemedical consultations in emergency situations in nursing homes?
- RQ2b: Which benefits are most relevant for geriatric patients and care personnel related to telemedical consultations in emergency situations in nursing homes?
- RQ3b: Which barriers and concerns are most relevant for geriatric patients and care personnel related to telemedical consultations in emergency situations in nursing homes?
- RQ4b: Which requirements are most relevant for geriatric patients and care personnel related to telemedical consultations in emergency situations in nursing homes?

3 Study I: Qualitative Interview Study

Within this section, the empirical procedure, including the structure and the specific contents of the interview study as well as the characteristics of the interview participants are presented.

3.1 Procedure and Structure of the Interview Study

Within the first part of the interviews, we introduced the participants to the overall project goal and lined out the content of the study. Subsequently, they provided their consent to the participation in the interview and their agreement with audio recordings. At the beginning, we asked the participants for some personal information, i.e., their age and gender. The participating nursing home residents also reported about their health situation as well as about their experiences and feelings connected to the life in the current nursing facility. In line with this, we asked the care personnel about their general professional experience in caring for geriatric patients and specifically related to the current professional everyday life in the specific nursing home. As a thematic transition to the topic of the project, we interviewed both groups of participants about their experiences with emergency situations in nursing homes: thereby, the participants described real past situations, existing processes, and potential difficulties. Subsequently, we provided a short descriptive scenario to the participants, explaining the concept of telemedical consultations in nursing homes (translated version, [16]):

"In the Optimal@NRW project, telemedical technology is being introduced and tested in various nursing homes in the region of Aachen. Once introduced, it will be possible for the on-site care personnel to request support in emergency situations via the central emergency number (116117) of the Association of Statutory Health Insurance Physicians. The trained staff at the center will decide whether the specific case is suitable for teleconsultation or whether another step must be taken.

If the requirements for a teleconsultation are met, a wheeled stand equipped with a camera, monitor, microphone, and specific medical technology equipment (for measuring blood pressure, oxygen saturation, pulse, and temperature) is pushed into the patient's room. Then, a specialist is available in a time period of maximum 10 minutes. The physician can communicate live with the patient and the care personnel and view the electronic patient file. Once the patient's medical history has been taken, the telemedicine specialist decides on the next course of action. If necessary, he or she can, for example, order the deployment of a specially trained mobile nurse to the nursing home, who can then carry out interventions on site, such as changing a catheter. Actions such as these can prevent a resident from being rushed to hospital, instead of being able to remain in their familiar environment. At the same time, long waiting times for the difficult-to-reach general practitioners or specialists should be avoided."

Following the scenario, we asked the participants to describe their first impressions related to the question if they can imagine using (or agree with) telemedical consultations in emergency situations in their respective nursing home. Further, we asked the participants if they associate potential advantages with the usage of telemedical consultations in their nursing home. In accordance with that, we also asked if they associate and connect potential concerns or barriers with using telemedical consultations in emergency situations. In the last part of the interview, we asked the participating nursing home residents and care personnel which specific wishes, needs, and requirements are important for them and should be addressed when the telemedical consultations are conceptualized, designed, and finally planned to be implemented in their nursing home. Finally, we gave the participants the opportunity to comment and give feedback on the topic or the interview itself, or to ask specific questions about the project.

Subsequent to the interviews, we transcribed the recorded audio files literally and analyzed them by means of qualitative content analysis [17]. In more detail, a deductive system of categories was derived for the data analysis based on the literature-driven interview guide. This deductive system of categories was then iteratively supplemented with inductive categories based on an analysis of the data material. The quotations were coded independently by the authors and indisputable quotations were included in the category system.

3.2 Characteristics of the Interviewed Persons

In the interview study, N = 28 participants took part (for details, see Fig. 1) of which 16 persons belonged to the care personnel, 11 persons were nursing home residents, and one person was an accompanying family member.

Starting with the care personnel, the participants were on average 40.4 years old (SD = 13.4) and most of them were female (n = 14). With more than 10 years of professional experience, the majority of this group reported to have a long-term experience in care; five participants indicated 1–5 years of professional care experience. The participating caregivers described to do their job with conviction and expressed satisfaction with their profession. In contrast, they also highlighted the intense burden in their everyday professional activities, in particular due to a lack of personnel and resulting time restrictions. As further relevant aspects, they pronounced a high individualism of the needs of their patients and that no two days are alike within their professional life.

As all residents of the participating nursing homes suffered from at least one chronic disease (see Fig. 1), we call this group of participants "geriatric patients" in this study. The mean age of the geriatric patients was 76.2 years (SD = 12.8), whereas the youngest person was 55 and the oldest 94 years. The majority of the participants was female (75%). With a mean of 8.5 years (SD = 6.0) the participants lived on average comparably long in the nursing homes. Among the reported chronic conditions were chronic diabetes, paralyses, chronic obstructive pulmonary disease (COPD), or cardiovascular diseases (CVD).

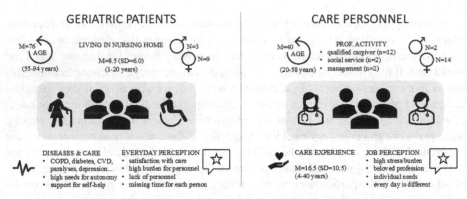

Fig. 1. Characteristics of the interviewees [16].

All geriatric patients reported that they were supported in their everyday life: thereby, the patients and their care personnel aim at a support for self-help and assistance in being as independent and autonomous as possible. Focusing on their living in the nursing home, the participants were on average satisfied with care and the respective care personnel. As opposed to that, the patients emphasized the high workload of the caregivers due to the lack of personnel and described also the resulting lack of time for the individual interaction (in particular, for social contact, conversations, etc.).

Discussing previous experiences with emergency situations, participants of both groups described that acute medical situations occur on a regular basis, and they stressed too long waiting times for physicians on call. In addition, the interviewees described that these circumstances frequently lead to hospital admissions, which in turn result in burden and frequent health deteriorations for the patients. Some of the participants highlighted that something must fundamentally change regarding healthcare supply and the underlying processes in nursing facilities in Germany.

3.3 Results of the Interview Study

In the following, key insights of the interview study are presented guided by the previously introduced research questions (RQ1a-RQ4a, see [16]).

General Perception of Telemedical Consultations (RQ1a). The telemedical consultations in emergency situations in nursing homes were generally positively perceived by both interview groups.

The participating care personnel evaluated the telemedical consultations to be a useful and beneficial approach. All of them intended to use telemedical consultations and they also appreciated the implementation of the telemedical care infrastructure within their nursing home. Only one of the participants added a skeptical comment regarding the accessibility and interaction with the telemedical physicians (see RQ3a). Moving to the perspectives of the geriatric patients, all of them showed a positive attitude towards the use of telemedical consultations in medically uncertain situations in their nursing home. Despite the overall positive perception, two of the respondents were also skeptical about the implementation of the technology in their everyday life and the potential resulting technical problems (see RQ3a). Nevertheless, all participating geriatric patients could easily imagine to use telemedicine in their nursing home. Further, they immediately started to weigh possible advantages against potential barriers and concerns.

Identification of Perceived Benefits (RQ2a). During the interviews, the participants overall mentioned 21 aspects referring to potential advantages of, and motives to, use telemedical consultations in their nursing home. As 13 of the 21 benefits were mentioned and discussed by at least two of the participants, these 13 perceived benefits were divided into three categories, namely the **general**, **patient-related**, and **personnel-related benefits** (see Table 1).

Table 1. Perceived benefits and their categories identified in the interview study [16].

Patient	Faster help in an emergency
	Shorter waiting times for medical treatment
	Avoidance of hospital admission or stay
	Avoidance of transport to the hospital
	Avoidance of stress and deterioration of health
Personnel	Reducing the workload of caregivers
	Quick decisions at the nursing homes
	Increase of safety for caregivers through medical decisions
	Flexibility in time and place
General	Higher sense of security
	Improved sense of care
	Improved doctor-patient communication
	Use of innovative technologies in care

Considering the category **general benefits,** the participants described that using telemedical consultations would give them a *higher sense of security* as faster advice of medical experts is enabled: *"It simply gives you more safety and a better feeling"* (Personnel, female, 24). Moreover, an *improved sense of care* as well as an *improved doctor-patient-communication* was associated with using telemedical consultations in the nursing homes: *"Maybe it will make residents feel better about the care they receive – here, in the nursing home, but also in conversations with physicians"* (Personnel, female, 34). As a last aspect in this category, it was also discussed that *the use of innovative technologies in care* is beneficial in order *"to move away from old and conventional conditions more and more"* (Personnel, female, 50 years).

Moving to the second category including **personnel-related benefits,** the geriatric patients described the expectation that using telemedical consultations would contribute to *reducing the workload of caregivers* and enable *flexibility in time and place:* *"It would be easier for and reduce efforts of, the care personnel, because it would be faster and they would be more flexible"* (Patient, female, 84). The participating care personnel pronounced the benefit of *quick decisions at the nursing homes* and explained that fast contact to medical experts would lead to an *increase of safety for caregivers though medical decisions:* *"In the future, it may bring relief in care, because responsibility can be handed over; when a doctor deals with it directly (without waiting time), the doctor takes responsibility and the decision"* (Personnel, female, 50).

Within the third category referring to **patient-related benefits,** the participants expressed the expectation that the use of telemedical consultations enables *faster help in emergencies* and *shorter waiting times for medical treatment.* The following two statements show that these aspects were relevant for the patients as well as the care personnel: *"Decisions are made here on site and, above all, help can be provided quickly"* (Patient, male, 84) and *"If a telemedical consultation would be guaranteed within 10 min, this would be so great and so much faster than calling a doctor and he had to come here first. Usually, we have been waiting many times longer"* (Personnel, male, 33). As a further very relevant aspect, more than half of the participants mentioned the *reduction* and *avoidance of hospital admissions or stays* as well as *avoidance of transport to the hospital* as relevant motives to use telemedicine in nursing homes. The following exemplary statement illustrates the relevance of these two beneficial aspects:

"Sometimes they lie in the emergency room for 6 h and then come back again – this could be avoided, and the residents could be spared the whole procedure (i.e., transport, stay). Especially for residents with dementia, or other cognitive impairments, staying in the facility is certainly always best" (Personnel, female, 26). In accordance with that, interviewees of both groups mentioned the *avoidance of stress and deterioration of health* and emphasized that reduced or avoided hospitalizations contribute to the wellbeing of the residents in nursing homes: *"Of course, I think that would save a lot of stress and health deterioration for our residents"* (Personnel, female, 58).

Identification of Perceived Barriers (RQ3a): The participants mentioned 15 different aspects related to perceived barriers and concerns when telemedical consultations are used in nursing homes. From these, 14 aspects were discussed by at least two participants. Therefore, these 14 potential barriers and concerns were classified into four categories related to **communicative, technological, handling,** as well as **data** management and **privacy concerns** (Table 2).

Table 2. Perceived barriers and their categories identified in the interview study [16].

Communicative concerns	Impersonal/Indirect Contact
	Distance to physicians providing treatment
	Inconvenient communication of complaints
	Lack of understanding of physicians due to the distance
Technological concerns	Immature, possibly deterrent technology
	Physicians not easy to understand
	Physicians not easy to recognize
	Technical failures (e.g., WLAN)
	Technical errors (e.g., pixelated display)
Handling concerns	Errors in operation (e.g., physicians, care personnel)
	Lack of availability of trained personnel
	Overstraining of care personnel
Data and Privacy Concerns	Insecure data transmission
	Invasion of privacy

The first category included **communicative concerns:** here, the participants described the concern of *impersonal or indirect contact* and thereby a feared *distance to the physicians providing treatment.* Two exemplary statements show that these concerns were relevant for the care personnel as well as the patients: *"It is just not face-to-face communication. Due to the distance, there is already the danger that the personality of the patient is not perceived in its entirety"* (Personnel, female, 50) and *"I am concerned that the doctor may not understand me (as usual), because he is less close"* (Patient, female, 82). In line with this, some of the participating patients indicated concerns that due to the distance *health complaints could be communicated inconveniently* by using telemedical consultations: *"I doubt whether I can describe it exactly how I feel, what I have and that it doesn't come across right if I say, for example, 'it's pressing there'"* (Patient, female, 82). Accordingly, both groups of participants described the concern of *a lack of understanding of the physicians due to the distance.*

Moving to the second barrier category including **technological concerns,** some participants of the care personnel indicated the concern that the *technology may have an immature, deterrent effect* on the patients; this was in particular mentioned focusing on patients suffering from dementia or other comparable cognitive impairments: *"For cognitively impaired residents in particular, the new equipment and also the conversation with the doctor via a monitor could have an initially deterrent effect"* (Personnel, female, 20). In addition, some of the geriatric patients described concerns that *the physicians are not easy to understand* and *not easy to recognize* within the telemedical consultations. In accordance with that, the greatest and most frequently mentioned concerns focused on specific technical problems. Here, specifically *technical failures (e.g., WLAN interruptions)* based on the infrastructure in the nursing homes and *technical errors (e.g., pixelated display)* referred to data transmission and the Internet connection were discussed: *"But if you have got a data connection that doesn't work before, which is pixelated, that you don't see the person properly like on TV, if it's raining, you've got the pixels. It could happen. And then you think, you're lying there, you want to tell him something, you can't see him properly and you think, does this have to be now? Why is that not possible and he should help me?"* (Relative of a patient, female, 57).

A further category of perceived barriers referred to **handling concerns**. Patients and care personnel expressed concerns about *errors in the operation* of the telemedical consultations – including potential errors on the side of the *physicians,* but also on the side of the responsible *care personnel: "I'm concerned that it won't work properly or much more that there won't be a person around to operate it properly"* (Patient, female, 82). Furthermore, most of the participating care personnel expressed concerns regarding a *lack of availability of trained personnel:* this was caused by previous experiences that new systems can often only be operated by one or a few trained colleagues in a nursing home, who are not always available on site. In accordance with that, some participants of the care personnel also feared an *overstraining of the care personnel* regarding the processes in interaction with the new technologies in particular at the beginning: *"And I think, depending on which caregiver colleague you have, it could be an overload. Because they're not used to it, it has to settle in [...]. They're nervous then thinking 'am I doing something wrong'?"* (Personnel, female, 58).

Finally, the last barrier category included **data and privacy concerns**. Within this category, a potential *insecure data transmission* and an *invasion of privacy* was mentioned. Here, it was striking that these well-known barriers in the field of other health-related technologies (e.g., [18]) were only sporadically mentioned by the participants of the present study focusing on using telemedical consultations.

Identification of Relevant Needs and Requirements (RQ4a): The participants mentioned overall 25 different aspects referred to specific needs and requirements. As 14 of these aspects were discussed by several participants, these aspects were subsequently classified in four categories, namely **introduction and training, trust-related conditions, technology-related conditions,** and **interaction with physicians** (Table 3).

Starting with the first category including aspects referred to **introduction and training**, almost all participants belonging to the care personnel emphasized the relevance of a *detailed technical introduction* as well as *regular technical trainings* on how to use the telemedical consultations correctly and how to behave in such situations adequately. In line with this, some participants also expressed to desire a *refreshment of specific medical trainings: "So in any case, a good introduction to the equipment must take place and not only once, but also repeatedly. That you are first of all well accompanied. That would be important"* (Personnel, female, 34).

Trust-related requirements characterized the second category of needs and requirements. Participants of both groups stressed that the *availability of trained staff* is a precondition for trust: *"There must be trained personnel and the technology must be operated 100%, of course everything must also fit technically"* (Relative of a patient, female,

Table 3. Identified need/requirements and their categories [16].

Introduction and training	Detailed technical introduction for staff
	Regular technical training for staff
	Refreshment of specific medical trainings for staff (e.g., medical parameters)
Trust	Availability of trained staff
	Trust in tele-physicians
	Ensure data privacy/system security
	Trust in the technology
Technology	Creation of technical requirements/ infrastructure (e.g., reliable WLAN)
	Appearance/design of technology
	Technical support and maintenance
Interaction with physicians	Tele-physicians must have enough time for consultations
	Understanding of tele-physicians for age-typical clinical pictures
	Empathy of the tele-physicians for the situation of the residents
	Patience of tele-physicians for residents and needs

57). In this regard, *trust in the technology* as well as *trust in the respective tele-physicians* were discussed to be relevant conditions as well. In comparison, the requirements of ensuring *data privacy and system security* were only occasionally mentioned.

Within the third category, **technology-related requirements** were focused. Here, the participants stressed that in particular the *technical infrastructure has to be created* and ensured. In more detail, most of these comments referred to the often poor WLAN connection in the nursing homes. In addition, the participants desired *technical support and maintenance* not only in the beginning but also continuously during the use of the telemedical consultations. Furthermore, participants of both groups discussed the *appearance and design* of the wheeled stand to be an important factor: here, it was highlighted that new technologies can have a deterrent effect, in particular to patients suffering from dementia. Therefore, the participants recommended to focus on unobtrusive and well-known designs.

The last category **interaction with physicians** included aspects mostly referring to the indirect contact between patients and treating tele-physicians. Based on partly negative previous experiences with physicians on call, the geriatric patients emphasized the necessity that the *tele-physicians must have enough time for the consultations* and *empathy for the residents' situations*: "Above all, it needs empathetic physicians who have time and act in the will and support of the residents" (Patient, female, 87). This requirement was specified by some comments of care personnel participants, adding that the tele-physicians should bring along *patience for the residents and their needs*: "*The physicians must have time for residents within the consultations, they must be skilled with geriatric-psychiatric residents and they have to take both, residents and their* *needs as well as the caregivers, seriously"* (Personnel, female, 55). Moreover, the care personnel participants stressed the importance of *an understanding of the tele-physicians for age-typical clinical pictures.*

4 Study II: Quantitative Survey Study

In the following, the empirical approach of the subsequent quantitative study is presented, starting with the concept and the structure of the applied survey. Then, the characteristics of the survey participants are described, followed by the presentation of the quantitative results.

4.1 Conception and the Structure of the Survey

Based on the interview study's results, we conceptualized in the next step the quantitative study in form of a survey. In order to keep the survey within a tolerable and reasonable extent, a compromise had to be found between including the identified categories (but not all identified single aspects) and reducing the length and complexity for the participants. As the group of care personnel represents the most decisive stakeholder when it comes to the decision, if a new technology or innovation is sustainably applied in such a sensible context as a nursing home, the quantitative study aimed at reaching a broad sample of care personnel across the participating nursing homes within the project. The geriatric patients were not addressed as the participation in the survey was too demanding and for the most part of them not feasible. In the following phases of the project and the subsequent studies, this sensible user group is therefore still to be addressed.

The survey started with a welcome of the participants and a short introduction into the topic. Subsequently, the participants were asked for some personal information, e.g., their age, gender, and educational level. Then the participants were asked to assess their state of health (answer options: min = 1 = "very bad"; max = 6 = "very well") and report whether they suffer from a chronic disease (answer options: yes/no). Considering private previous experience in care, the participants indicated if they have been the caregiver for a close family member (answer options: yes/no). Addressing their professional experience, the participants indicated the duration of working in their (current) institution (answer options: <1 year, 1–3 years, 5–10 years, >10 years) and they shortly described their current occupation (open comment field).

In a second part of the survey, the concept of telemedical consultations was explained to the participants using a descriptive scenario (based on the scenario in Sect. 3.1) in addition to an illustration of the technical equipment.

Subsequent to this information, the participants evaluated their *Attitude towards Telemedical Consultations* measured by 3 items (Cronbach's α = .96) as well as their *Intention to use Telemedical Consultations* also measured by 3 items (Cronbach's α = .79). All single items of these and the following constructs were assessed on six-point Likert scales (min = 1 = "I strongly disagree"; max = 6 = "I strongly agree") and are presented in Fig. 2. Based on the identified perceived benefits of using telemedical consultations (see Table 1), 10 relevant items were selected covering the three categories of benefits. Thus, the participants evaluated the *Perceived Benefits* of using telemedical consultations based on 10 items (Cronbach's α = .95). All these single items are presented in Fig. 3. Considering the perceived barriers of using telemedical consultations (see Table 2), again 10 relevant items were selected covering the four previously identified categories of barriers. Therefore, the participants assessed the *Perceived Barriers* of using telemedical consultations based on 10 items as well (Cronbach's α = .92). All these single items are presented in Fig. 4. In accordance with the perceived benefits and barriers, the needs and requirements of using telemedical consultations were also operationalized based on the previously identified factors (see Table 3). Here, 11 relevant items were selected covering the four categories of needs and requirements. The participants evaluated the *Needs and Requirements* based on 11 items (Cronbach's α = .96) and all items are presented in Fig. 5. At the end of the survey, the participants had the opportunity to provide feedback to the survey and the project on an optional basis.

4.2 Characteristics of the Survey's Participants

The survey was made available both online and as a paper-and-pencil version in the time period from November 2021 to January 2022. Overall, N = 145 participants from 12 different nursing homes took part in the study. Partly, the surveys were not filled out completely. However, to acknowledge the effort and time spent on their participation—despite the burden of caregiving—all participants were included in the analysis. However, this is the reason for the varying reported number of responses.

The mean age of the participants was 38.2 years (SD = 1.25; min = 19; max = 65) and the majority (73.9%) was female (22.5% male, 3.5% diverse). The majority of the sample indicated to live together with at least one other person (42.0%), or with several persons (40.6%), while a smaller proportion indicated to live alone (17.4%). Asked for their health status, most of the participants assessed their health status to be good (46.4%) or very good (21.0%), whereas 25.4% reported a rather good health status. Minorities of the respondents assessed their health as rather bad (5.8%) or bad (1.4%). In line with this, one third of the participants indicated to suffer from a chronic disease (30.9%). Asked for previous private experience in care, 31.7% of the participants confirmed to have a family member in need of care, while 60.6% indicated to have already been the caregiver for a family member in need of care. Asked for the duration of their professional experience in the current institution, the answers were very balanced: 23.7% worked less than 1 year, 28.9% between 1 and 3 years, 21.5% between 5 and 10 years, and 25.9% more than 10 years in the respective nursing home.

4.3 Results of Quantitative Study

Due to the varying numbers of answers provided, data was predominantly analyzed descriptively (means (M) and standard deviations (SD)). To analyze the relationships between the evaluated constructs, correlation and regression analyses were conducted.

Acceptance of Telemedical Consultations (RQ1b). Figure 2 shows the evaluations of the participants' *Attitude towards Telemedical Consultations* (M = 4.6; SD = 1.2) as well as their *Intention to use Telemedical Consultations* (M = 4.5; SD = 1.0), indicating

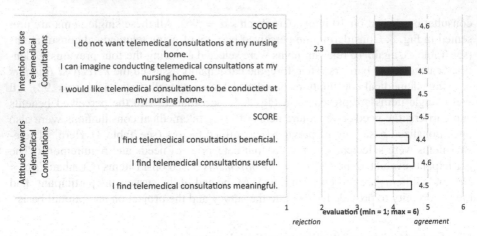

Fig. 2. Acceptance of using telemedical consultations in nursing homes (N = 131).

overall positive, affirming assessments. With regard to the *Attitude towards Telemedical Consultations* the three single items were evaluated similarly positively with means higher than the mean of the scale. Considering the *Intention to use Telemedical Consultations* both positive items received clear agreeing values above the mean of the scale. Instead, the negative item "I do not want telemedical consultations at my nursing home" was clearly rejected (M = 2.3; SD = 1.3).

Perceived Benefits (RQ2b). Figure 3 illustrates the quantitative evaluation of the *Perceived Benefits* (M = 4.5; SD = 1.0) of using telemedical consultations, which was overall quite positive. Starting with the **patient-related benefits**, all five items were assessed equally positive, e.g., "Avoiding transport to the hospital" (M = 4.7; SD = 1.1) or "faster help in case of emergencies" (M = 4.6; SD = 1.2). Moving to **personnel-related benefits**, "Increase of safety for caregivers through medical decisions" (M = 4.8; SD = 1.1) and "Quick decisions on site" (M = 4.7; SD = 1.0) were evaluated quite positive, while "Reducing the workload of caregivers" (M = 4.1; SD = 1.3) was less relevant, but still assessed rather positively. In comparison, the items referring to **general benefits** were assessed as less relevant, but still positively by the participants, e.g., "Improved sense of care" (M = 4.1; SD = 1.3).

Perceived Barriers (RQ3b). The evaluation of the *Perceived Barriers* (M = 3.7; SD = 1.0) is presented in Fig. 4 and was circulating around the mean of the scale.

Starting with the **communicative concerns**, "Indirect contact..." (M = 3.8; SD = 1.3) as well as a "Lack of understanding" (M = 3.6; SD = 1.3) were evaluated on a rather neutral level of values. Compared to that, **technological concerns** played a more relevant role and were evaluated more affirmatively, e.g., "Technical Failures (e.g., Wan)" (M = 4.3; SD = 1.4). With regard to **handling concerns**, concerns related to "Errors in operation" (M = 3.9; SD = 1.3) received slight agreements, while fears regarding an "Overstraining of care personnel" (M = 3.5; SD = 1.3) were evaluated neutrally. Finally, the results concerning **data and privacy concerns** revealed slight rejections of an "Insecure data transmission" (M = 3.4; SD = 1.2) and an "Invasion of privacy" (M

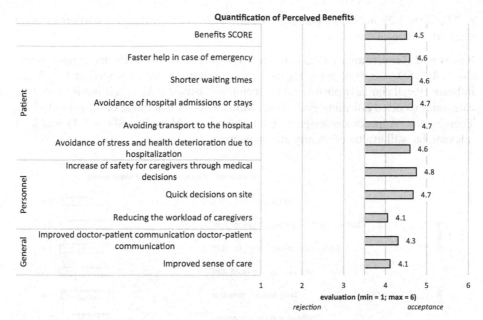

Fig. 3. Quantified perceived benefits of using telemedical consultations (N = 132).

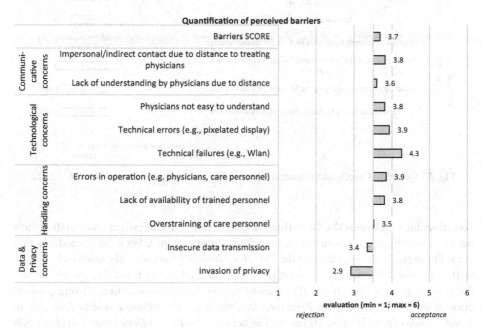

Fig. 4. Quantified perceived barriers of using telemedical consultations (N = 130).

= 2.9; SD = 1.2), indicating that these aspects do not represent severe barriers of using telemedical consultations.

Needs and Requirements (RQ4b). The evaluations of the *Needs and Requirements* (M = 4.9; SD = 0.9) of using telemedical consultations are presented in Fig. 5 and indicate overall similarly positive and agreeing assessments. All single items of the four categories received affirming evaluations within a very small range of means (4.6–5.0). Thereby, the "Appearance/design of the technology" (M = 4.6; SD = 1.1) was least relevant, but still evaluated clearly affirmatively.

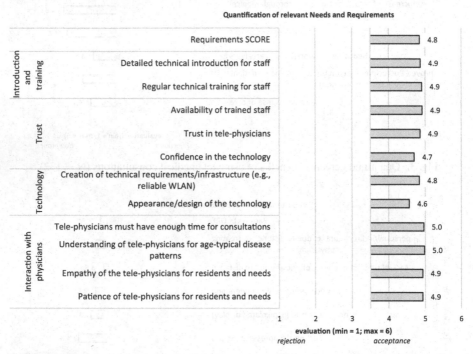

Fig. 5. Quantified needs and requirements of using telemedical consultations (N = 124).

Relationships Between the Investigated Constructs. To investigate the relationships between the investigated constructs, correlation analyses have been conducted in a first step. These analyses revealed that the *Perceived Benefits* were slightly negatively related to the *Perceived Barriers* ($\rho = -.19$; p < .05) and moderately related to the *Needs and Requirements* ($\rho = .48$; p < .01) of using telemedical consultations. Strong positive correlations resulted between *Perceived Benefits* and the *Attitude towards Telemedical Consultations* ($\rho = .70$; p < .01) as well as between *Perceived Benefits* and the *Intention to use Telemedical Consultations* ($\rho = .67$; p < .01). In terms of content, this means that the more beneficial care personnel in nursing facilities perceived the teleconsultation the higher was their attitude towards and their intention to use it. Interestingly, *Perceived Barriers* were only negatively related to the *Attitude towards Telemedical Consultations*

($\rho = -.20$; p < .05). The *Needs and Requirements* were moderately correlated with the *Attitude towards Telemedical Consultations* ($\rho = .43$; p < .01) as well as with the *Intention to use Telemedical Consultations* ($\rho = .46$; p < .01). Thus, the respondents' willingness to use telemedicine was clearly linked to perceptions of given requirements and needs in the nursing context. Furthermore, not surprising was the strong positive correlation between the *Attitude towards Telemedical Consultations* and the *Intention to Use Telemedical Consultations* ($\rho = .84$; p < .01) meaning that the more positive professional caregivers thought about telemedicine consultations, the more they wanted to use them.

In addition to the correlation analyses, regression analyses were calculated. The results in Fig. 6 demonstrate that 49.3% (adj. $r^2 = .493$) of the variance of the *Attitude towards Telemedical Consultations* can be explained by the constructs *Perceived Benefits* ($r = .76$; p < .01) as well as *Needs and Requirements* ($r = .20$; p < .01). Hence, *Perceived Benefits* and the *Needs and Requirements* represent the key predictors for the Attitude towards Telemedical Consultations. In a second step, the analyses revealed that 74.3% (adj. $r^2 = .743$) of the variance of the *Intention to use Telemedical Consultations* can be explained by the *Attitude towards Telemedical Consultations* ($r = .65$; p < .01). Therefore, the *Attitude towards Telemedical Consultations* represents the decisive predictor for the *Intention to use Telemedical Consultations*.

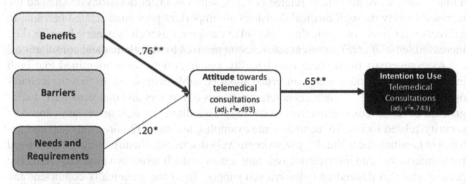

Fig. 6. Regression analyses: relationships between the constructs (N = 124).

5 Discussion

In the following, we discuss the key results of the qualitative interview study as well as the quantitative survey study. Subsequently, we present the limitations of the empirical procedure and ideas for future work.

5.1 Insights of the Empirical Approach

Our interview study and the respective results show that both investigated user groups, the geriatric patients and the care personnel, are open-minded and have overall positive attitudes towards using telemedical infrastructure in nursing homes. Our subsequent quantitative study quantified and validated these outcomes for the group of professional caregivers: the measurements clearly prove a positive attitude towards telemedical consultations as well a high intention to use telemedical consultations in nursing homes.

In line with previous research on technology acceptance in healthcare (e.g., [18, 19]), the evaluations, perceptions, and opinions are related to, and based on, the specific technology-, person-, and context-related benefits and barriers or concerns of using telemedical applications in nursing homes. Confirming previous findings, e.g., [20, 21], our results reveal that both investigated stakeholder groups differed in their priorities and depth of detail related to the perceived benefits and barriers.

In more detail, our interview study enables to identify concrete categories of perceived benefits (divided in general, personnel- and patient-related aspects) when telemedical consultations are used in acute situations in nursing homes. Giving an example, the participating geriatric patients mentioned rather generic benefits, such as a potential reduction of the care personnel's workload and thus a relief of the burden of their professional everyday life. Compared to that, the care personnel named the perceived benefits of the usage of telemedical consultations in nursing homes very precisely, i.e., faster decisions at the nursing homes and an increase of their safety through medical decisions enabled by the quick consultation of (tele-)medical experts. Beyond the identification of perceived benefits, our quantitative study focusing on professional caregivers revealed a high relevance of all patient-related benefits, whereas faster decisions on site and the increased safety through medical decisions are important personnel-related benefits. In a direct comparison, reducing the workload of caregivers as well as generic benefits (i.e., increased sense of care) represent less relevant motives to use telemedical consultations.

As counterpart to the perceived benefits, our interview study identified that both investigated user groups were concerned about possible disadvantages that the technology can bring along. Thereby, concrete categories of barriers and concerns were distinguished covering communicative, technology-, handling- as well as privacy- and data security-related facets. To mention some examples, technical requirements and competence in handling the technology were intensively discussed. Unsurprisingly, the demand for uninterrupted and interference-resistant access to the Internet is a major concern. The participants also desired an uninterrupted support from the technically competent and accordingly trained personnel. Other relevant concerns refer to the potential communication difficulties resulting from the distance to the treating tele-physicians. In addition to the identification of these barriers, the quantitative study provided knowledge about the relevance of the perceived barriers: technological concerns represented the most relevant barriers and played a decisive role for the acceptance of telemedical consultations, while communicative, handling, and most strikingly data and privacy concerns were considered less important.

Beyond the identified and quantified perceived benefits and barriers, our interview study also revealed specific relevant needs and requirements of using telemedical consultations and applications in nursing homes, covering the areas introduction and training, technology, interaction with physicians, and trust. Taking trust as an example and confirming previous research on trust as a prerequisite for technology acceptance in healthcare [22, 23], both investigated user groups differently prioritisized the needs and requirements. The participants required a proper technical training and an accessible technical support from a technically competent staff. Beyond that, an appropriate technological infrastructure was required in such care facilities in order to build trust in these novel ways of communication. As further relevant requirements, empathy, patience, and sensitivity for the situation of the nursing home's residents from the treating physicians were assessed as even more vital in the comparably indirect telemedical settings than in the direct doctor-patient interactions. Our quantitative study confirms the relevance of all identified needs and requirements by evaluations at a comparably high value level.

As a last aspect, our quantitative analyses provided insights into the relationships between the attitude towards and acceptance of telemedical consultations on the one, and the perception of benefits, barriers, needs and requirements on the other hand. Besides strong correlations between all discussed constructs, the results revealed that the attitude towards telemedical consultations can be predicted by the perception of benefits as well as the perception of needs and requirements. In addition, the intention to use telemedical consultations is predicted by the attitude towards telemedical consultations. Interestingly, according to outcomes benefits as well as needs and requirements were considered more relevant for the acceptance of telemedical consultations than the perceived barriers. These results provide a good basis for the communication and information concepts, but also for the implementation of, and interaction phases with the telemedical infrastructure. The high relevance of beneficial aspects as well as needs and requirements should be considered, and future users (patients and personnel) should be transparently informed about the technology. Thereby, the beneficial and requirement-related aspects should be explained in a comprehensible way. Although the perceived barriers were evaluated as less relevant, they should also be taken seriously and be considered in terms of transparent and clear explanations and information.

5.2 Limitations and Ideas for Future Research

A first limitation of the present research refers to the fact that the participants of both studies solely envisioned the use of the telemedical infrastructure having not real experiences with the technology at this time. Therefore, it is to assume that the attitudes, reported evaluations, and statements made could significantly differ from the actual use behavior [24]. In addition, so far we focused only on the perspectives of patients (qualitatively) and care personnel (qualitatively and quantitatively), however, the telemedical setting requires the triad between patient, care personnel, and treating physician. Thus, for a purposeful and trouble-free use of the telemedical consultations the perspective of treating physicians should be also appropriately addressed in the future research to uncover potential additional issues.

Based on the knowledge gained from both presented studies, concrete strategies for future research on the acceptance of telemedical applications can be derived. In addition to the scenario-based approaches, the different stakeholders' real interaction within the telemedical setting would provide convincing outcomes relevant to the implementation. Applying multi method approaches, which consist of observations, interviews, and surveys, seems to be most promising to get insights into the opinions, existing difficulties, and process flows depending on the respective user perspective, i.e., patient, care personnel, physician. Here, the consideration of all relevant stakeholders is highly recommended to do justice to the specific requirements and needs of each specific user group. Moreover, acceptance-related empirical studies should be iteratively performed in all relevant phases of the technology's development, implementation, and evaluation to enable comparisons (pre- and post-implementation) and allow user-centered adaptions /adjustments of the technical applications. In further steps, the in the project participating health insurers are involved in order to realize a sustainable integration of telemedical services in the health care system. Beyond that, the long-term optimization of data management should not be missed, and an appropriate privacy policy should be elaborated on the basis of the knowledge accumulated from these measures and our future empirical studies.

Acknowledgements. The authors thank all participants – residents and care personnel of the different nursing homes – for their patience and openness to share opinions on a novel technology approach in healthcare. Furthermore, the authors want to thank Anna Rohowsky for research assistance. Beyond that, the authors thank the Optimal@NRW research group. This work was funded by the German joint federal committee "Innovationsfond" (grant number: 01NVF19015).

References

1. Jacobs, K., Kuhlmey, A., Greß, S., Klauber, J., Schwinger, A.: Pflege-Report 2018: Qualität in der Pflege. [Care Report 2018: Quality in Care]. Springer Nature (2018)
2. Sundmacher, L., Fischbach, D., Schuettig, W., Naumann, C., Augustin, U., Faisst, C.: Which hospitalisations are ambulatory care-sensitive, to what degree, and how could the rates be reduced? Results of a group consensus study in Germany. Health Policy **119**(11), 1415–1423 (2015)
3. Theou, O., et al.: What do we know about frailty in the acute care setting? A scoping review. BMC Geriatr. **18**(1), 1–20 (2018)
4. Wootton, R., Craig, J., Patterson, V.: Introduction to Telemedicine. CRC Press (2017)
5. Cook, D.J., Augusto, J.C., Jakkula, V.R.: Ambient intelligence: technologies, applications, and opportunities. Pervasive Mob. Comput. **5**(4), 277–298 (2009)
6. Al-Shorbaji, N.: The world health assembly resolutions on eHealth: eHealth in support of universal health coverage. Methods Inf. Med. **52**(06), 463–466 (2013)
7. Amkreutz, J., Lenssen, R., Marx, G., Deisz, R., Eisert, A.: Medication safety in a German telemedicine centre: Implementation of a telepharmaceutical expert consultation in addition to existing tele-intensive care unit services. J. Telemed. Telecare **26**(1–2), 105–112 (2020)
8. Felzen, M., et al.: Utilization, safety, and technical performance of a telemedicine system for prehospital emergency care: observational study. J. Med. Internet Res. **21**(10), e14907 (2019)
9. Czaplik, M., et al.: Employment of telemedicine in emergency medicine. Methods Inf. Med. **53**(2), 99–107 (2014)
10. Flórez-Revuelta, F., Mihailidis, A., Ziefle, M., Colonna, L., Spinsante, S.: Privacy-aware and acceptable lifelogging services for older and frail people: the PAAL project. In: 2018 IEEE 8th International Conference on Consumer Electronics-Berlin (ICCE-Berlin), pp. 1–4. IEEE (2018)
11. Ohligs, M., Stocklassa, S., Rossaint, R., Czaplik, M., Follmann, A.: Employment of telemedicine in nursing homes: clinical requirement analysis, system development and first test results. Clin. Interv. Aging **15**, 1427 (2020)

12. Kollmann, T.: Akzeptanz innovativer Nutzungsgüter und Systeme: Konsequenzen für die Einführung von Telekommunikations- und Multimediasystemen. [Acceptance of innovative consumer goods and systems: consequences for the introduction of telecommunication and multimedia systems] Bd. 239. Springer (1998)

13. Davis, F.D.: Perceived usefulness, perceived ease of use, and user acceptance of information technology. MIS Q. 319–340 (1989)

14. Venkatesh, V., Morris, M.G., Davis, G.B., Davis, F.D.: User acceptance of information technology: toward a unified view. MIS Q. 425–478 (2003)

15. Rahimi, B., Nadri, H., Afshar, H.L., Timpka, T.: A systematic review of the technology acceptance model in health informatics. Appl. Clin. Inform. **9**(03), 604–634 (2018)

16. Offermann, J., Wilkowska, W., Schaar, A.K., Brokmann, J., Ziefle, M.: Needs, requirements, and technology acceptance using telemedical consultations in acute medical situations in nursing homes. In: Proceedings of the 8th International Conference on Information and Communication Technologies for Ageing Well and e-Health, pp. 105–116. SciTePress (2022)

17. Mayring, P.: Qualitative content analysis: theoretical foundation, basic procedures and software solution. Klagenfurt (2014). https://nbn-resolving.org/urn:nbn:de:0168-ssoar-395173

18. Peek, S.T., Wouters, E.J., Van Hoof, J., Luijkx, K.G., Boeije, H.R., Vrijhoef, H.J.: Factors influencing acceptance of technology for aging in place: a systematic review. Int. J. Med. Informatics **83**(4), 235–248 (2014)

19. Offermann-van Heek, J., Wilkowska, W., Brauner, P., Ziefle, M.: Guidelines for integrating social and ethical user requirements in lifelogging technology development. In: 4th International Conference on Information and Communication Technologies for Ageing Well and e-Health (ICT4AWE 2019), pp. 67–79 (2019)

20. Jaschinski, C., Allouch, S.B.: An extended view on benefits and barriers of ambient assisted living solutions. Int. J. Adv. Life Sci **7**(2), 40–50 (2015)

21. Offermann-van Heek, J., Ziefle, M.: They don't care about us! care personnel's perspectives on ambient assisted living technology usage: scenario-based survey study. JMIR Rehabil. Assist. Technol. **5**(2), e10424 (2018)

22. Montague, E.N., Winchester, W.W., III., Kleiner, B.M.: Trust in medical technology by patients and healthcare providers in obstetric work systems. Behav. Inf. Technol. **29**(5), 541–554 (2010)

23. Wilkowska, W., Ziefle, M.: Understanding trust in medical technologies. In: Proceedings of the 4th International Conference on Information and Communication Technologies for Ageing Well and e-Health (ICT4AWE 2018), pp. 62–73 (2018)

24. Ajzen, I., Fishbein, M.: Understanding Attitudes and Predicting Social Behavior. Prentice-Hall, Englewood Cliffs

Digital Health and e-health

Categorization of Health Determinants into an EHR Paradigm Based on HL7 FHIR

Athanasios Kiourtis[1]([⊠]), Argyro Mavrogiorgou[1], Spyridon Kleftakis[1], Dimosthenis Kyriazis[1], Francesco Torelli[2], Domenico Martino[2], and Antonio De Nigro[2]

[1] Department of Digital Systems, University of Piraeus, Piraeus, Greece
{kiourtis,margy,spiroskleft,dimos}@unipi.gr
[2] Engineering Ingegneria Informatica, SpA - R&D Laboratory, Rome, Italy
{Francesco.Torelli,Domenico.Martino,Antonio.Denigro}@eng.it

Abstract. Healthcare platforms are included in multiple domain-related systems which however produce and provide individual and unlinked data to other systems, with high heterogeneity among them. The concept of mapping data from healthcare platforms to other citizens' daily data could create advantages in identifying and finding better decisions, strategies or guidelines against multiple diseases. In detail, in the current environment where there exist multiple data sources producing hundreds of megabytes of data, the creation of a baseline that aggregates and correlates clinical information, avoiding uncertainties, is mandatory. The current paper presents a new Electronic Health Record (EHR) paradigm, the Holistic Health Records (HHRs), as a form of health records that aggregate data from multiple sources and can provide a complete overview of a citizen, containing several health determinants. This information may be produced by several platforms and devices, at different times of the patient's life, including data related to the daily activities, the social behavior, the vital signs, the personal examination, or the treatment of a citizen. Several standardization organisms define healthcare standards towards an interoperable healthcare ecosystem, with HL7 Fast Healthcare Interoperability Resources (FHIR) being the standard that best suits the purpose of the HHRs. Consequently, the HHRs and the models that finally construct this new EHR paradigm, are based on HL7 FHIR, including data related with the citizens' roles, the healthcare organizations, results deriving from diagnosis and clinical findings, as well as daily habits. The main goal of the HHR model is to facilitate and guarantee interoperability, being constructed based on existing FHIR libraries, having an additional goal to be also used as an independent component that can be tailored and adjusted for not only exchanging health data, but also categorizing it and classifying it into similar groups.

Keywords: CrowdHEALTH · HL7 FHIR · Holistic health records · Interoperability · Health determinants · Classification · Personalized healthcare

L. A. Maciaszek et al. (Eds.): ICT4AWE 2021/2022, CCIS 1856, pp. 299–323, 2023.
https://doi.org/10.1007/978-3-031-37496-8_16

1 Introduction

The evolution of services in healthcare creates a plethora of devices, platforms and frameworks that, one independently from the others, produce and provide information, data, and knowledge on the citizen's life [1]. The concept of mapping clinical information with other citizens' life data would create several advantages and benefits for better decision making and for identifying outcomes of prevention strategies, diseases, and efficiency of clinical pathways [2]. The challenge is to merge the data that is available for exploiting the advantages of community knowledge, by constructing the Holistic Health Records (HHRs), an extension of Electronic Health Records (EHRs), containing data of any type and category, that is relevant to a citizen's overall health (i.e. medical, nutritional, lifestyle, social care data, etc.). Despite that thousands of medical data models exist [3], these are targeting mainly on the integration of data from clinical trials. More general interoperability data models (e.g. OpenEHR [4], HL7 Fast Healthcare Interoperability Resources (HL7 FHIR) [5] are sufficiently general and extensible to cover multiple needs, but the latter do not promise a solution to heterogeneity, as through them it may be represented the same information using different data structures or different coding systems.

The data model of the HL7 FHIR is surrounded by many interoperability artefacts composed of a set of modular components called "resources". These represent discrete information units with specified purpose and target, describing the information that can be collected for each different type of clinical information. Currently, there exist several resources for constructing medical knowledge structuring from a patient, an adverse reaction, a procedure, and an observation, among many others. In the context of HL7 FHIR, the multiple types of resources can be categorized in six major categories: (a) Clinical: content of clinical record, (b) Identification: supporting entities involved in the care process, (c) Workflow: management of the healthcare process, (d) Financial: resources that support the billing and payment parts of FHIR, (e) Conformance: resources that manage specification, development and testing of FHIR solutions, and (f) Infrastructure: general functionality and resources for internal FHIR requirements. The overall content of the resources can be structured in formats such as XML, JSON or Turtle, allowing also additional formats. As a result, it can be obtained information structured based on the FHIR resource data model, and represented in one of these formats, resulting to information which can be interpretable by both humans and machines. Within this standard, 119 other resources (apart from the patient resource) are defined at different maturity levels. To this context, HL7 aims to define and limit the structures used for the exchange of clinical information.

Regarding the different coding systems, while a terminology can refer to several different things, in healthcare it is associated with the "language" used to code entries in Electronic Health Records (EHRs) [6] including LOINC [7], SNOMED-CT [8], ICD-10 [9], or ICD-9 [10], among others. Most people encounter medical terminologies at some point in their lives – whether it is as physicians, medical purchasers, or patients. In the world of EHRs, terminology is one of the key parts for achieving real interoperability between healthcare systems and integrating their data. For instance, in the case that it has to be sent information between two systems, for the data to be usable, these systems have to talk in the same language, meaning that the codes from one system must be interpretable and have compatibility with the codes from the other system. While combining data from multiple systems cannot be very hard, in the case that the coding systems cannot be mapped to one another, this leads to the creation of locked data [1]. Since there exist several standards, a lot of research is performed to link these vocabularies so that the movement from one to the other can be easier. To this end, there is work that has been done and is ongoing, such as mappings between ICD-9 and ICD-10, LOINC and CPT [11], or LOINC and SNOMED CT.

In this context, it should be noted that medical information is typically represented following some specific standards. The SNOMED-CT terminology is an ontology that defines (some) concepts, such as, some diseases in terms of their cause, the part of the body they affect and how they can be diagnosed. It also includes some food categories, sport categories or activities of daily living. The Open Biomedical Ontologies (OBO) consortium [12] is an initiative trying to integrate the multiple ontologies developed in the biomedical domain, which also includes ontologies formalizing patient medical care and EHRs. The International Classification of Functioning, Disability and Health (ICF) [13] is an ontology classifying health and health-related domains from a body perspective, a personal activities perspective and a societal perspective. It classifies according to the body structure (i.e. eye, ear, digestive systems, etc.), the body function (i.e. mental, voice, etc.), activities and participations and the environmental context. Thus, it contains medical categories as well as some social categories as part of the activities, participations, and environmental domains. All concepts are linked to the ICD code in the ICD terminology. The National Cancer Institute Thesaurus (NCIT) [14] is a reference thesaurus covering biomedical concepts and inter-concept relationships. As part of that, it also includes medical categories, categories for physical activities, social activities, and behavioural categories. However, a major problem is the success of using ontologies in many domains, as it leads to the development of many different not necessarily linked ontologies and taxonomies. This creates in practice the problem of interoperability, both at the taxonomic and the semantic levels. To overcome that problem, major effort is provided from initiatives, such as OBO and BioPortal [15]. It is also the motivation for the OntoHub [16] repository, which behind the scenes attempts to utilize alignment techniques from formal methods for the ontology domain. The Medical Subject Headings (MeSH) [17] is a vocabulary maintained by the US National Library of Medicine (NLM) [18]. It is a hierarchically organized terminology of biomedical information contained in NLM database, including MEDLINE®/PubMed® [19]. It is often combined information following the RxNorm [20], as well as the LOINC standard for medical laboratory observations. Therefore, the mere adoption of interoperability standards is not sufficient to query health data coming from various health data sources and systems, in a uniform, efficient, complete, and unambiguous way.

In this manuscript, it is presented the data integration approach in the form of HHRs that has been adopted by CrowdHEALTH [21]. CrowdHEALTH is a digital health-care system aiming to exploit big data techniques, applied to extended health records and collective health knowledge (i.e. clustered records), to evaluate healthcare gover-nance policies. One of the pillars of the CrowdHEALTH system is the development and exploitation of the HHRs. HHRs are intended to provide an integrated view of the patient, including all health determinants. Such health-related data may be produced by different human actors or systems, in different moments of a patient's life, and include both i) medical data, associated with regular patientcare or a part of a clinical program, and ii) non-medical data that may have an impact on the patient's health status. HHRs potentially include: (a) social and lifestyle data collected by either the patient or other individuals (e.g. family members, friends), (b) social care data collected from social care providers, (c) physiological and environmental data collected by medical devices and sensors, (d) clinical data coming from healthcare information systems and produced by healthcare professionals (e.g. primary care systems and electronic medical records), (e) laboratory medical data, and (f) nutrition data.

It should be mentioned that the overall work is an extension of our work in [22] where in the current manuscript, it has been given a better explanation of the combination among the HHR model and the most used Health Data models from International Standards. Furthermore, additional UML Conceptual models of the HHR models have been specified, regarding the modelling of information related with identifiers, activities, organizations, and conditions. Nevertheless, due to page limitations additional references are being provided for more models that are supported for the HHR modeling. To this end, regarding the evaluation and experimentation of this work, more information has been provided regarding the HHR manager library, splitting it into the explanation of the library per se and the HHR manager generator, where both of them aim to develop the corresponding models.

The rest of this document is structured as follows. Section 2 introduces similar data models and describes the HHR model, its goal and the approach followed to realize it, aiming at satisfying various data requirements, while Sect. 3 reports the experimentation, the evaluation and the development steps followed towards the creation of the HHR model, through an easily followed example. To this end, Sect. 4 includes an overall discussion of the current results, including our conclusions and next steps.

2   Method

2.1   Health Data Models from International Standards

HL7 FHIR

The data model of the HL7 FHIR [5] standard revolves around a series of interoperability artefacts composed of a set of modular components called "Resources". These resources are discrete information units with defined behavior and meaning and describe what information can be collected for each type of clinical information.

HL7 RIM

The HL7 Reference Information Model (RIM) [23] model is intended to be used as a reference for the creation of information models aimed at creating information storage systems of any situation related to the environment of health services, such as patient diagnoses, sanitary material, costs for treatments and information concerning the personnel of a health organization.

i2b2 CRC

The i2b2 Clinical Research Chart (CRC) [24] model is designed to store clinical trial data, medical records, and laboratory tests, as well as many other types of clinical information. Following an approach like HL7 RIM, the acts or facts in this case form the main element of this star model, forming a central table surrounded by other tables that provide additional dimensions.

OMOP CMD

The Observational Medical Outcomes Partnership Common Data Model [25] (OMOP CMD) is oriented to the analysis of disparate observational databases, having the objective of transforming data contained between these databases in a common format and as a common representation (terminologies, code systems, etc.). Once the data is transformed into a common format, this would allow for systematic analysis using an analytical standard library created specifically for that common format.

2.2 Main Principles of the HHR Model

The goal of the CrowdHEALTH personalized healthcare system is the development of a set of data analysis tools that can be applied to different use cases, possibly merging data coming from different contexts. Therefore, there is the need to define one integrated model for HHRs, both combining and tackling several points of the models defined in Sect. 2.1, to guarantee the possibility to apply these tools to all produced data. For these reasons, firstly the HHR model must represent in a consistent way all the data required by the specific use cases. Secondly, the model is intended to be a seed for future extensions including types of data that are not currently required but are considered likely to be used soon or are useful to exemplify how the model can be extended in the future. Thirdly, the model is defined using existing models as a reference, with the HL7 FHIR standard having been selected as the main reference for the definition of the HHR model. It should be noted that despite that the standard is still under development and can represent mainly clinical data, it already has the ability to represent data that is not necessarily clinical, such as information coming from environment sensors or related to the social behavior of the citizen. Moreover, due to the usage of the HL7 FHIR resources and the definition of a flexible extension mechanism, the FHIR model is conceived from the fundament to be applicable in different contexts. Moreover, CrowdHEALTH also considers ontologies at the state of the art, useful to qualify entity types that correspond to specializations or abstractions of entities represented by FHIR elements. Fourthly, the HHR model is designed at conceptual level and in parallel mapped with existing standards. The model is provided both in a semiformal format, using UML, and in a completely formal format, using the HHR mapping language (an XML mapping language) that was created in the context of CrowdHEALTH. The HHR mapping language allows the simple expression of the structure of the model and its mapping to FHIR and to existing or new terminologies. Several constraints are imposed to the designer of the HHR model to guarantee the feasibility of a direct mapping to FHIR. The reason for not directly using the selected reference standard is to untie the HHR model from choices related only to the FHIR implementation (for instance to simplify the implementation of restful services) and make explicit in the model some aspects that are implicit in FHIR, so to ease the usage of the HHR model independently from FHIR. Therefore, the HHR model has as a goal to be easily implementable on top of existing FHIR implementations, and it is also intended to be easily implementable using different technologies.

2.3   Organization of the HHR Model

As described in the previous section, the HHR model is described in a semi-formal way using UML. The overall model is divided in several packages to simplify the representation and the description of the reported information. Each package collects information related to a specific topic (e.g. the representation of the information characterizing a Person, clinical Conditions of patients or Measurements performed on Persons). For each fragment, the description of each entity and its relationships with the other entities in the fragment is reported. Although the model is split in several packages, its classes belonging to different packages have always different names, to reduce the risk of misunderstanding and enable implementations that put all classes in a single software package.

2.4   Level of Abstraction and Scope of the HHR Model

Each class of the HHR model can be represented by a resource type or a data type of the FHIR model, with the difference that the HHR model is designed at an ontological level and is more specialized than the FHIR model. Through that, the multiplicity constraints on the UML associations and attributes do not represent integrity constraints, as in the case of FHIR, but represent real world existence constraints. For instance, if an attribute has minimum multiplicity equal to 1, this does not imply that the value of that attribute must be mandatorily stored or transmitted when exchanging data, but only implies that at least one value of that attribute always exists in the world, and this information is not stored in any information system or not transmitted. All the attributes of the entities in the HHR model are not mandatory, i.e. their values are not required to be stored or transmitted for each data transmission occurrence. Another aspect is the usage of abstract classes that have no direct corresponding type in FHIR but correspond to super-types of FHIR resource types. Such classes are introduced to make explicit some semantic commonalities that are implicit in the FHIR model. Moreover, to represent ontological distinctions that cannot be expressed with standard UML, a specific stereotype and pattern is adopted. For example, classes of entities (e.g. Patient) that correspond to roles of instances of other classes (e.g. Person), are marked with the stereotype <role> and use the standard relation "player" to associate the entity (e.g. the person) that plays the role. If needed, implementations of the HHR model may exploit the explicit representation of roles and accept to assign instances of a certain role as a value of attributes whose type is not that role, but it is the type of the instances that may play that role (e.g. accepting a Practitioner as value of an attribute expecting a Person). However, this cannot be realized for the vice versa scenario (i.e. it is forbidden to assign a Person to an attribute expecting a Practitioner). When a class C has numerous subclasses, but these subclasses add no specific attributes or constraints, then the subclasses are reified. Each subclass is represented by an item of an enumeration (stereotype <enum>) and a mandatory attribute of the class C (with name Ctype) is used to represent the specific subclass of the instance. For example, the subclasses of the class Condition correspond to values of the enumeration ConditionType and the specific subclass of a Condition instance is represented by the value of the attribute named conditionType. The fact that the HHR model is more specialized than the FHIR model is also evident in several aspects. The most important aspect in the HHR model is the absence of classes and elements that are present in FHIR, since they are not needed by the current CrowdHEALTH use cases. Moreover, an HHR class that corresponds to a certain FHIR resource class may have explicit subclasses that are not represented as distinct resource classes in FHIR. Differently from the addition of new attributes, usually the introduction in the HHR model of these explicit subclasses does not require a corresponding FHIR extension. The instances of all such HHR subclasses correspond to instances of the same FHIR resource class, and their semantic type is distinct by assigning a specific value, chosen from specific terminologies to a "category" or "code" attribute of the resource class. The values of these attributes are fixed by the HHR model, to assure that the same type of data is always represented using the same terms from the same terminologies. In other terms, the HHR model explicitly represents concepts that are needed by the CrowdHEALTH use cases and either are implicit in FHIR or need a FHIR extension.

As mentioned above, a few constraints are imposed to the HHR model to guarantee an easy mapping with FHIR and with specific coding systems. The main constraint is that any leaf element of the HHR model (i.e. any class, attribute or association that does not have subclasses or specializations) must correspond to exactly one (resource or data) type of the FHIR model, i.e. all possible instances of an HHR class must represent the same entities of possible instances of only one corresponding FHIR class. Another constraint is that each instance of an HHR class must correspond to exactly one instance of the FHIR model. On the other hand, any non-leaf element of the HHR model, is considered ontologically "abstract" (i.e. all its representable instances or values must be instances or values of some subclass). This is intended to avoid the usage of instances of non-leaf classes to represent unintended entities. Implementations may impose the instantiation of only leaf classes. As HHR classes are conceptual, advanced implementations may also allow to instantiate non-leaf classes of the HHR model, in order to allow to represent entities whose type is not completely known, possibly allowing to specify a more specific type in a second moment (i.e. allowing the same instance to conceptually move from a superclass to a subclass when more information is available). Although the semantics of the HHR elements are usually more specific than the ones of the FHIR model, to make the mapping more evident, the name of the most general HHR element that is mapped to a specific FHIR element usually takes the same name of the corresponding FHIR element. In any case, different names are chosen when the semantics of the HHR element are specific and would be misleading to adopt the same name with FHIR. The detailed specialization of the HHR model, with respect to more general-purpose standards, has the advantage of reducing the ambiguity of the model and simplifying its comprehension, thus mitigating the risk that different standard elements are used to represent the same type of information. The final version of the HHR model aims to represent the information enabling the execution of all the use cases of the CrowdHEALTH system.

2.5 Steps Followed to Define the HHR Model

Following the development approach of the CrowdHEALTH project, the development of the HHR model followed a multi-cycles process, producing two different versions of the HHR model aligned with corresponding versions of the use case requirements. In each development cycle, different tasks have been performed.

1. As a first step, the use case partners had to describe the information that should be stored and analysed using the CrowdHEALTH tools, focusing on the data needed for the first version of their use case implementation. A specific template was provided to each use case to perform this description where they created and described a UML conceptual diagram representing the type of entities and relationships described by their data source (abstracting from implementation details of the actual database scheme). It was also described each attribute of each entity and the corresponding cardinality and value constraints. In the second cycle this description has been in some case produced by extending the one produced during the first cycle, and in some other case, starting the process from scratch to obtain a better model.
2. Afterwards, different analysts have been assigned to each use case, to clarify ambiguity issues related to their data source and to express a mapping of their dataset scheme to the FHIR model, to disambiguate the semantics of each type, relationship and attribute. The mapping was expressed using specific tables and the FHIRPath language.
3. As a third step, the conceptual models that were constructed by the use cases were merged in a unique HHR model. Different conceptual classes that different use cases had mapped to the same FHIR classes or to FHIR classes with similar semantics have been merged in a unique HHR class, or in different subclasses of a same abstract HHR class. The same analyses have been performed for attributes and associations.
4. Then, the formalization of the mapping to FHIR happened, using the same semi-formal approach used for the mapping of data source conceptual schemes.
5. The last step was to define the HHR model and the mapping to FHIR using the formal XML language specified by the CrowdHEALTH project.

The resulting specification distinguish general purpose concepts that are included in the HHR model, and extensions to the HHR model required by specific use cases. The extensions of the HHR model are formalized in the same way of the HHR model but are not considered mandatory parts of the HHR model, because they represent information that is meaningful only to specific cases and does not need to be exchanged in a standardized way with other organizations.

2.6 Health-Related Aspects Covered by the HHR Model

The data types that are covered by the HHR model belong to nine different categories. In particular:

1. Physical activities including information related with workouts, biodata and fitness tests performed by a person or groups of persons.
2. Lifestyle data including information related with sleep patterns, substances consumption such as alcohol, tobacco or recreational drugs.
3. Social data which are related to social interactions, such as the emotion, the number of the contact in the phone or the number of exchanged multimedia items.
4. Events concerning episodes of care, hospitalizations, clinical procedures, laboratory tests and care plans.
5. Medication data that have to do with prescription, request, and assumption of medication.
6. Condition information consisting of symptoms, diagnosis, allergies, and intolerances that a specific patient or group of patients suffer.
7. Nutrition information with data regarding the food and beverage intake.
8. Administrative information concerning demographics and administrative information about an individual or group of individuals. It also includes data about the educational level, occupational status or assurance of individuals.
9. Measurement information and simple assertions about a patient, device, or other subject. It also includes collective health measurements about a group of persons sharing common characteristics.

2.7 UML Conceptual Model

The conceptual HHR model is described using UML class diagrams. The overall model is divided in several packages to simplify the representation and the description of the reported information. Each package collects information related to a specific topic, e.g. the representation of the information characterizing a Person, clinical Conditions of patients or Measurements performed on Persons. For each fragment, the description of each entity and its relationships with the other entities in the fragment is reported. All attributes of the entities in the HHR model are not mandatory, i.e. their values are not required to be stored or transmitted for each data transmission.

The following subsections present some UML packages of the HHR model. Since all the HHR models cannot be defined and specified in the context of this paper due to page limitations, more information can be found in [27, 28], listing additional models such as the Person model, the Episode of care model, the Measurement model, or the Quantitative measures models containing laboratory test measures, fitness measures, or heart rate and blood pressure measures, among others.

Identifier. All entities of the HHR model inherit from IdentifiedEntity, which represents any entity that can be identified using a string id that is unique within a given Identifier-System. As shown in Fig. 1, an IdentifiedEntity has at least one Identifier representing a numeric or alphanumeric string that is associated with a single entity within a given identifier system, and each identifier is generated by one system. The acknowledged systems in the HHR model are listed in the coded class IdentifierSystem representing a standard to associate a unique id to each entity belonging to a specific context. Each identified entity may have only one identifier per IdentifierSystem and it is not possible that two identified entities share the same identifier belonging to the same IdentifierSystem.

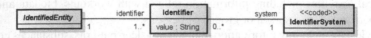

Fig. 1. Identifier model.

Activity. Planned or performed activities recorded in the HHR model are instances of PersonOrGroupEvent. Each event has an EventStatus, and each specialization of PersonOrGroupEvent may use a specialized set of status. More instances of Person-OrGroupEven can be grouped in a CollectionOfEvents having an instance of Group as subject. The category of the members belonging to the collection of events can be set with the PersonOrGroupCategory enumeration. The activity model shown in Fig. 2, Fig. 3, Fig. 4, and Fig. 5 describe three specializations of PersonOfGroupEvent, namely Procedure, MedicationEvent and MedicationDispense.

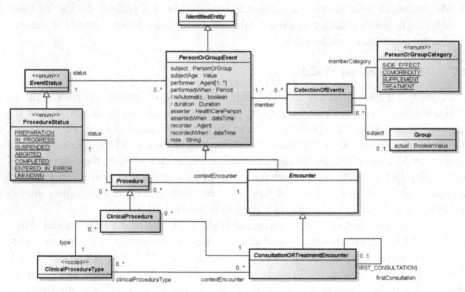

Fig. 2. Activity Model (part 1 out of 4).

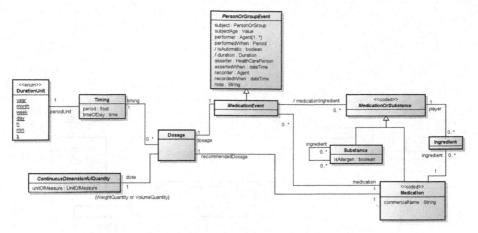

Fig. 3. Activity Model (part 2 out of 4).

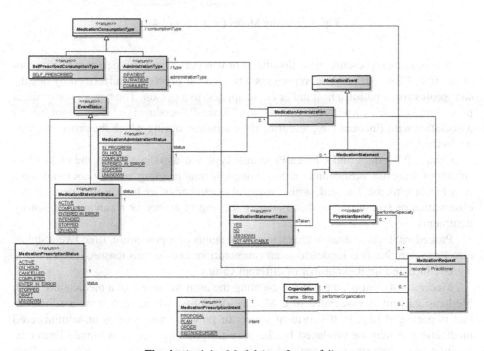

Fig. 4. Activity Model (part 3 out of 4).

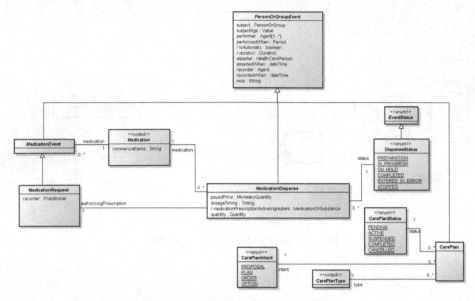

Fig. 5. Activity Model (part 4 out of 4).

A Procedure represents any action that is or was performed on a person while its specialization, ClinicalProcedure, represents any medical procedure performed by healthcare professional within a hospital or clinic applied to a person. The type of the medical procedure is specified with the coded class ClinicalProcedureType. Procedure has an association with Encounter representing the encounter during which the procedure was performed.

ClinicalProcedure and ClinicalProcedureType are associated with the class ConsultationORTreatmentEncounter representing a formal meeting, usually not requiring a creation of a medical record, with a medical doctor or other healthcare operators for observation or monitoring or discussion or seeking of advice or receiving ambulatory treatments.

ProcedureStatus is used to characterize the status of a procedure. Like EventStatus, also ProcedureStatus is modelled as an enumeration, and for this reason, it can assume a predefined and limited number of different values.

MedicationEvent is an event representing the administration of a medication. Each MedicationEvent is associated to a Medication entity, which represents a substance that is packaged (e.g. in the form of tablets or powder) and used as an administered medication. It may be produced by the hospital pharmacy or by a brand. The composition of a Medication is specified by one or more instances of the class Ingredient where the player is a MedicationOrSubstance. The dosage that is recommended from the official documentation of the Medication is represented by means the association recommendedDosage with the class Dosage that has an association with Timing and ContinuousDimensionfulQuantity: Timing specifies an event that may occur multiple times inside a DurationUnit time frame while ContinuousDimensionfulQuantity represents the amount of medication per dose, it can be a weight or a volume quantity. A

Substance is a pure substance (i.e. a form of matter that has constant chemical composition and cannot be separated into components by physical separation methods) or a homogeneous mixture (i.e. a material that has the same proportions of its components throughout any given sample). A Substance has a definite composition, specified by zero or more ingredients, which are other substances.

The entity MedicationEvent is specialized by MedicationStatement and MedicationAdministration. MedicationStatement represents an assertion, by some individual (the asserter), that a specific medication has been prescribed (also not necessary taken) or has been taken (also without a prescription). MedicationAdministration represents an administration of a medication asserted by an individual that belongs to the organization that provides it. Respectively, MedicationStatementStatus and MedicationAdministrationStatus represents the status of those entities. The type of the medication administration is represented with SelfPrescribedConsumptionType class while AdministrationType indicates where the medication that is expected to be consumed or administered; both shares the same super class MedicationConsumptionType. A MedicationRequest is an order or request for both supply of the medication and the instructions for administration of the medication to a patient/person, it can be authorized by a performer with a specific PractitionerSpecialty. A performer may have several specialties, but only one is used for the prescription (therefore it is not possible, in general, to derive the PractitionerSpecialty, from the specialties of the performer). The enumeration MedicationPrescriptionIntent is used to set the intend of the prescription while the association performerOrganization describes the Organization of the role played by the Practitioner that performed the MedicationRequest, of course a Practitioner by play different roles belonging to different organizations.

Another specialization of PersonOrGroupEvent is MedicationDispense indicating that a medication product is to be or has been dispensed for a named person/patient. This includes a description of the Medication product (supply) provided and the instructions for administering it. The MedicationDispense is the result of a pharmacy system responding to a MedicationRequest order. Its status is represented by the DispenseStatus enumeration.

A PersonOrGroupEvent can be also a CarePlan describing the intention of how one or more practitioners intend to deliver care for a particular patient, group or community for a period of time, possibly limited to care for a specific condition or set of conditions. CarePlan is used to represent both proposed plans (for example, recommendations from a decision support engine or returned as part of a consult report) as well as active plans. Its current status is specified by the association status and may be one of the values in the CarePlanStatus enumeration. The level of the authority/intentionality of the care plan can be described through the association "intend" with CarePlanIntent indicating the level of authority/intentionality associated with the care plan and where the care plan fits into the workflow chain while the CarePlanType specifies the kind of the plan (e.g. "home health", "psychiatric", "asthma", "disease management", "wellness plan", etc.).

Organization. A person is a student when he or she attends a School. The Grade enumeration lists all the possible grade of school handled by the HHR model. Since the school degree of a student is expected to evolve, the same person may correspond to several instances of Student (that is a PersonInTime), each one related to a specific school degree.

A school belongs to one and only one Municipality and a municipality belongs to one and only one Region. A MedicalDepartement belongs to one and only one CenterDepartment and a centre department consists of several medical departments. School, Municipality and MedicalDepartment share the same superclass NestedOrganization, this means that they can be part of another organization. The superclass of NestedOrganization, Region and CenterDepartement is Organization that represents a formally or informally recognized grouping of people or organizations formed for the purpose of achieving some form of collective action, it includes companies, institutions, corporations, departments, community groups, healthcare practice groups, etc.

Details and position information for a physical place where services are provided and resources and participants may be stored, found, contained, or accommodated are represented by the class Location (Fig. 6).

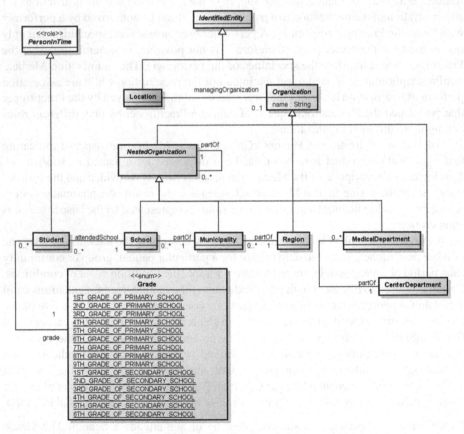

Fig. 6. Organization model.

Condition. A PersonOrGroupEvent is the record of an automatic or manual activity or observation or request of an activity, that is performed on a person or group (e.g. the administration of a medication to a patient) or that produces information about a person or group (e.g. the calculation of the BMI of a person). It is not required that the event is directly related to a healthcare service. If the event is a request to perform an activity, then the attributes of this type of entity does not refer to the requested activity (that does not exist yet at the moment of the request), but to the requesting action, e.g. the performer of a MedicationRequest is different from the performer of the MedicationAdministration (see section Activity).

The HHR model introduces several kinds of events (Fig. 7). A Condition is a statement about an objective state of a patient. The statement may be done by the patient itself or by a group of persons or by a practitioner. Condition is distinct from a PersonOrGroupObservation (see Measurement section) because it refers to a persistent state, while a PersonOrGroupObservation refers to a particular instant in time.

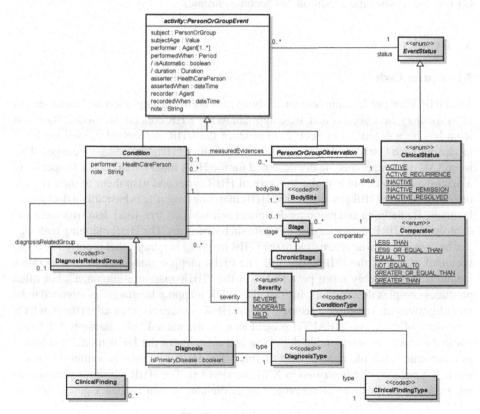

Fig. 7. Condition model.

Condition has two subclasses: ClinicalFinding and Diagnosis, having an association-end "type" with ClinicalFindingType and DiagnosisType respectively. The last two coded classes share the same superclass CondionType. An instance of ClinicalFindingType represents a statement about a persistent objective status of a patient. A DiagnosisType is a statement that is the result of a cognitive process, i.e. it is the interpretation of a set of measures and/or clinical findings. Each Condition can be associated to zero or one DiagnosisRelatedGroup representing a patient classification system that standardizes prospective payment to hospitals and encourages cost containment initiatives.

The status of the clinical condition of the subject (PersonOrGroup) is specified by the association status and may be one of the values in the ClinicalStatus enumeration.

The evidence at the base of the Condition is represented by the class PersonOrGroupObservation. The current severity of the Condition of the patient is specified by the association severity and may be one of the values in the Severity enumeration.

The class BodySite represents the anatomical location where the Condition manifests itself while the entity Stage specifies its stage or grade. Stage is specialized in ChronicStage when the condition has become chronic.

3   Results

3.1   Source Code

The HHR Manager Java implemented library, allows the instantiation and modification of in-memory Java objects that are compliant to the HHR conceptual model. Based on what has been described in Sect. 2, to produce the HHR conceptual model, the HHR model has been first formalized using a language called "HHR mapping language". This is an XML language, specifically designed for the HHR model, that allows to specify in a machine-interpretable way the structure of HHR types and map them to the structure of corresponding FHIR resources. The HHR mapping language is basically a declarative language for defining and mapping document oriented (i.e. tree-like) data structures and exploits the FHIRPath language to navigate such structures. The HHR mapping language can be considered as an alternative to the FHIR mapping language, that is currently being specified as part of the FHIR standard. The FHIR mapping language is an imperative language and arguably more powerful than the "HHR mapping language", but often produces complex descriptions. Instead, the "HHR mapping language" is intended to be more lightweight. The current prototype of the HHR Manager is released on the Artefacts repository of the CrowdHEALTH project as a jar file named "hhr-manager-1.3.5.jar", while the machine-interpretable definition and mapping of the HHR model is released as a separate XML file named "hhr_to_fhir". The HHR Manager is written in Java 8, while the mapping file is written in XML version 1.0. The HHR Manager generator is released on the repository of the project as jar file named "hhr-manager-generator".

3.2 HHR Manager Library

The hhr-manager library provides several interfaces to instantiate, serialize and de-serialize java objects representing personal and health data, but it neither includes any kind of data storage mechanisms, nor it shares any data with external services. Therefore, personal data security and privacy management is delegated to the specific components that use the library. The library consists of four main packages:

- eu.crowdhealth.hhr.model: the definition of the HHR Manager API (HHRFactory in the above picture), i.e. a set of public Java interfaces and enumerations corresponding to the conceptual types defined by the HHR conceptual model.
- eu.crowdhealth.hhr.impl: the implementation of the HHR Manager API.
- eu.crowdhealth.hhr.serializer: the definition of the APIs to serialize/deserialize the HHR JAVA object in XML representation and vice versa.
- eu.crowheath.hhr.exceptions: the management of unwanted or unexpected events

The HHR Manager API is a Java representation of the HHR model: each class of the HHR model corresponds to a homonymous Java interface or Java class. Each attribute of a class of the HHR model corresponds to a couple of get and set methods of the HHR API, according to the JavaBeans conventions.

Classes of the HHR model with stereotype <coded> or <enum> corresponds to enumerations, i.e. to classes that have a predefined (i.e. defined at static time) set of instances, each one having a specific name. In particular the classes with stereotype <enum> corresponds to Java Enum (i.e. their instances are defined within a Java), while the classes with stereotype <coded> are represented by Java interfaces which instances are defined in a separate xml file having the same name of the interface and stored in a common directory, usually called "extensions" (but it may have whatever name). Therefore, while the instances of <enum> classes are fixed, the instances of <coded> classes can be configured by editing the corresponding files.

The HHR model, and its Java representation, uses values from enumerations to represent non-Instantiable concepts or to represent conceptual classes that is not convenient to represent as Java classes. HHRFactory (Fig. 8) is an interface implemented by the singleton class ConcreteHHRFactory, which unique instance is obtained by means of the static method getInstance(...). It is aimed to create Java objects compliant to the HHR model.

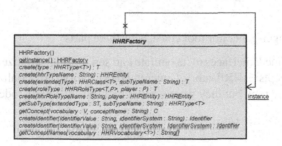

Fig. 8. HHR Factory class.

An implementation of HHRFactory is a singleton class which unique instance is obtained by means of a public static method. Any conceptual class of the HHR model or of an extension of the HHRModel (defined by means of the HHR mapping language) is represented by a Java interface I and is reified as an instance of HHRType denoted by the static attribute I.cclass. Some conceptual types are not represented as classes in the HHR model, but as values of a type-class (i.e. a class inheriting from HHRType). HHRTypes instances are used instead of conceptual classes when there are several types that share a same structure, and it is not convenient to represent them as different classes because they are too many or they are context dependent (custom types). Some HHRType is a kind of HHRConcept. Each instance of HHRConcept belongs to a vocabulary. Some vocabulary is represented by a Java Enum, while vocabularies that are too big to be represented as Java Enum are represented as Java Interfaces which instances are defined using a specific portion of the HHR mapping language by files stored in the directory "extensions". Any vocabulary is represented by the reification (V.cclass) of the type V having the concepts of the vocabulary as instances. The invocation HHFactory.getConcept(V.cclass, name) returns the concept having the specified Name and belonging to the vocabulary V. When V is an Enum, then V.name returns the same concept.

3.3 HHR Manager Generator

The hhr-manager library is the output of another developed tool called "hhr-manager-generator". It takes as an input the hhr-to-fhir xml file defining the structure of all classes, attributes and enumerations included in the HHR model and produces in output the java code of the hhr manager library (Fig. 9).

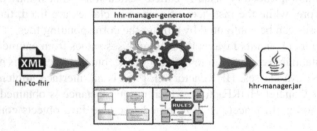

Fig. 9. The hhr-manager-generator tool [22].

The hhr-manager-generator tool consists of three parts:

- A set of predefined interfaces to instantiate and serialize/de-serialize the HHR objects and HHR concepts (HHRFactory, ConcreteHHRFactory and Serializer). They are not produced by the tool, but they were written by hands and hard-coded.

6. The implementation of a set of rules to generate the source code (of abstract and concrete java classes, java interfaces, java enumerations, attributes, getter, and setter methods). There is a set of rules for each kind of tag of the hhr-maping-language.
7. The implementation of a set of rules aiming to add JAXB annotations to serialize/de-serialize HHR objects to/from XML documents.

The hhr-manager-generator works in two phases (Fig. 10): in the first phase a parser analyses the definition of the HHR model given as input (hhr-to-fhir.xml) expresses using the hhr mapping language and builds a hierarchical tree structure. The structure of the tree is then navigated and the rules for generation of source code and JAXB annotations are applied.

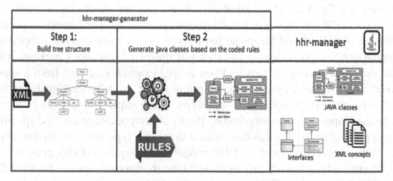

Fig. 10. Functionality of the hhr-manager-generator [22].

The output is the generation of the hhr-manager library containing the source code of Java classes, the interfaces to instantiate and serialize/de-serialize hhr objects and standard xml files for the concepts included in HHR model. Thanks to the hhr-manager-generator tool it is easy to update the source code of the hhr-manager whenever new classes, new attributes (or changes to the existing ones) are added to the HHR model expressed by the input file hhr-to-fhir.xml.

The introduction of this new tool allows to each use case (or other stakeholder) to extend the HHR model by editing the file hhr-to-fhir.xml and generate the corresponding hhr-manager library. Therefore, the developer of a use case may choose to use just the provided XML file describing the final version of the HHR model or can add it whatever extensions extension is needed.

Moreover, if some use case requires just to add new instances to some coded class, then it is not needed to re-generate the HHR manager. The distinct files that defined the instances of the <coded> classes are loaded and interpreted at runtime, therefore the developer of the use case has just to extend the content of these files.

3.4 Working Environment

The HHR Manager depends on a standard java virtual machine that supports Java 8 and can be imported in any compatible project. Similarly, the mapping file may be read with any XML parser compatible with XML version 1.0. Also, the hhr-manager-generator requires a virtual machine supporting Java 8. The overall evaluation and testing were performed on a platform that supports dynamic resource allocation based on the application requirements [26].

3.5 HHR to FHIR Mapping Example

This section reports an example of usage of the HHR mapping language. It shows how to map the class CarePlan of the HHR model. It maps the HHR class CarePlan to the homonymous FHIR resource type CarePlan. An instance of HHR CarePlan is converted to an instance of FHIR CarePlan, its attributes type, intent and status are mapped respectively to the attributes type, intend and status of the FHIR resource CarePlan. It should be noted that, when a class (like CarePlan, in this example) inherits from a supertype (PersonOrEvent, in this example), the mapping of all the inherited attributes may be specified within the definition of the supertype. If the supertype inherits from another supertype the mapping is also inherited by the its supertype and so on. The specification of the mapping of an HHR class ends where there is a type without any supertype. In the case of the class CarePlan of the HHR model, the mapping to FHIR ends in the class IdentifiedEntity which has not any supertype (the inheritance chain is IdentifiedEntity, PersonOrGroupEvent, CarePlan).

The attribute identifier of the HHR class CarePlan is mapped to the attribute identifier of the FHIR type CarePlan. The mapping of this attribute is contained in the tag <class> of the HHR conceptual class IdentifiedEntity. Note that this HHR conceptual class has no correspondent FHIR type (indeed the tag-attribute fhirName is empty). More in details the value attribute of HHR Identifier is mapped to the value attribute of FHIR identifier while the attribute system of the HHR class Identifier is mapped to the attribute system of the FHIR type Identifier. Note that isMultipleValue = "true" so there can be more than one value for the attribute identifier.

The HHR class Agent has no corresponding FHIR type and therefore the fhirName is set to the empty string. It is an abstract class having as superclass IdentifierEntity.

Also, the HHR class PersonOrGroupEvent has no corresponding FHIR type, and its attributes are mapped within the tags <class> of the subclasses.

The attribute performer of HHR abstract type Agent is mapped to the attribute performer.actor of the target FHIR resource type. Note that isMultipleValue = "true" so there can be more than one instance of the attribute performer. The attribute subject (of HHR abstract type PersonOrGroup) is mapped to the FHIR attribute subject of the target resource. The attribute note is mapped to the FHIR attribute comment. The remaining attributes are mapped to FHIR extensions of the target FHIR resource, each one having a specific StructureDefinition.

- asserter (of type HHR abstract class HealthCarePerson) which StructureDefinition is defined at http://hl7.org/fhir/StructureDefinition/asserter
- isAutomatic (of HHR type boolean) which StructureDefinition is defined at http://hl7.org/fhir/StructureDefinition/is-automatic
- performedWhen (of HHR type Period) which StructureDefinition is defined at http://hl7.org/fhir/StructureDefinition/performed-when
- assertedWhen (of HHR type dateTime) which StructureDefinition is defined at http://hl7.org/fhir/StructureDefinition/asserted-when
- recorder (of HHR type Agent) which StructureDefinition is defined at http://hl7.org/fhir/StructureDefinition/recorder
- recordedWhen (of HHR type dateTime) which StructureDefinition is defined at http://hl7.org/fhir/StructureDefinition/recorded-when
- subjectAge (of HHR type depending on the kind of value set in subjectAge) which StructureDefinition is defined at http://hl7.org/fhir/StructureDefinition/subject-age
- duration (of HHR type Duration) which StructureDefinition is defined at http://hl7.org/fhir/StructureDefinition/duration

The player of the role class PersonInTime is of type Person. PersonIntime is an abstract class inheriting from IdentifiedEntity that has not corresponding FHIR type. The role class HealthCarePerson is an abstract and that inherits from PersonInTime role class. The class CarePlan is mapped to the homonymous FHIR type CarePlan. The HHR attribute type is an instance of CarePlanType and it is mapped to the attribute category of the target FHIR type CarePlan. The HHR attribute intent is a mandatory attribute mapped to the FHIR attribute intent and it can be set with any of the instances of the CarePlanIntent enum. Finally, the HHR attribute status is a mandatory inherited attribute mapped to the FHIR attribute status and it can be set with any of the instances of the CarePlanStatus enum. In Fig. 11, it is provided the final content of the mapping of the CarePlan class of the HHR model, based on the current description.

```
<hhr-to-fhir>
        <class hhrName="IdentifiedEntity" fhirName="" isAbstract="true" >
        <attribute hhrPath="identifier" hhrType="Identifier" isMultipleValue="true" />
        </class>
    <class hhrName="Identifier">
        <attribute hhrPath="value" hhrType="String" />
        <attribute hhrPath="system" hhrType="IdentifierSystem" />
        </class>
        <class hhrName="Agent" fhirName="" isAbstract="true" hhrSupertype="IdentifiedEntity"/>
        <class    hhrName="PersonOrGroupEvent"    hhrSupertype="IdentifiedEntity"    isAbstract="true"
                fhirName="">
        <attribute   hhrPath="performer"   hhrType="Agent"   isMultipleValue="true"   isAbstract="true"
fhirPath="performer.actor" />
        <attribute        hhrPath="asserter"        hhrType="HealthCarePerson"        isAbstract="true"
fhirExtension="http://hl7.org/fhir/StructureDefinition/asserter" />
        <attribute                     hhrPath="isAutomatic"                     hhrType="boolean"
fhirExtension="http://hl7.org/fhir/StructureDefinition/is-automatic" />
        <attribute hhrPath="subject" hhrType="PersonOrGroup" isAbstract="true" />
        <attribute hhrPath="performedWhen" hhrType="Period"
                        fhirExtension="http://hl7.org/fhir/StructureDefinition/performed-when"
                />
        <attribute              hhrPath="assertedWhen"              hhrType="dateTime"
fhirExtension="http://hl7.org/fhir/StructureDefinition/asser-when" />
        <attribute              hhrPath="recorder"              hhrType="Agent"
fhirExtension="http://hl7.org/fhir/StructureDefinition/recorder" />
        <attribute              hhrPath="recordedWhen"              hhrType="dateTime"
fhirExtension="http://hl7.org/fhir/StructureDefini/recorded-when" />
        <attribute        hhrPath="subjectAge"        hhrType="Range|Duration"        isAbstract="true"
fhirExtension="http://hl7.org/fhir/StructureDefinition/subject-age" />
        <attribute              hhrPath="duration"              hhrType="Duration"
fhirExtension="http://hl7.org/fhir/StructureDefinition/duration" />
        <attribute hhrPath="status" hhrType="EventStatus" isAbstract="true" />
        <attribute hhrPath="note" hhrType="String" fhirPath="comment" />
        </class>
    <role hhrName="PersonInTime" fhirName="" hhrPlayer="Person" hhrSupertype="IdentifiedEntity"
            isAbstract="true" />
    <role hhrName="HealthCarePerson" fhirName="" hhrSupertype="PersonInTime" isAbstract="true"/>
    <class hhrName="CarePlan" hhrSupertype="PersonOrGroupEvent" fhirName="CarePlan" >
        <attribute hhrPath="type" hhrType="CarePlanType" fhirPath="category" />
        <attribute hhrPath="intent" hhrType="CarePlanIntent" fhirPath="intent" fhirMandatory="true"
/>
        <attribute hhrPath="status" hhrType="CarePlanStatus" isInherited="true" fhirPath="status"
fhirMandatory="true" />
        </class>
        <coded hhrName="CarePlanType" fhirName="CodeableConcept" />
        <enum    hhrName="CarePlanStatus"        hhrSupertype="EventStatus"        fhirName="code"
                fhirCodingSystem="http://www.crowdhealth.eu/hhr-t/consultation-or-treatment-
                encounter-type">
        <instance hhrName="PENDING" fhirCode="pending" fhirCodeDisplay="Pending" />
        <instance hhrName="ACTIVE" fhirCode="active" fhirCodeDisplay="Active" />
        <instance hhrName="SUSPENDED" fhirCode="suspended" fhirCodeDisplay="Suspended" />
        <instance hhrName="COMPLETED" fhirCode="completed" fhirCodeDisplay="Completed" />
        <instance hhrName="CANCELLED" fhirCode="cancelled" fhirCodeDisplay="Cancelled" />
        </enum>
    <enum hhrName="CarePlanIntent" fhirName="code" fhirValueSet="care-plan-intent">
        <instance hhrName="PROPOSAL" fhirCode="proposal" fhirCodeDisplay="Proposal" />
        <instance hhrName="PLAN" fhirCode="plan" fhirCodeDisplay="Plan" />
        <instance hhrName="ORDER" fhirCode="order" fhirCodeDisplay="Order" />
        <instance hhrName="OPTION" fhirCode="option" fhirCodeDisplay="Option" />
        </enum>
</hhr-to-fhir>
```

Fig. 11. Mapping of the CarePlan class of the HHR Model [22].

4 Discussion

HHRs are structured health records that may include several types of information that are relevant to a patient's health status, such as laboratory medical data; clinical data; lifestyle data collected by the patient or related people; physical activities data; social care data; physiological and environment data collected by medical devices and sensors; nutrition data. Currently, many data models have been specified for representing the aforementioned data, but there is no single model that covers in an integrated way all the needs of CrowdHEALTH use cases.

In general, aggregating information and also bypassing ambiguities is of crucial importance. Various standards and best practices have been defined over the years with this purpose. Among them, HL7 FHIR is the specification more tailored to the needs of the current research. It has been selected as a ground base for the HHR model, because it is considered easier to implement than previous standards, covers very well the clinical aspects of human health and has a good extension mechanism that allows adding information models for aspects not yet covered by the model. Hence, it has a high coverage of clinical data and high flexibility in its extension mechanism that allows the modelling of not yet supported clinical data types. FHIR can deal with multiple requirements in order to more efficiently represent and exchange clinical data, according also to the requirements set by CrowdHEALTH. Nevertheless, it also has some drawback in the cases of data integration and analysis, since it allows data representation with various Resource types, creating the risk of non-homogeneous representations which cannot be easily aggregated and analysed. Another drawback is that it may hide crucial conceptual distinction that are based on choosing right codes for semantic representation. Consequently, in real-life applications, FHIR has to be surrounded by specifically tailored constraints and rules, in order to guarantee and make more efficient the overall interoperability paradigm. Nevertheless, FHIR is not able to cover some of the Crowd-HEALTH's requirements, lacking a specific representation of information that is present in the analysed use cases dataset.

For these reasons, a new model, the HHR model, has been designed and tailored to the CrowdHEALTH use cases. The HHR model has been obtained by first producing a separate conceptual data model for each CrowdHEALTH use case, then clarifying their semantics with a preliminary mapping to the FHIR standard and finally merging the separate models in a unique HHR conceptual model. A coherent mapping to FHIR has therefore been defined with respect to the merged conceptual model, to guarantee that different teams adopt the same FHIR representation (as FHIR allows different representations for the same information). Although based on FHIR, the HHR model is designed at a higher conceptual level, making explicit several concepts that are implicit in the FHIR standard, other than extending it by adding missing concepts. These extensions have as a goal to add details to health-related events, including the specification of who assert and/or perform an event during an episode of care and when it occurs, indicating if the performer is an automatic agent, the age (or range of age) of the subject at the time the event occurs, the date when a person is registered into the system.

Since FHIR also requires suitable coding systems, such as ICD-10, LOINC or SNOMED CT, the latter have been adopted in the cases that they have been considered of crucial importance. Considering the limitations of SNOMED CT due to its terms of license, only ICD-10 and LOINC were actually used and adopted as standard terminologies and the concepts which were not covered by these terminologies have been represented with a custom made terminology, being defined by CrowdHEALTH.

By maintaining both a conceptual and a logical view, the HHR model aims firstly to guarantee the interoperability and the possibility to implement it on top of existing FHIR libraries, and it is also intended to be usable independently from FHIR (and its future evolutions), being applicable also for different purposes than only exchanging health data (e.g., it can be more suitable than FHIR as data schema for Object Oriented local APIs).

To conclude, CrowdHEALTH healthcare system integrates a wide set of mechanisms enabling data acquisition from different sources, cleaning, aggregation, and transformation into structures that capture all health determinants, the so-called HHRs. These HHRs reflect currently 2 million records and 700,000 streams of everyday activities, obtained from more than 200,000 users, while the system is expected to exploit the current 75 million measurements from 1 million people. It is within our future goals to continuously update this object-oriented model equivalent to a FHIR profile expressed both in a human oriented format and in a machine-oriented format, for supporting additional data entities, and finally representing more kinds of information, including social activities and lifestyle information, as well as real-time workout or daily activities [27, 28].

Acknowledgment. The research leading to the results presented in this paper has received funding from the European Union's funded project CrowdHEALTH under Grant Agreement no 727560. The research has been also co-financed by the European Union and Greek national funds through the Operational Program Competitiveness, Entrepreneurship, and Innovation, under the call RESEARCH – CREATE – INNOVATE (project code: DIASTEMA - T2EDK-04612).

References

1. Mavrogiorgou, A., Kiourtis, A., Kyriazis, D.: Plug'n'play IoT devices: an approach for dynamic data acquisition from unknown heterogeneous devices. In: Barolli, L., Terzo, O. (eds.) CISIS 2017. AISC, vol. 611, pp. 885–895. Springer, Cham (2018). https://doi.org/10.1007/978-3-319-61566-0_84
2. Kiourtis, A., Nifakos, S., Mavrogiorgou, A., Kyriazis, D.: Aggregating the syntactic and semantic similarity of healthcare data towards their transformation to HL7 FHIR through ontology matching. Int. J. Med. Inform. **132**, 104002 (2019)
3. Geßner, S., et al.: The portal of medical data models: where have we been and where are we going? In: Studies in Health Technology and Informatics, pp. 858–862. IOS Press (2017)
4. openEHR. https://www.openehr.org/. Accessed 19 July 2021
5. HL7 FHIR. https://www.hl7.org/fhir/. Accessed 19 July 2021
6. Kiourtis, A., Mavrogiorgou, A., Menychtas, A., Maglogiannis, I., Kyriazis, D.: Structurally mapping healthcare data to HL7 FHIR through ontology alignment. J. Med. Syst. **43**(3), 62 (2019)
7. LOINC. https://loinc.org/. Accessed 19 July 2021
8. SNOMED CT. http://www.snomed.org/. Accessed 19 July 2021
9. ICD-10 Version: 2016. https://icd.who.int/browse10/2016/en. Accessed 19 July 2021
10. ICD-9 Data. http://www.icd9data.com/. Accessed 19 July 2021

11. What is CPT. https://www.aapc.com/resources/medical-coding/cpt.aspx. Accessed 19 July 2021
12. Smith, B., et al.: The OBO Foundry: coordinated evolution of ontologies to support biomedical data integration. Nat. Biotechnol. **25**, 1251–1255 (2007)
13. Kiourtis, A., Mavrogiorgou, A., Kyriazis, D.: Aggregating heterogeneous health data through an ontological common health language. In: 10th International Conference on Developments in eSystems Engineering, pp. 175–181 (2017)
14. Zhe, H.E., Geller, H.: Preliminary analysis of difficulty of importing pattern-based concepts into the National Cancer Institute thesaurus. Stud. Health Technol. Inform. 228–389 (2002)
15. Noy, N.F., et al.: BioPortal: ontologies and integrated data resources at the click of a mouse, Nucleic acids research. Nucleic Acids Res. 170–173 (2009)
16. Mossakowski, T., Kutz, O., Codescu, M.: Ontohub: a semantic repository for heterogeneous ontologies. In: Proceedings of DACS. CiteSeer (2014)
17. Lipscomb, C.E.: Medical subject headings (MeSH). Bull. Med. Libr. Assoc. **265** (2000)
18. Lindberg, C.: The unified medical language system (UMLS) of the national library of medicine. J. Am. Med. Rec. Assoc. 40–42 (1990)
19. Fontelo, P., Liu, F., Ackerman, M.: ask MEDLINE: a free-text, natural language query tool for MEDLINE/PubMed. BMC Med. Inf. Decis. Making **5** (2005). https://doi.org/10.1186/1472-6947-5-5
20. Liu, S., et al.: RxNorm: prescription for electronic drug information exchange. IT Prof. 17–23 (2005)
21. Kyriazis, D., et al.: CrowdHEALTH: holistic health records and big data analytics for health policy making and personalized health. Stud Health Technol. Inform. 19–23 (2017)
22. Kiourtis, A., Mavrogiorgou, A., Kyriazis, D., Torelli, F., Martino, D., De Nigro, A.: Holistic health records towards personalized healthcare. In: Proceedings of the 7th International Conference on Information and Communication Technologies for Ageing Well and e-Health (ICT4AWE 2021), pp. 78–89 (2021)
23. Pérez-Rey, D., et al.: SNOMED2HL7: a tool to normalize and bind SNOMED CT concepts to the HL7 reference information model. Comput. Methods Programs Biomed. **149**, 1–9 (2017)
24. Gardner, B.J., et al.: Incorporating a location-based socioeconomic index into a de-identified i2b2 clinical data warehouse. J. Am. Med. Inform. Assoc. **26**(4), 286–293 (2019)
25. Papez, V., et al.: Transforming and evaluating electronic health record disease phenotyping algorithms using the OMOP common data model: a case study in heart failure. J. Am. Med. Inform. Assoc. (2021)
26. Diastema project. https://diastema.gr/. Accessed 19 July 2021
27. CrowdHEALTH D3.1 - Health Record Structure: Design and Open Specification v1. https://www.crowdhealth.eu/sites/default/files/crowdhealth/public/content-files/deliverables/CrowdHEALTH_D3.1%20_Holistic_Health_Record_Design_Open_%20Specification%20v1.1.pdf. Accessed 19 July 2021
28. CrowdHEALTH D3.3 Health Record Structure: Software prototype v1. https://www.crowdhealth.eu/sites/default/files/crowdhealth/public/content-files/deliverables/CrowdHEALTH_D3.3%20Health%20Record%20Structure%20Software%20prototype%20v1.1.pdf. Accessed 19 July 2021

Multi-task Neural Networks for Pain Intensity Estimation Using Electrocardiogram and Demographic Factors

Stefanos Gkikas[1]($\boxtimes$)(iD), Chariklia Chatzaki[1](iD), and Manolis Tsiknakis[1,2](iD)

[1] Department of Electrical and Computer Engineering, Hellenic Mediterranean University, Estavromenos, 71410 Heraklion, Greece
gikasstefanos@gmail.com
[2] Institute of Computer Science, Foundation for Research and Technology-Hellas, Estavromenos, 70013 Heraklion, Greece

Abstract. Pain is a complex phenomenon which is manifested and expressed by patients in various forms. The immediate and objective recognition of it is a great of importance in order to attain a reliable and unbiased healthcare system. In this work, we elaborate electrocardiography signals revealing the existence of variations in pain perception among different demographic groups. We exploit this insight by introducing a novel multi-task neural network for automatic pain estimation utilizing the age and the gender information of each individual, and show its advantages compared to other approaches.

Keywords: Pain recognition · ECG · Deep learning · Age · Gender

1 Introduction

Pain according to Williams and Craig [3] is *"a distressing experience associated with actual or potential tissue damage with sensory, emotional, cognitive and social components"*. As a biological mechanism, pain facilitates the identification of harmful situations by the activation of primary sensory neurons releasing prostanoids molecules and growth factors in the spinal cord [19]. The two main types of pain are acute and chronic, where their main difference is related to the duration; the pain is considered as acute when is present less than three months and probably accompanied with clear physiological damage, while chronic when persist beyond the normal healing time [23]. Pain affects people in a major degree, provoking a plethora of daily life challenges, especially in chronic pain condition, which often leads to mental health problems e.g. anxiety, depression and sleep related problems [13]. In addition, there are various collateral negative effects, associated with opioid and drug overuse, addiction and poor social behavior relationships [19]. Pain is a serious issue concerns the whole society, since the consequences of it constitute clinical, economic and social constraints [6]. Especially in health care systems, more than 50% of the patients in hospitals are experience painful conditions, requiring large resources of medical and nursing stuff [5]. An important body of research indicates discrepancies regarding to pain manifestation and

L. A. Maciaszek et al. (Eds.): ICT4AWE 2021/2022, CCIS 1856, pp. 324–337, 2023.
https://doi.org/10.1007/978-3-031-37496-8_17

sensation in people of different gender and age, which increases the complication of pain management. In the meta-analysis of Riley et al. [17] refer that females demonstrate an elevated sensitivity for a variety of pain stimulus, while in the psychological review research [2] the author deduced that females perceive increased irritation and pain in more areas of the body than males. Furthermore, alterations in pain sensation, presented in the study [9] among elderly and youth population as well.

In clinical settings, self-report is the gold standard for the evaluation of presence and intensity of pain, by rating scales and questionnaires. Nevertheless, this process is high labor-intensive, and the constant patient supervision is impracticable. In addition, the pain assessment is further intricate and demanding regarding to patients with communicational limitations, mental deficiency, severe illness, or infants [26]. Sufficient and impartial pain assessment is required, in order to provide the essential medical management to those in pain and prevent additional heath problems. The estimation of pain is derived from the interpretation of behavioural and physiological responses; the behavioural responses includes facial expressions, body-head movements and vocalizations, while the physiological are the electrical flow generated from neurochemical activities which provoke the sympathetic nervous system, something that can be manifested and perceived in the physiological signals [20] e.g. electrocardiography (ECG), electromyography (EMG) and skin conductance response (GSR).

This study is founded on our previous work [8] investigating the variations of pain manifestation among different demographic groups, exploiting ECG signals. Furthermore, we extend our study by adopting neural networks as the main machine learning model, and propose a novel multi-task learning (MTL) neural network which exploits the demographic information by estimating the age and the gender beyond the pain level, in order to develop an improved automatic pain estimation system. The remaining of this paper is organised as follows: in Sect. 2 we present the related work, in Sect. 3 we describe the process of the feature extraction and the development of the neural network, Sect. 4 presents the conducted experiments and findings, and finally Sect. 5 concludes the paper.

2   Related Work

An important number of published research studies, founded on the utilization of biosignals in order to analyse the pain manifestation [13,25]. A major reason of the preference of biosignals instead of vision modalities e.g. facial expressions, is related to circumstances where subdued lightning, facial occlusions or even face absence occur, especially in clinical settings where the conditions are far from being perfect. Furthermore, in several occasions people exhibit exaggerated symptoms through facial expressions and body posture in order to elicit self-interest [18].

Utilizing ECG, EMG and electrodermal activity (EDA), researchers in [12], extracted various handcrafted features including skewness, standard deviation and QRS complexes, performing multi-level classification through a Random Forest (RF) classifier. Similarly, Amirial et al. [1] utilized ECG, EMG and EDA, where several features extracted from the time and frequency domain. By developing a Radial Basis Function (RBF) Neural Network, they achieved accepted results, while in [14] the authors designed a Recurrent Neural Network (RNN), feed it with the extracted R peaks and interbeat Intervals (IBIs) from ECG signals. Regarding to multi-task learning approaches, Lopez-Martinez and Picard [13] proposed a multi-task neural network utilizing ECG and EDA signals, where beyond the pain estimation the model predicts the identity of the person. In a follow-up study of the same authors [15] extended their work by adding visual modality, and furthermore, clustering subjects into different profiles according to their physiological and behavioural responses.

Recently, plethora of Deep Learning (DL) methods have been adopted in automatic pain estimation field, since in some cases their results are superior than traditional feature engineering and classical machine learning. The research of Wang et al. [25] utilized EEG potentials and an Autoencoder (AE) encoding the raw data to a compressed format, and classified them with a Logistic Regressor (LR) classifier, while Yu et al. [27] developed a framework which was consisted of five convolutional modules in order to analyse three classes of pain, namely no pain, moderate and severe based on EEG signals. Thiam et al. [22] designed deep 1D Convolutional Neural Networks employing ECG, EMG and GSR, experimenting with unimodal approaches, as well as multimodal fusion techniques. Interestingly, the authors in [11] proposed a framework to compute pseudo heart rate gain from videos through a 3D convolutional neural network (CNN). Utilizing the pseudo physiological modality achieved high performance in binary and multi-class classification setting.

However, to the best of our knowledge, extremely limited work has been conducted on the automatic pain estimation research taking into consideration demographic factors. The authors in [10], employing numerous biosignals such as EDA, respiration rate and diastolic blood pressure, as well as facial action units, revealed alterations in pain sensation among males and females. Similar are the findings in [21], where the conducted experiments which founded on a hybrid CNN-LSTM model and the utilization of ECG and EDA, indicating variations between the gender. Finally, our previous work [8], beyond the gender differences reveled even higher variations including the factor of age.

3   Methods

This section describes the employed pain database, the signal processing algorithm and feature extraction method, as well as the design of the multi-task neural network.

3.1   Dataset Details

In this study we employed the publicly available *BioVid Heat Pain Database* [24], which combines (1) frontal facial videos, (2) electrocardiogram, (3) electromyogram and (4) skin conductance level, recorded from 87 subjects (44 males, 43 females, age 20–65). Currently, the BioVid Heat Pain Database, is the only publicly available database which in-corporates the age and gender of the subjects. By subjecting heat stimulus on the right arm by a thermode, data were collected since the pain threshold (the temperature for which the participant's sensing changes from heat to pain) and pain tolerance (the temperature at which the pain becomes intolerable) for each subject were determined. Based on the specific thresholds, 5 pain intensities defined: No pain (NP), mild pain (P1), moderate pain (P2), severe pain (P3), very severe pain (P4). The subjects were stimulated 20 times for each intensity, thus generating 100 samples for every modality. The sampling frequency of ECG recordings is equal 512 Hz. In this work we employed the pre-processed with a Butterworth band-pass filter ECG samples ($87 \times 100 = 8700$) from Part A of the *BioVid*.

3.2   ECG Processing and Feature Extraction

An ECG signal reflects the electrical activity of the heart during time, where cardiac muscles depolarize and repolarize during a cardiac cycle. The cardiac cycle describes the undergoing activity from the beginning of one heartbeat to the beginning of the next, which in an ECG complex consists of a PQRST complex. The P wave indicates atrial depolarization, while the QRS complex represents ventricular depolarization and contraction. The T wave describes repolarization of ventricles. Consequently, the ECG analysis prerequisites the decomposition of the PQRST complex (see Fig. 1). By the accurate detection of R wave, which is the most prevalent peak in the complex, we are capable to calculate the heart rate (HR) and the heart rate variability (HRV), which is related with the time interval between consecutive R waves, called as RR interval or Interbeat interval. In this study, we adopt the Pan-Tompkins Algorithm [16] for the QRS detection. The specific algorithm is widely used and evaluated over the years, with the results supporting its efficiency even in noisy and low-quality data [7]. The synthesis of the algorithm emerges in two stages: the pre-processing and the decision; the pre-processing deals with removing noise and artifacts, as well as smoothing the signal and increasing the QRS slope, while the decision, encompass the initial QRS detection based on adaptive thresholds, a search back for missed QRS complexes, and a process for T wave discrimination. The basic flow diagram of Pan-Tompkins algorithm as well as the pre-process procedure applied in raw ECG presented in Fig. 2 and Fig. 3 respectively.

Following the accurate detection of R waves, the inter-beat intervals (IBIs) were estimated, and the most important relevant features were extracted. Particularly, the mean of IBIs, the root mean square of successive differences (RMSSD), the standard deviation of IBIs (SDNN), the slope of the linear regression of IBIs, the ratio of SDNN to RMSSD, and the heartbeat rate, were calculated as in detail described in our previous work [8].

3.3   Neural Network

Our proposed neural network trained in two different settings; with single-task learning (STL) and multi-task learning (MTL), where the latter beyond the pain estimation it involves the simultaneous training of age and/or gender estimation.

Single-Task Neural Network. The proposed neural network consists of two sub-networks; the encoder which is mapping the original feature vectors into a higher dimensional space, and the task-specific classifier. Our method employs fully-connected (FC) layers for both the encoder and the classifier, each one defined as follows:

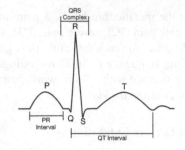

Fig. 1. The PQRST complex.

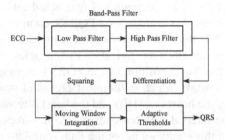

Fig. 2. The flow diagram of the pre-processing procedure of the Pan-Tompkins algorithm [8].

$$z_i(s) = b_i + \sum_{j=1}^{n_{in}} W_{ij}s_j \quad \text{for} \quad i = 1, .., n_{out} \tag{1}$$

where z_i is the outcome of the linear aggregation of incoming inputs s_j, and each input is weighted by W_{ij} and biased by b_i. Every layer of the encoder is followed by a non-linear activation function, namely rectified linear unit (ReLU) defined as:

$$\sigma(z) = \begin{cases} 1, & z \geq 0 \\ 0, & z < 0 \end{cases} \tag{2}$$

while the classifier' layers are connected without nonlinearity. The encoder consists of 4 FC layers with 256, 512, 1024 and 1024 neurons respectively, while the classifier consists of 2 layers with 1024 and n neurons, where n is the number of the corresponding pain classes. In Table 1, we list the hyper-parameters of our network.

Table 1. Training hyper-parameters used in our method.

Epochs	Optimizer	Learning rate	LR decay	Weight decay	Warmup epochs	Label smooth	EMA
300	AdamW	1e-3	cosine	0.1	50	0.1	✓

Multi-task Neural Network. The specific machine learning method is founded on the principle of sharing representations between related tasks, enabling the model to generalize better on the original task, i.e. pain estimation. In this settings, we retained

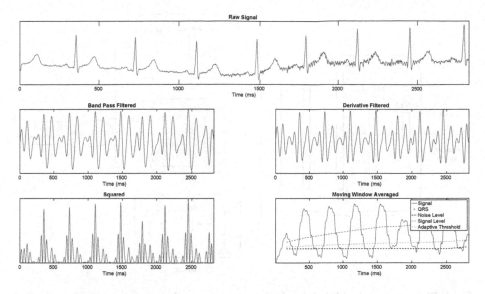

Fig. 3. ECG pre-processing with Pan-Tompkins algorithm [8].

the identical encoder and pain classifier, while we added two auxiliary networks, for age and gender estimation respectively. Figure 4 presents the architecture of proposed MTL neural network. The objective of the network is the minimization of the three losses, simultaneous. We adopt and extend the proposal of [4] regarding the multi-task learning loss, in which learned weights multiple the loss functions by considering the homoscedastic uncertainty of each task:

$$L_{total} = [e^{w1}L_{Pain} + w_1]c_1 + [e^{w2}L_{Age} + w_2]c_2 + [e^{w3}L_{Gender} + w_3]c_3 \quad (3)$$

where L is the corresponding loss, w the weights and c the coefficients which restrain the L_{Age} and L_{Gender} in order to influence the learning procedure into the pain estimation task. We mention that all the tasks addressed as classification problems, adopting the *cross-entropy* loss with label smoothing:

$$L_D = -\sum_{\delta \in D} \sum_{i=1}^{n_{out}} p(i|x_\delta) \log[q(i|x_\delta)] \quad (4)$$

where D is the pain database, $p(i|x_\delta) = 1 - \epsilon$ and $p(i \neq i_\delta|x_\delta) = \epsilon/(n_{out} - 1)$ is the distribution over the components i of the ground truth, and $q(i|x_\delta)$ is the distribution over the components i of the networks' output.

4 Experiments and Results

4.1 Demographic Groups

Utilizing the single-task neural network (ST-NN) we conducted the first body of experiments related to the influence of demographic factors. Specifically, adopting the idea

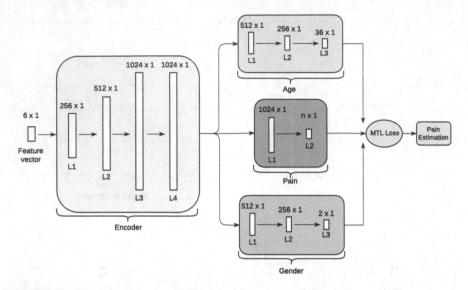

Fig. 4. Illustration of the MTL network. The output vectors' size of the network is: for Pain classifier $nx1$ where n the number of pain estimation tasks (i.e. 2 for binary classification, 5 for multi-class classification), for Age classifier 36×1 where 36 is equal to the number of possible values of subjects' age, for Gender classifier 2×1 where 2 the number of possible values (i.e. males, females).

of [8] we developed five schemes; (1) basic scheme, utilizing all the subjects of the database, (2) gender scheme, dividing the subjects into males and females, (3) age scheme, based on the subjects' age forming three groups i.e. *20–35, 36–50, 51–65*, and (4) gender-age scheme combining the gender and age of the subjects, creating six groups i.e. *Males 20–35, Females 20–35, Males 36–50, Females 36–50, Males 51–65, Females 51–65*. We note that all the experiments of this study conducted in binary and multi-class classification settings. In particular: (1) NP vs P1, (2) NP vs P2, (3) NP vs P3, (4) NP vs P4 regarding the binary classification and finally (5) multi-class pain classification, utilizing all the available pain classes of the database.

Table 2 presents the classification results of Basic scheme, utilizing all the subjects of the database. For the multi-class pain classification we achieved 29.43%, while the accuracy on NP vs P1 attained 61.15% and reaching up to 68.82% on NP vs P4. We observe that as the pain intensity raise, the performance scores increased as well, revealing the challenges to recognise the low magnitude of pain severity. According to the gender scheme (see Table 3) there are clear differences among males and females, especially in higher pain intensities. Specifically, in NP vs P4 females attained 69.48% over 66.48%, while the two genders present 1.63% variance in total, exhibiting that females characterized by a higher pain sensitivity. Figure 5a outlines the classification differences among the gender. On the age scheme (see Table 4), and particularly on NP vs P4 the group *20–35* presents 72.58% over 66.29% and 64.91% from the groups *36–50* and *51–65* respectively, while in lower pain intensities the differences are less noticeable. Nevertheless, the specific scheme reveals that the factor of age influences the pain manifestation, especially for older population. Figure 5b depicts the results of age scheme.

In the last scheme, dividing the subjects into additional number of groups, we are able to study them in a more precisely manner, and obtain and better understanding about the correlation of gender and age with the pain sensation. In Table 5 we observe that in task NP vs P4 the group *Females 20–35* achieved the highest accuracy with 71.67%, exceeding the group *Males 51–65* by 11% which obtained the minimal performance, and described as the least sensitive group. Similar are the observations on the multi-class classification, as well as in the remaining pain tasks, where *Females 20–35* and *Males 51–65* presented the uppermost and the minor pain estimation accuracies respectively. This corroborates that females defined with elevated pain manifestation, while males, especially seniors possess diminished sensation. We mention that in some cases e.g. *Males 20–35*, *Males 36–50* despite the fact the pain intention in increased, the classification accuracy is diminished, something also observed in [8]. An possible interpretation would be the accustomation of the subjects in pain situations, especially in low intensities. Figure 5c visualize the performances of the gender-age scheme.

Table 2. Classification results of the Basic Scheme, reported on % accuracy.

Group	Algorithm	Task				
		NP vs P1	NP vs P2	NP vs P3	NP vs P4	MC
All	ST-NN	61.15	62.87	65.14	68.82	29.43

ST-NN: single-task neural network NP: no pain P1: mild pain P2: moderate pain P3: severe pain P4: very severe pain MC: multi-classification

Table 3. Classification results of the Gender Scheme, reported on % accuracy.

Group	Algorithm	Task				
		NP vs P1	NP vs P2	NP vs P3	NP vs P4	MC
Males	ST-NN	60.40	63.24	63.18	66.48	28.61
Females	ST-NN	60.87	62.15	66.98	69.48	30.59

Table 4. Classification results of the Age Scheme, reported on % accuracy.

Group	Algorithm	Task				
		NP vs P1	NP vs P2	NP vs P3	NP vs P4	MC
20–35	ST-NN	61.58	64.08	66.08	72.58	31.07
36–50	ST-NN	60.52	61.38	64.05	66.29	29.59
51–65	ST-NN	61.70	60.80	62.50	64.91	27.82

4.2 Augmentation of Feature Vectors

Based on the observations from the previous section regarding the influence of demographic factors in pain manifestation, we investigate the functional exploitation of

Table 5. Classification results of the Gender-Age Scheme, reported on % accuracy.

Group	Algorithm	Task				
		NP vs P1	NP vs P2	NP vs P3	NP vs P4	MC
Males 20–35	ST-NN	62.83	62.33	65.5	71.33	29.73
Males 36–50	ST-NN	61.79	60.00	59.64	64.11	27.14
Males 51–65	ST-NN	59.50	58.67	57.33	60.67	26.07
Females 20–35	ST-NN	63.17	63.17	66.83	71.67	31.53
Females 36–50	ST-NN	59.50	61.00	65.83	67.00	29.13
Females 51–65	ST-NN	60.96	60.96	59.23	63.27	27.69

subjects' demographic information. We conducted a set of experiments utilizing the ST-NN and the feature vectors which augmented by the expansion of them with demographic elements. Specifically, the original feature vectors, consisting of six features (see Sect. 3.2), expanding by an additional feature (i.e. the subjects' gender or age), or two additional features (the subjects' gender and age). In this manner, utilizing the new set of features we carried out the identical experiments related to pain estimation tasks. Table 6 presents the classification results, where we observe increased performances adopting the approach of augmented feature vectors. In particular, the most effected type of augmentation is the combination of Gender and Age feature, which improved the mean pain estimation performance by 0.55%, while the utilization of them individually, enhanced the classification accuracy, but in a lower degree.

Table 6. Comparison of classification results adopting the feature augmentation approach, reported on % accuracy.

Group	Algorithm	Aux.	Task				
			NP vs P1	NP vs P2	NP vs P3	NP vs P4	MC
All	ST-NN	–	61.15	62.87	65.14	68.82	29.43
All	ST-NN	F(G)	61.44	63.19	65.00	68.79	29.68
All	ST-NN	F(A)	61.21	62.67	65.66	69.57	29.71
All	ST-NN	F(GA)	61.09	63.48	66.21	69.54	29.86

Aux: Auxiliary information -: original feature vectors F(G): feature vectors with the additional feature of gender F(A): feature vectors with the additional feature of age F(GA): feature vectors with the additional features of gender and age

4.3 Multi-Task Neural Network

The final set of experiments conducted in a multi-task learning manner, utilizing the proposed MT-NN described in Sect. 3.3. The classification performances of MT-NN with the additional tasks of (1) gender estimation, (2) age estimation and (3) gender & age estimation simultaneously, are presented in Table 7. The results of the previous approaches based on the ST-NN method, are presented as well in Table 7. We observe that the additional task of gender estimation performed inferior compared to others

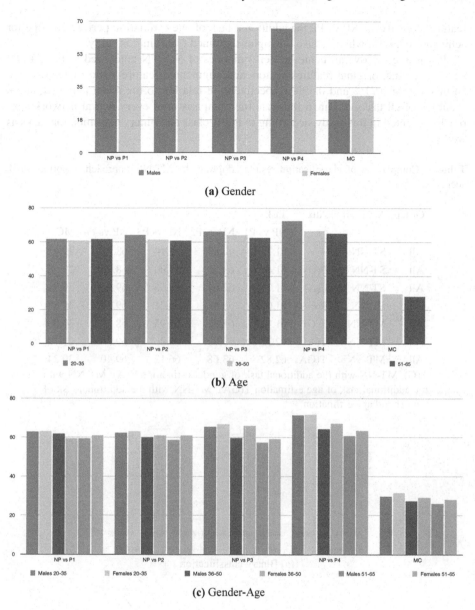

(a) Gender

(b) Age

(c) Gender-Age

Fig. 5. Classification results on different Schemes.

tasks, while the combination of gender & age achieved the highest performance in four of the five tasks. Specifically, in the multi-class classification attained 30.24%, while in NP vs P1 62.82% which are the greatest results compared to every presented method in this study. Similarly, in NP vs P3 and NP vs P4 outperformed the gender and age additional tasks, however underperformed to ST-NN approaches with the augmented features. Finally, in NP vs P2 the additional task of age estimation performed superior achieving 63.97%, which is also the highest attained result in this study.

Regarding the overall achieved performances of MT-NN compared to the ST-NN approaches (i.e. original features vectors and augmented feature vectors), we observe an increase of 0.71% and 0.39% respectively, in relation to the mean pain estimation accuracy of all tasks. Figure 6 illustrate the comparison of every neural network approach presented in this study, according to multi-class and binary classification tasks as well.

Table 7. Comparison of classification results adopting the MT-NN approach, reported on % accuracy.

Group	Algorithm	Aux.	Task				
			NP vs P1	NP vs P2	NP vs P3	NP vs P4	MC
All	ST-NN	–	61.15	62.87	65.14	68.82	29.43
All	ST-NN	F(G)	61.44	63.19	65.00	68.79	29.68
All	ST-NN	F(A)	61.21	62.67	65.66	69.57	29.71
All	ST-NN	F(GA)	61.09	63.48	66.21	69.54	29.86
All	MT-NN	T(G)	61.72	63.39	65.95	68.99	30.00
All	MT-NN	T(A)	62.72	63.97	65.40	69.28	29.79
All	MT-NN	T(GA)	62.82	63.68	66.12	69.40	30.24

T(G): MT-NN with the additional task of gender estimation T(A): MT-NN with the additional task of age estimation T(GA): MT-NN with the additional task of gender and age estimation

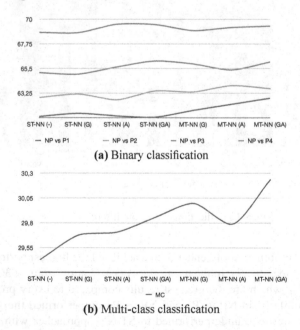

(a) Binary classification

(b) Multi-class classification

Fig. 6. Comparison of classification performances adopting different neural networks approaches.

4.4 Comparison with Existing Methods

Finally, in this section we compare our accomplished results utilizing the MT-NN employed the additional tasks of gender and age estimation, with corresponding studies which utilized the electrocardiography signals of the Part A of *BioVid* database with all 87 participants, and followed the same evaluation protocol i.e. leave-one-subject-out (LOSO) cross validation for the purpose of an equitable comparison. The results depicted in Table 8, including studies utilizing hand-crafted features and classic machine learning algorithms [8,26], *end-to-end* deep learning approaches [11,22], and methods combining hand-crafted features with deep learning classification algorithms [14]. Our method exploiting the carefully designed ECG features, followed by the high-dimensional mapping from the encoder with the combination of the multi-task learning neural networks, was able to outperform other approaches in every pain estimation task, either in binary or multi-class classification setting.

Table 8. Comparison of studies which utilized *BioVid*, ECG signals and LOSO cross validation.

Study	Task				
	NP vs P1	NP vs P2	NP vs P3	NP vs P4	MC
Gkikas et al. [8]†	52.38	52.78	55.37	58.62	23.79
Huang et al. [11]*⊙	–	–	–	65.00	28.50
Martinez and Picard [14]*	–	–	–	57.69	–
Thiam et al. [22]*	49.71	50.72	52.87	57.04	23.23
Wernel et al. [26]†	48.70	51.60	56.50	62.00	–
This study*	62.82	63.68	66.12	69.40	30.24

†:hand-crafted features and classic machine learning *: end-to-end deep learning
*: hand-crafted features with deep learning classification algorithms ⊙: pseudo heart rate gain extracted from visual modality

5 Conclusion

This work explored the application of multi-task learning neural networks for automatic pain estimation based on electrocardiography signals. Utilizing the Pan-Tompkins algorithm for the detection of QRS complexes we extracted essential features related to IBIs. Several experiments conducted in order to investigate the relation of gender and age with the pain manifestation, revealing the great influence of them to pain perception. Furthermore, we proposed two methods in order to exploit the demographic information enhancing the pain estimation results. First, the original feature vectors augmented with the subjects' demographic elements which indeed improved the classification accuracy. Second, the multi-task learning neural network integrating the pain estimation task with the gender and age estimation as well. The latter demonstrated superior results compared to previous presented methods in this paper, as well as to other related studies. This suggests that extracted domain specific features combined with properly designed deep learning architectures and demographic factors are able to accomplish great results.

In summary, we suggest that clinical pain management tools need to be designed in such a way so that patients' demographic information, which clearly influence pain manifestation, are included. However, from the machine learning viewpoint, it is evident that additional research efforts are needed, in order to achieve reliable and accurate estimations, especially when multi-level pain assessment is concerned and to enhance clinical adoption of such tools. In future work, we will focus on the exploration and use of additional biosignals, e.g. EMG or GSR, in both a unimodal and multimodal setting as well.

References

1. Amirian, M., Kächele, M., Schwenker, F.: Using radial basis function neural networks for continuous and discrete pain estimation from bio-physiological signals. In: Schwenker, F., Abbas, H.M., El Gayar, N., Trentin, E. (eds.) ANNPR 2016. LNCS (LNAI), vol. 9896, pp. 269–284. Springer, Cham (2016). https://doi.org/10.1007/978-3-319-46182-3_23
2. Bartley, E.J., Fillingim, R.B.: Sex differences in pain: a brief review of clinical and experimental findings. Br. J. Anaesth. 111(1), 52–58 (2013). https://doi.org/10.1093/bja/aet127, https://pubmed.ncbi.nlm.nih.gov/23794645, https://www.ncbi.nlm.nih.gov/pmc/articles/PMC3690315/
3. de C Williams, A.C., Craig, K.D.: Updating the definition of pain. Pain 157, 2420–2423 (2016). https://doi.org/10.1097/j.pain.0000000000000613
4. Cipolla, R., Gal, Y., Kendall, A.: Multi-task learning using uncertainty to weigh losses for scene geometry and semantics. In: 2018 IEEE/CVF Conference on Computer Vision and Pattern Recognition, pp. 7482–7491 (2018). https://doi.org/10.1109/CVPR.2018.00781
5. Cordell, W.H., Keene, K.K., Giles, B.K., Jones, J.B., Jones, J.H., Brizendine, E.J.: The high prevalence of pain in emergency medical care. Am. J. Emerg. Med. 20, 165–169 (2002). https://doi.org/10.1053/ajem.2002.32643
6. Dinakar, P., Stillman, A.M.: Pathogenesis of pain. Semin. Pediatr. Neurol. 23, 201–208 (2016). https://doi.org/10.1016/J.SPEN.2016.10.003
7. Fariha, M.A.Z., Ikeura, R., Hayakawa, S., Tsutsumi, S.: Analysis of pan-tompkins algorithm performance with noisy ECG signals. J. Phys. Conf. Ser. 1532, 12022 (2020). https://doi.org/10.1088/1742-6596/1532/1/012022
8. Gkikas., S., Chatzaki., C., Pavlidou., E., Verigou., F., Kalkanis., K., Tsiknakis., M.: Automatic pain intensity estimation based on electrocardiogram and demographic factors, pp. 155–162. SciTePress (2022). https://doi.org/10.5220/0010971700003188
9. Hadjistavropoulos, T., Craig, K.D.: A theoretical framework for understanding self-report and observational measures of pain: a communications model. Behav. Res. Therapy 40, 551–570 (2002). https://doi.org/10.1016/S0005-7967(01)00072-9
10. Hinduja, S., Canavan, S., Kaur, G.: Multimodal fusion of physiological signals and facial action units for pain recognition, pp. 577–581. Institute of Electrical and Electronics Engineers Inc. (2020). https://doi.org/10.1109/FG47880.2020.00060
11. Huang, D., et al.: Spatio-temporal pain estimation network with measuring pseudo heart rate gain. IEEE Trans. Multimed. 24, 3300–3313 (2022). https://doi.org/10.1109/TMM.2021.3096080
12. Kächele, M., Thiam, P., Amirian, M., Schwenker, F., Palm, G.: Methods for person-centered continuous pain intensity assessment from bio-physiological channels. IEEE J. Sel. Top. Signal Process. 10, 854–864 (2016). https://doi.org/10.1109/JSTSP.2016.2535962

13. Lopez-Martinez, D., Picard, R.: Multi-task neural networks for personalized pain recognition from physiological signals, vol. 2018-Janua, pp. 181–184. Institute of Electrical and Electronics Engineers Inc., January 2017. https://doi.org/10.1109/ACIIW.2017.8272611

14. Lopez-Martinez, D., Picard, R.: Continuous pain intensity estimation from autonomic signals with recurrent neural networks, vol. 2018, pp. 5624–5627 (2018). https://doi.org/10.1109/EMBC.2018.8513575

15. Lopez-Martinez, D., Rudovic, O., Picard, R.: Physiological and behavioral profiling for nociceptive pain estimation using personalized multitask learning. In: Neural Information Processing Systems (NIPS) Workshop on Machine Learning for Health. Long Beach, USA (2017)

16. Pan, J., Tompkins, W.J.: A real-time QRS detection algorithm. IEEE Trans. Biomed. Eng. **BME-32**, 230–236 (1985). https://doi.org/10.1109/TBME.1985.325532

17. 3rd Riley, J.L., Robinson, M.E., Wise, E.A., Myers, C.D., Fillingim, R.B.: Sex differences in the perception of noxious experimental stimuli: a meta-analysis. Pain **74**, 181–187 (1998). https://doi.org/10.1016/s0304-3959(97)00199-1

18. Rohling, M.L., Binder, L.M., Langhinrichsen-Rohling, J.: Money matters: a meta-analytic review of the association between financial compensation and the experience and treatment of chronic pain. Health Psychol. **14**, 537–547 (1995). https://doi.org/10.1037/0278-6133.14.6.537

19. Khalid, S., Tubbs, R.S.: Neuroanatomy and neuropsychology of pain. Cureus **9** (2017). https://doi.org/10.7759/CUREUS.1754

20. Stewart, G., Panickar, A.: Role of the sympathetic nervous system in pain, December 2013. https://doi.org/10.1016/j.mpaic.2013.09.003

21. Subramaniam, S.D., Dass, B.: Automated nociceptive pain assessment using physiological signals and a hybrid deep learning network. IEEE Sens. J. **21**, 3335–3343 (2021). https://doi.org/10.1109/JSEN.2020.3023656

22. Thiam, P., Bellmann, P., Kestler, H.A., Schwenker, F.: Exploring deep physiological models for nociceptive pain recognition. Sensors **19**, 4503 (2019). https://doi.org/10.3390/s19204503

23. Turk, D.C., Melzack, R.: The measurement of pain and the assessment of people experiencing pain, pp. 3–16 (2011). https://psycnet.apa.org/record/2011-03491-001

24. Walter, S., et al.: The biovid heat pain database: data for the advancement and systematic validation of an automated pain recognition, pp. 128–131 (2013). https://doi.org/10.1109/CYBConf.2013.6617456

25. Wang, J., et al.: An autoencoder-based approach to predict subjective pain perception from high-density evoked EEG potentials, vol. 2020-July, pp. 1507–1511. Institute of Electrical and Electronics Engineers Inc. (2020). https://doi.org/10.1109/EMBC44109.2020.9176644

26. Werner, P., Al-Hamadi, A., Niese, R., Walter, S., Gruss, S., Traue, H.C.: Automatic pain recognition from video and biomedical signals, pp. 4582–4587. Institute of Electrical and Electronics Engineers Inc. (2014). https://doi.org/10.1109/ICPR.2014.784

27. Yu, M., et al.: Diverse frequency band-based convolutional neural networks for tonic cold pain assessment using EEG. Neurocomputing **378**, 270–282 (2020). https://doi.org/10.1016/j.neucom.2019.10.023

The Influence of Culture in the Adoption and Use of Mobile Applications in the Management of Non-communicable Disease

Mariam Jacobs-Basadien and Shaun Pather[✉]

Department of Information Systems, University of the Western Cape, Cape Town, South Africa
{mjacobsbasadien,spather}@uwc.ac.za

Abstract. Mobile health (m-health) applications have been widely recognised in healthcare literature in recent years as tools for delivering effective and efficient interventions to patients with chronic conditions such as diabetes. Understanding m-health acceptance for diabetes management, in particular, is critical as it impacts on the achievement of development goals, including the United Nations' SDG 3. Previous research argued that individuals' culture persuasions have an influence on diabetics patients' decisions to adopt and use mobile applications for diabetes self-management. This research assesses typical low income communities through an integrated lens of culture concepts and technology adoption. The paper presents evidence that Hofstede's cultural dimensions, and the Unified-theory of Acceptance and Use of Technology 2, are relevant conceptual avenues to investigate the phenomena of mobile application adoption for diabetes self-management. The locus of the discussion is set in South Africa, more specifically, the Cape Flats in the Western Cape Province.

Keywords: South African · Mobile health (m-health) · Diabetes self-management · Culture · Technology adoption

1 Introduction

In the last two decades, disparities with respect to accessibility to and availability of the internet have reduced, due to technological advances and lower-cost access to broadband internet [1]. The prevalence of Information and Communication Technology (ICT) and infrastructure is greater than it was a decade ago. Mobile technologies are no longer limited to specific demographics, as they are made increasingly affordable to all in developing countries. Globally, there are estimated to be 5.3 billion internet users [2]. In Africa, there are a total of approximately 601.32 million internet users [3], 41,19 million of which are South African users [4]. In South Africa (SA), 77.5% of internet users can access the internet from anywhere, of which 89.1% reside in the Western Cape [5]. Furthermore, 69.4% of people in the Western Cape can access the internet from their mobile phones [5].

L. A. Maciaszek et al. (Eds.): ICT4AWE 2021/2022, CCIS 1856, pp. 338–361, 2023.
https://doi.org/10.1007/978-3-031-37496-8_18

The South African Government has developed a South African National Infrastructure Plan (NIP) consisting of 18 Strategic Integrated Projects (SIPs) to improve the social and economic infrastructure across provinces. The knowledge SIP comprising SIP 15 involves increasing access to "communication technology" by integrating the network into rural areas [6]. Access to broadband internet has also greatly improved with several local government public Wi-Fi programmes, and public access centres, e.g. The Smart Cape programme of the City of Cape Town. The improved access to hardware and the internet provides an opportunity for technology to address various social ills as well as providing patients with the ability to access health care information [7].

ICT such as mobile health (m-health) applications can help people manage their chronic conditions [8]. Mobile health (m-health) has emerged as an aspect of electronic health (e-health) and received recognition in healthcare literature in recent years. M-health applications is defined as a software that provides health services to individuals through mobile technologies such as smartphones and tablets [9].

There are several examples in the literature of the role of ICT on health-related matters. It was found that m-health technologies can assist patients to adhere to diet regimes (for example, sending reminders when medication must be administered) and control blood pressure and glucose levels [10].

Diabetes mellitus, a global health problem affects people of all ages. 6.7 million deaths are attributable to diabetes [11]. People living with diabetes come from both low and middle income nations [12]. South Africa is one of the African countries with a high prevalence of diabetes [13]. It accounts for high morbidity and mortality rates and is the second leading cause of death [14]. Furthermore it shows that approximately 45% of the South African population are not screened for diabetes [15, 16]. Out of 9 provinces, the Western Cape has the third highest prevalence of diabetes [17]. The risk factors associated with diabetes are comprised of,—but are not restricted to—tobacco use, alcohol consumption and unhealthy eating [18]. These risk factors could lead to complications such as cardiovascular disease, amputations, and blindness [19]. Therefore, it is imperative that diabetic patients follow guidelines such as the seven self-care behaviour activities of the American Association of Diabetes Educators (AADE).

There is evidence that mobile applications are an ideal platform for delivering effective and efficient interventions, which can help decrease Non-Communicable Disease (NCD) risk factors [20]. However, for individuals to self-manage their conditions, they have to first accept and use the technology [21].

Technology adoption is described as the acceptance or the first use of a technology [22]. It has been stated that users must first make use of technology, such as m-health applications, before the sought-after results can be attained [23]. Technology acceptance is widely investigated and understood in the Information Systems (IS) literature. Of the models for user acceptance, many researchers have applied the Unified-theory of Acceptance and Use of Technology (UTAUT) (e.g., [24–26]) and the Technology Acceptance Model (e.g., [27–29]) to investigate technology adoption problems. Of the several technology adoption problems, research indicates that a link exists between technology adoption and culture. Culture can either enable technology acceptance [30] or hinder technology adoption [31].

Several authors [32–36] asserted that culture have an influence on the adoption of technology. Furthermore literature indicates that socio-cultural factors in the healthcare sector affect the adoption of m-health services [37]. This indicates that the relationship between culture and technology use is an established area in IS research [27, 32, 38].

Jacobs-Basadien and Pather [8] developed a framework to understand the role of culture in the adoption of m-health applications for management of disease. This paper revisits that framework and examines and assess the conceptual framework in relation to the literature review on culture and technology adoption. The literature is examined to look for further evidence to uphold the framework developed by Jacobs-Basadien and Pather [8]. Moreover, this paper will examine an instance of culture of marginalised communities and interrogate the concepts of culture and technology adoption to further understand the conceptual framework.

The remainder of the paper is organised as follows: Sect. 2 provides reviews on extent literature of diabetes mellitus, culture viz. South African culture and localised culture. Section 3 concludes this research paper.

2 Literature Review

2.1 Defining Diabetes Mellitus

Diabetes mellitus is defined as an atypically high level of sugar glucose in the blood. Diabetes occurs either when the body produces insufficient insulin (which is made by the pancreas), or where there is inadequate sensitivity of cells in the body to use the insulin it produces [39]. The two types of diabetes are diabetes type 1 and diabetes type 2. Type 1 diabetes mellitus (T1DM), commonly known as juvenile diabetes as well as insulin-dependent diabetes mellitus (IDDM) is described as an autoimmune disease where the pancreas produces little or no insulin [39]. It typically develops more quickly than other forms of diabetes and occurs in children and youths. Patients with type 1 diabetes are required to administer insulin medication daily as the body cannot function without insulin [40]. On the other hand, type 2 diabetes mellitus (T2DM) formerly known as adult-onset diabetes, but which of late has been diagnosed in children [39], is a chronic condition in which the body ineffectively uses the insulin. The pancreas makes insulin, yet the body is unable to use the glucose-controlling hormone, which results in the pancreas being unable to produce as much insulin as the body requires [39].

Self-management is an essential part of diabetes management. Self-management is defined as the process whereby patients are actively involved in the long-term care of managing their chronic condition [41–43]. Diabetes self-management (DSM) refers to actions taken by the patient in regulating diabetes mellitus– that is its treatment– and disease escalation prevention [44].

There are several risk factors associated with diabetes, and these include inter alia age, ethnicity, socio-economic status and lifestyle factors [39]. These factors are prevalent in minority racial/ethnic populations, where the prevalence of diabetes is high [45]. Although the pervasiveness of diabetes varies with socio-economic status, the disparities can be worsened by the poor lifestyles adopted by individuals [46].

Lifestyle activities such as healthy eating, physical activity and sufficient sleep are imperative in order to prevent the onset of Type 2 diabetes [47]. Unhealthy lifestyles are among the reasons for the high prevalence of diabetes in South Africa, with type 2 diabetes being over 90% of all cases [46]. This is because people from lower socio-economic groups have factors such as their socio-economic status and a lack of knowledge that increases the prevalence of diabetes [48]. In addition, limited access to healthy food is another of the challenges faced by people of low socio-economic status, and this situation increases their chances of developing diabetes.

In South Africa, the pervasiveness of T2DM may be attributed to unhealthy lifestyle factors [49] and negative attitudes toward diabetes [50] as well as to the beliefs and behaviours of others influencing the health behaviours of individuals [51]. Therefore, patients need to be able to implement self-care practices in their daily lives, as morbidity and mortality are preventable through medication adherence and risk factor modification [37].

Proper diabetes management improves the quality of life and may prevent diabetes complications and early fatalities [39]. Effective interventions are essential characteristics of diabetes care [52]. For the patient, self-managing their condition is multi-dimensional and requires a range of activities [53].

The American Association of Diabetes Educators (ADA) has identified seven behavioural activities that diabetes patients should follow to improve their health outcomes. These seven behaviours are: healthy eating, being active, health monitoring, taking prescribed medication, problem-solving, healthy coping, and reducing risks. These have been identified as the seven essential behaviours for improving diabetes self-management [19]. Adhering to these self-care behaviour activities can positively impact the quality of life of type 2 diabetic patients. However, integrating them into a patients' life can become challenging and often difficult to maintain long term. To assist with this, self-management programs for type 2 diabetes are available through smartphone technologies.

2.2 Advantages of m-Health Applications for Diabetes Self-management

The use of ICT has become increasingly popular in recent years for medical self-care. Numerous technological advances have emerged to address health-related issues of patients [54]. M-health is defined as "medical and public health practice supported by mobile devices such as mobile phones, patient monitoring devices, personal digital assistants (PDAs), and other wearable devices" [6, p. 6].

Many m-health applications exist today that offer options to support self-management activities. Many of these applications are free, while others require a once-off or monthly subscription fee [53]. Research indicates that diabetes applications support patients in improving their knowledge regarding their condition and include awareness of diabetes complications and competencies for their self-management [55].

Medical interventions and self-management are vital to ensure the well-being of patients that suffer from NCDs [56]. Diabetes self-management is crucial for patients as it facilitates the prevention of diabetes complications. Healthcare provided via mobile applications provides countless benefits when applied to patients with diabetes [57]. M-health applications are especially advantageous in developing countries because they require low start-up costs, and mobile applications are even affordable to people residing in more impoverished areas [58].

The usage of m-health applications has the potential of improving the self-management of patients with type 2 diabetes as it enables them to adhere to self-care activities [59]. Diabetes self-management improves health outcomes by providing lifestyle modifications such as diet, exercise and medication adherence. All these activities can be improved through mobile applications since m-health helps a user to achieve lifestyle modification [57]. Even though patients have the required knowledge and skills to cope with diabetes [44], they may acquire more knowledge from m-health applications and thus be provided with continuous motivation [60].

The clinical benefit that diabetes self-management provides to patients is that it empowers patients to engage in managing their condition, thereby promoting self-efficacy [61]. Self-efficacy has been found to influence self-care behaviours of patients. Individuals– and in this context– diabetes patients are likely to partake in activities they perceive to encompass high self-efficacy. It is, therefore, imperative to develop self-efficacy to improve adherence to self-care activities.

M-health applications can also provide patients with better decision making, including insulin administration [41]. M-health applications are used to provide patient care, better decision making, access to health and general health services, enhance clinical diagnosis and treatment adherence, as well as many other benefits that can help patients manage their daily activities associated with living independently [9].

Many researchers have identified that m-health applications can provide patients access to their health information at any time and any place and can therefore reduce the time and cost associated with dealing with chronic conditions [61–64]. Additionally, remote access to care provides the opportunity for patients living in rural and limited resourced areas to connect to quality individualised care [65]. This entails that m-health applications are readily available without the constraint of a geographical barrier [66].

M-health applications can augment medical resources that are available in healthcare facilities [63]. For example, blood glucose data can be collected, analysed, stored and be presented to the patient in real-time [66], making health information readily available for diabetic patients [41]. Another benefit of m-health applications relates to health education [62]. M-health applications provide better health outcomes by providing patients with increased knowledge about their condition [67]. M-health applications can create a smart environment where patients can engage in the management of their health, which supports the transition from clinic-centric to patient-centric healthcare [66]. Fundamentally, the adoption of m-health can improve the self-care activities that patients undertake, such as exercise, food intake, blood sugar levels and their health behaviours [68].

2.3 Models and Theories of Individual Acceptance

Technology adoption is well-established in IS research. Several models exist that assess the variables that influence the adoption of technologies [69]. It was argued that individuals' reactions to using information technology (IT) is driven by their intention to use IT which then determine their actual use of IT [70]. Figure 1 illustrates a framework that underline the eight user acceptance models.

The eight models include the theory of reasoned action (TRA), theory of planned behaviour (TPB), technology acceptance model (TAM), the model of PC utilisation,

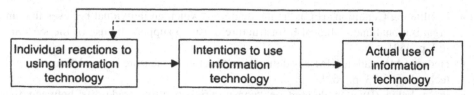

Fig. 1. Basic Concepts Underlying User Acceptance Models (Source: [70], p. 427).

motivational model, combination of TAM and TPB, Social cognitive theory and the Diffusion of innovation theory.

The four most widely used user acceptance models (Fig. 2) in the area of m-health include Theory of Reasoned Action (TRA), Technology Acceptance Model (TAM), Theory of Planned Behaviour (TPB), Unified-theory of Acceptance and Use of Technology (UTAUT) and UTAUT2 [8].

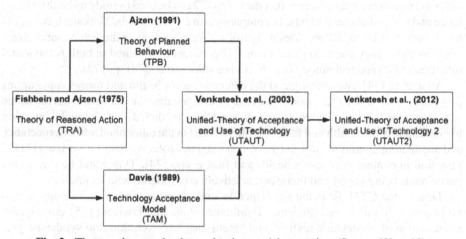

Fig. 2. The prominent technology adoption models over time (Source: [8], p. 38).

Unified-Theory of Acceptance and Use of Technology 2. Venkatesh, Thong and Xu [71] revised the UTAUT model to come up with the UTAUT2. In this revised model, the authors introduced three new constructs: Hedonic Motivation, Price and Habit, and they excluded voluntariness of use from the moderating variables. The core constructs of the UTAUT2 model are defined below:

- Performance Expectancy (PE): "is the degree to which an individual believes that using the system will help him or her to attain gains in job performance" [67, p. 447].
- Effort Expectancy (EE): "is the degree of ease associated with the use of the system" [67, p. 450].
- Social Influence (SI): "is the degree to which an individual perceives that important others believe he or she should use the new system" [67, p. 451].

- Facilitating Conditions (FC): "is the degree to which an individual believes that an organisational and technical infrastructure exists to support the use of the system" [67, p. 453].
- Hedonic Motivation (HM): is defined as "the fun or pleasure derived from using a technology" [73, p. 161].
- Price Value (PV): is defined as "consumers' cognitive trade-offs between the perceived benefits of the applications and monetary costs for using them" [73, p. 161].
- Habit (HT): "the extent to which people tend to perform behaviours automatically because of learning" [73, p. 161].

Researchers have assessed the behavioural intention for m-health adoption behaviour [25, 72, 73]. Hoque and Sorwar [25] found that the constructs of UTAUT have an influence on users' behavioural intention to adopt m-health services. Baptista and Oliveira [73] merged UTAUT2 and Hofstede's cultural dimensions and the results indicate that these models combined can investigate the acceptance of mobile applications. This provides the researcher with evidence that the UTAUT2 can be used to study m-health acceptance and use of diabetes patients. In comparison to earlier models, Venkatesh et al. [71] have stated that UTAUT2 provides a significant improvement in the behavioural intention and technology use field of research. "The variance explained in both behavioural intention (74%) and technology use (52%) are substantial" [73], p. 172].

Yuan et al. [74] have investigated the determinants of health and fitness applications grounded on the UTAUT2 model. The results indicate that the constructs performance expectancy, hedonic motivation, price value and habit predicted an individuals' intention to continuously use health and fitness applications. On the other hand, effort expectancy and facilitating conditions did not have a substantial role in affecting an individuals' intention to continuously use a health and fitness app [74]. This could be due to the participants being young and therefore, relatively comfortable with technology.

Despite the UTAUT2 being developed to understand consumer technology acceptance better, it still faces criticisms. Tamilmani, Rana and Dwivedi [75] employed a combination of "systematic review" and "meta-analysis" techniques to synthesise previous research that utilised UTAUT2. By systematically reviewing 650 articles, no more than 147 (22%) employed at best only one UTAUT2 construct. The outstanding 503 (77%) articles did not cite UTAUT2 in any significant way [75, 76]. Even though cultural factors play a role in technology adoption, it is overlooked in many of the models for user acceptance. The UTAUT2 model has been critiqued for not including cultural variables and lacks cultural awareness in non-Western countries [69]. Therefore, when studying culture with technology adoption, many authors extend the models by including cultural models such as Hofstede's cultural dimensions.

2.4 Conceptualising Culture

Researchers have investigated culture and the role of cultural differences in the adoption and acceptance of information technology. Research indicates that cultural backgrounds play an imperative role in affecting the uptake and use of technology [27, 77, 78]. In addition, cultural beliefs are factors that influence technology acceptance and use [79].

To address the concept of culture, it needs to be conceptualised. The concept of culture is quite broad and as such difficult to delineate. It comprises a range of definitions provided by various anthropologists.

There are various definitions of culture provided by various anthropologists. One hundred and sixty-seven interpretations of culture have been developed [80]. Definitions of culture by anthropologists date back to the 1800s as being inclusive of "knowledge, beliefs, art, morals, law, custom, and any other capabilities and habits acquired by man as a member of the society" [81, p. 1]. Culture can be viewed as crucial in clarifying how individuals differ from social groups. Moreover, culture is no more just a set of values. Culture may vary in its value orientations [82]. Rohner [86, p. 119] describes culture as "the totality of equivalent and complementary learned meanings maintained by a human population, or by identifiable segments of a population, and transmitted from one generation to the next". He further mentions that an entire society does not precisely share cultural meaning. Two people from the same society may have different explanations for the same occurrence or share the same explanation with other people from a given society but not with each other [83]. Culture can also be perceived as thoughts and behaviours that distinguish one person from another or shared by a group of individuals which can impact their daily lives [84]. Each group of people conveys a set of shared cognitive programs that represent their group culture. Hofstede defines culture as the collective programming of the mind which distinguishes the members of one human group from another" [83, p. 13].

Hofstede's Cultural Dimensions. Hofstede [84] developed a model to measure work-related values based on the data collected from IBM units between 1967 and 1973. The data consisted of 116,000 survey responses from seventy-two distinct countries in twenty languages. The survey was not initially aimed at studying cross-cultural differences. In his analysis, however, Hofstede identified variations in how respondents from different parts of the world responded to specific groups of questions. Furthermore, Hofstede (1980) developed an index model and presented four cultural values of culture: Power Distance, Individualism versus Collectivism, Masculinity versus Femininity, and Uncertainty Avoidance. Hofstede then included Long-Term versus Short-Term Orientation as a fifth dimension [85]. He later added Indulgence versus Restraint as a sixth dimension [86]. Hofstede has addressed culture by focusing merely on disparities between cultures [84]. Additionally, Hofstede associates the notion of culture with assessing the 'value orientation characteristic' of persons from diverse nations [87].

The six constructs by Hofstede, Hofstede and Minkov [86] are defined below:

- Power distance (PD) – "extent to which the less powerful members of institutions and organisations within a country expect and accept that power is distributed unequally" (p. 61).
- Individualism-collectivism (IDV) – "refers to societies in which the ties between individuals are loose: everyone is expected to look after him or herself and his or her immediate family. Collectivism as its opposite pertains to societies in which people from birth onward are integrated into strong, cohesive in-groups, which throughout people's lifetime continue to protect them in exchange for unquestioning loyalty" (p. 92).

- Masculinity-femininity (MAS) – Masculinity refers to a "society in which emotional gender roles are clearly distinct" (p. 519). Femininity is seen as a "society in which emotional gender roles overlap: both men and women are supposed to be modest, tender, and concerned with the quality of life" (p. 517).
- Uncertainty avoidance (UA) – "the extent to which the members of a culture feel threatened by ambiguous or unknown situations" (p. 191).
- Long-term orientation - Short-term orientation (LTO) – "the fostering of virtues oriented toward future rewards—in particular, perseverance and thrift." (p. 239). Short-term orientation "the fostering of virtues related to the past and present—in particular, respect for tradition, preservation of face, and fulfilling social obligations" (p. 239).
- Indulgence-restraint (IR) – Indulgence refers to a "society that allows relatively free gratification of basic and natural human desires related to enjoying life and having fun" (p. 519). Restraint refers to a "society that suppresses gratification of needs and regulates it by means of strict social norms" (p. 521).

Hofstede's culture framework has been extensively studied in the areas of Information Systems and Information Technology studies (e.g., [30, 77, 88, 89]). These studies suggest that a significant relationship exists amongst national culture and the rate of technology adoption and acceptance. Despite the criticism, Hofstede's [84, 86] cultural model is applicable to study technology uptake and use for health. The model is useful in understanding which cultural dimension has a link with technology acceptance.

Culture can be a facilitating condition or an inhibiting condition as it affects people's attitudes and beliefs. Mutunda [90] suggests that culture is rooted in the many traditions and practices which are focused on family and different ethnicities. The African culture, however, goes beyond the six dimensions that are described in the Hofstede model. In Africa, culture emerges as spiritual beliefs [91], respect for authority and the elders, communal life, and tradition [92]. Previous studies have ascertained that culture plays a central role in health-related behaviours [93, 94]. Jia et al. [93] postulate that culture affects people's behaviour and thinking, and therefore influences health management behaviour. Also, findings by Levesque and Li [94] suggest that culture has a significant impact on health conceptions, which in turn influence health practices. It is imperative therefore to study the influence of culture on the acceptance of an m-health application. Culture is, therefore, one of the factors that will be discussed to provide answers for diabetes self-management.

2.5 Culture in Relation to Diabetes Management

It has been observed from the findings discussed above [93] that cultural influences play a vital role in determining people's attitudes and beliefs hence, culture has an effect on attitudes and beliefs regarding diabetes self-management. Diabetic patients' perceptions, religion, cultural beliefs and values may hinder the proper use of insulin in particular racial and ethnic minority groups [95], and may influence self-management of diabetes. Cultural influences may have a direct impact on patients' self-management behaviour via the perception of health management of their condition and how an informed decision is made [96, 97]. Cultural factors may include cultural health beliefs [97, 98] and dietary preferences [98]. These factors have been shown to influence diabetes self-management of culturally diverse populations [99]. Despite self-management having a positive impact on a patients' overall health outcome [100], successfully managing diabetes solely depends on the patients' willingness to perform self-management activities daily. The self-management behaviour is influenced by the patients' culture and practices, including health-seeking behaviour and understanding of the condition [96, 101]. Therefore, culture must be understood in the context being studied. Research indicates that culture is unique to geography and may not be viewed in isolation [72]. Therefore, culture in South Africa will be discussed to provide context to this study.

2.6 South African Culture

South Africa, known as a Rainbow Nation Country, is seen as a diverse and complex nation consisting of various values, norms, and belief systems. As in any geography, traditions and practices are based on the belief systems of the citizens. The belief in, and people's perceptions about the traditions and practices play an important role in the cultural orientation of individuals, which is conveyed from one generation to the next [102], and these cultural orientations have a strong influence on behaviour and behavioural intention [103]. Understanding culture in a South African context is an important consideration in this study.

Culture and ethnic diversity is a challenging phenomenon in the healthcare sector, particularly in low and middle income countries (LMICs) [104]. South Africa is a culturally diverse country and may have a good appreciation of the effects of culture on healthcare management. It is therefore vital to look at a holistic view of culture in South Africa. South Africa is characterised by diversity requiring sensitivity towards culture [104]. The cultural backgrounds influence patients' choices, and it is crucial for healthcare providers to understand the influence of culture [105]. A study carried out by Abdulrehman et al. [106], for example, has found that cultural influences play a vital role in diabetes self-management, especially in low resource areas.

Patients' culture may determine how they define health, identify ailment, and seek treatment. As culture dramatically influences health, the perceptions of people regarding healthcare and health seeking behaviour, it is important to consider cultural factors when designing health promotion studies [107]. In South Africa, the healthcare sector lacks culturally appropriate communication strategies to address healthcare concerns to encourage awareness and self-management [104]. Therefore, "it cannot be assumed that m-health interventions developed in one culture can simply be translated into another culture without consulting the cultural context in which they should operate" [113, p. 295]. As such, an m-health intervention employed in a developed country can not necessarily be successfully implemented within a developing country without taking into consideration cultural differences [108] because cultures may vary between the countries [109].

Understanding patients' self-management, cultural and value systems is a significant factor for constructing effective self care interventions that could ultimately influence self-care behaviours, i.e. their diet and exercise choices [110]. Culture may influence diabetes self-management [111]. Research indicates that culture and socio-economic status shapes diabetic patient eating patterns [112].

The preceding section has provided context to the study. It presented insight into South Africa, the culture and beliefs of this population. The succeeding section will discuss the localised culture viz. the Cape Flats.

2.7 Culture in the Cape Flats

While the previous section looked at South African culture in general, this section is a presentation of the Cape Flats culture. The society is predominantly of the "Coloured" race [113]. The impact of culture may be significant, especially amongst populations such as those with diverse ethnic backgrounds, which hold unique health behaviours that may differ from the cultural norms of the general population [114].

In South Africa, racial and ethnic minorities who are marginalised, disadvantaged and mistreated socially, economically, culturally are deemed as categories of poverty. In addition, people from diverse racial/ethnic groups may share comparable cultural values due to living with similar lifestyles and socio-economic circumstances [115]. Further research has found that older adults survive off social grants which are used to support their relatives. This shows that they cannot afford to purchase food items that are suitable for diabetic patients [116]. As such, people with limited or no income are restricted in terms of food choices and are more susceptible to eating unhealthy meals [117].

Research based on culture in the Cape Flats has found that "the Coloured community is a separate racial grouping with its own identity and its own culture" [118, p. 83]. This serves as evidence that there are cultural differences amongst ethnic groups. The customs and practices of people are based on their convictions [34]. Sachdeva et al. [111] have found that perception about diabetes is influenced by tradition, customs and ethos [111].

In the Cape Flats area, there is a strong (influential) culture of religious activities [119]. Research indicates that participation in these religious activities appears to be more evident amongst Muslims than adherents to other religions [119]. Also, it is more prominent amongst the senior citizens as compared to the younger population [119]. Studies suggest that culture and religion have a strong influence on different health behaviours [120].

Culture can also play an essential role in the foods that people choose to eat. Dietary habits and practices are influenced by culture and religion, as well as economic conditions [111]. Individuals stated that their ethnic or religious background influenced their choice of healthy foods [117]. A study based on diabetes in the Cape Flats found that although patients follow a healthy diet and healthy techniques of making meals, the participants found it expensive and time-consuming to cook more than one meal at a time. This is due to the rest of the family refusing to eat food that they regard as diabetic food [116]. In addition to this, many participants mentioned that they eat healthy during the week and would indulge on weekends.

A study based on the food choices in the Cape Flats area has found that people in Khayelitsha and Mitchells Plain are not exercising because they live in unsafe communities. It was found to be unsafe to walk around for exercising or to visit the clinic early in the morning [117]. This is consistent with a study conducted in another marginalised community, Bishop Lavis. It was found that diabetic patients in Bishop Lavis are unable to partake in physical activity due to crime [116]. This indicates that low-income communities have a high level of crime which inhibits physical activity. Crime, especially cybercrime influences the confidence and the use of mobile applications by users [121]. Therefore, failure to understand the setting where a specific technology is intended to be implemented similarly indicates failure of the technology adoption process [78].

2.8 Cultural Values on an Individual Level

Numerous studies have investigated the relationship between culture and technology. Many of these studies have just operationalised cultural value orientations at the national or organisational level [122]. Most of the literature focuses on the influence of culture on technology acceptance at a national or organisational level [123]. In contrast, there has been scant literature published concerning the effects of culture on an individual level. There appears to be a consensus that cultural values from a national level cannot be used to determine individual values [31, 124].

Hofstede's cultural model was operationalised by Dorfman and Howell [125] to study culture at an individual level. Research conducted by Srite and Karahanna [126] followed this recommendation by testing the model in two studies on computing technology acceptance (one on the use of personal computers (PCs), and another on personal digital assistants). It was found that "social norms are stronger determinants of intended behaviour for individuals who espouse feminine and high uncertainty avoidance cultural values" [89, p. 679]. The findings illustrate that people's cultural values affect their technology acceptance [126].

An example of another study that integrated culture and the Technology Acceptance Model (TAM) is that of Tarhini et al. [77]. The authors combined Hofstede's cultural dimensions [84], and the Technology Acceptance Model by Davis [127] to investigate the research problem. They assessed the effect of individual-level culture on the acceptance of e-learning tools. Subjective norms were added to the TAM to overcome the limitations posed by using TAM in a developing country. The authors found that perceived ease of use and perceived usefulness to be important factors of behavioural intention and the use of e-learning for both the British and Lebanese students. In terms of cultural dimensions, it was found that there is a stronger relationship among users with high collectivistic cultures [77]. This is due to Individualism/collectivism, which moderates the relationship between subjective norms and behavioural intention. In addition, this study found that British and Lebanese students are likely to be persuaded by the sentiments of their teachers and classmates when deciding whether or not to accept technology [77]. As such, it provided evidence that culture plays a role in technology acceptance.

Teo and Huang [35] investigated espoused cultural values and the behaviour intention of lecturers to use technology in Chinese universities. Hofstede's four cultural dimensions were assessed at the individual level, "as technology acceptance was considered an individual concern" [31, p. 1]. The results indicated that the extended TAM model was suitable to understand the role of cultural values in describing the behavioural intention of educators. The study found that educators' behavioural intention was affected by their subjective norms and their espoused cultural values [35].

A more recent study has examined the influence of cultural values at an individual level. Sun, Lee and Law [32] have investigated cultural values at an individual level in the context of the hotel industry. It has found that two of Hofstede's key constructs collectivism and long-term orientation have been positively correlated to perceived usefulness and perceived ease of use. "While national culture is a macro-level phenomenon, the acceptance of technology by end-users is an individual-level phenomenon" [80, p. 308]. The cultural characteristics from an individual's national culture may be influenced by their ethnicity, social groups and religion that each have their own unique culture [128]. Therefore, conceptualising culture at the individual level manifests the multi-layered cultural values accumulated in the self.

2.9 Technology Adoption Versus Culture

To understand how users', accept new technology, such as mobile applications, it is necessary to understand the many variables that affect an individual's decision. The factors that affect technology uptake and use are an individual's attitudes towards using the technology, the ease of use associated with the new technology and socio-cultural factors [37].

Technology adoption is a cultural matter just as it is a cognitive process of reaching a decision [129]. It has been found that cultural beliefs are a crucial factor in technology acceptance [79]. Individualism-collectivism is found to be one the most explored cultural dimensions in technology adoption [122]. The literature indicates that cultural factors have a significant role in ICT acceptance [30, 88]. This is due to technology being often used in cultural contexts of users. Im, Hong and Kang [129] indicate that culture plays an essential role in technology adoption, as cultural factors are significant in explaining IT usage behaviour [124]. Research indicates that cultural dimensions may influence how people perceive technology [130]. Lin [131] indicates that the influence of Hofstede's power distance is related to social influence in the Unified-theory of Acceptance and Use of Technology model. Therefore, it is crucial to review technology adoption models to identify a suitable model that could be used in health and culture research.

Research indicates that the Unified-theory of Acceptance and Use of Technology model was unable to predict usage. It was found that behavioural intention did not translate into the usage of ICT. Other factors such as facilitating conditions could affect uptake and usage [132]. This is consistent with recent research that has found that uptake of diabetes self-management applications is low [133] and continued use is also low [134], possibly due to other factors affecting adoption such as culture [135], It was found that cultural beliefs are fundamental for technology acceptance and use [79]. Research shows that low health literacy is related to poorer health outcomes [136] and thus has a significant impact on people's ability to self-manage their condition [137]. Therefore, interventions such as "A Patient-centred communication style that incorporates patient preferences, assesses literacy and numeracy, and addresses cultural barriers to care" [138, p. S5] should be addressed to improve health outcomes.

Several researchers (e.g., [139–141]) state that cultural influences need to be taken into account when researching technology acceptance as the way people use Information Systems is influenced by their culture [30, 129]. Srite and Karahanna [126] support this by stating that cultural values act as a significant moderator in technological acceptance. The acceptance and user behaviour towards technology can be influenced by cultural, individual differences and social influences [142]. Furthermore, it has been found that people's cultural beliefs are a key factor for technology uptake and adoption [79], and cultural backgrounds can also influence technology acceptance [78, 143].

Within the context of diabetes and diabetes self-management, there are a host of factors that influence self-management of diabetes such as religious, social factors as well as cultural values and beliefs, all of which influence how people understand and treat their condition [106]. Concerning technology acceptance, in certain cultures, people are more family-oriented and thus have a negative view on technology, as it is seen as a potential threat to family and social life. As South Africa is an individualistic society [144], the social pressure to perform a certain behaviour is relatively less than in a collectivist society [145]. For example, technology uptake and usage are acted upon within a cultural and social context and these influences how people behave towards technology [78].

Many authors have investigated the effect of cultural values using the Technology Acceptance Model constructs' [28, 77, 126]. Thowfeek and Jaafar [146] have indicated that in feminine cultures, individuals are expected to be mindful of the opinion of others as they are deemed more people-oriented. Hoque and Bao [28] have explored the impact of culture on the adoption of electronic health services in Bangladesh. This study used items from Davis [127] and incorporated Hofstede's cultural dimensions. It found that perceived usefulness is a significant factor of e-health adoption in Bangladesh. In contrast, it found that perceived ease of use appeared to have no significant effect on adoption of e-health [28].

In terms of culture, this study also found that power distance and masculinity have a significant influence on the intention to use e-health. This indicates that people who have a high position in an organisation, with enough money and power have better access to e-health services in Bangladesh. In addition, the adoption of e-health was significantly influenced by people who form part of a masculinity culture. It has also been found that uncertainty avoidance and collectivism have no significant effect on the intention to use e-health. This suggests that in public and private hospitals, electronic health is not well developed to face impending uncertainties. Additionally, it can be assumed that people (Bangladeshis) are independent and are not loyal to a group. Restraint was found to have a significant negative relationship with intention to use e-health adoption decision [28]. Tarhini et al. [80, p. 321] found that power distance, masculinity–femininity, uncertainty avoidance and individualism–collectivism "were found to be significant moderators of this relationship". This result supports the view formulated by Srite and Karahanna [89, p. 697] that "social environment is a significant conduit via which culture manifest and impacts individual behaviour".

A study on the relationship between culture and technology acceptance found that low power distance and low levels of uncertainty avoidance but a high individualist culture, tend to adopt and accept new technology quickly [147]. The author further revealed that people in countries with a high masculinity score give more consideration to achieving their goals, as success is important to them. This indicates that they are presumed to have a stronger inclination to adopt new technology. In contrast, countries with cultures that score high in power distance, collectivism and uncertainty avoidance, tend to resist accepting new technology [148].

A recent study by Petersen et al. [135] used the Technology Acceptance Model to identify the impediments to ICT adoption of diabetes self-management. It was found that socio-cultural factors are some of the factors that hinder the ICT adoption of diabetes self-management. The authors further recommended that culture in the use of m-health acceptance for diabetes self-management could be explored in future research. On the other hand, irrespective of the possible influence on the acceptance of information technology, culture has not been foremost in technology acceptance research, particularly in low-middle income countries [88].

The succeeding section provides studies that have used technology adoption models together with cultural models. This is executed to identify which models and methodologies were used in previous studies in order to identify the methodology most suited for this research problem. This section supports the research objective of this study which seeks to derive a framework that defines the concept of culture.

A Synthesis of Previous Research on Culture and Technology. Table 1 represents the user acceptance models that have been used together with cultural models in different research contexts.

Table 1. Studies on culture and technology in different contexts (Source: Adapted from Jacobs-Basadien and Pather [8]).

Author	Constructs used in this study	Methodology and models used
Sun, Lee and Law [32]	Individual-level Culture Hofstede cultural dimensions Perceived usefulness and Perceived ease of use	TAM Hofstede cultural dimensions Questionnaire
Zhang, Weng and Zhu [33]	Performance expectancy Effort expectancy Social influence Perceived risk Trust Hofstede's cultural dimensions	UTAUT Hofstede's cultural dimensions Questionnaire
Yavwa and Twinomurinzi [34]	Performance expectancy Effort expectancy Social influence Facilitating conditions Spirituality, Communalism, Respect Behavioural intention, E-filing usage and E-payment usage	UTAUT Questionnaire
Huang and Teo [35]	Hofstede cultural dimensions Perceived ease of use Perceived Usefulness Attitude towards use Behavioural intention	Extended TAM Hofstede cultural dimensions Questionnaire

(*continued*)

Table 1. (*continued*)

Author	Constructs used in this study	Methodology and models used
Lu, Yu, Liu and Wei [36]	Hofstede's cultural dimensions Perceived effort expectancy Perceived performance expectancy Perceived mobile Social influence Perceived privacy protection	Espoused cultural dimension of Hofstede UTAUT Questionnaire
Tarhini et al. [77]	Individual-level culture Perceived ease of use Subjective norms Behavioural Intention	TAM Questionnaire
Lai et al. [122]	Long-term orientation Collectivism Power Distance Uncertainty avoidance Performance expectancy Effort expectancy Social influence Hedonic Motivation Facilitating conditions	Hofstede cultural dimensions UTAUT2 Survey
Baptista and Oliveira [73]	UTAUT2 Hofstede cultural dimensions Behavioural intention Use behaviour	UTAUT2 Hofstede cultural dimensions Questionnaire
Hoehle, Zhang and Venkatesh [149]	Uncertainty avoidance Perceived usefulness Perceived ease of use Perceived usefulness	Collected data from consumers using ICT in four countries, Hofstede cultural dimensions
Al-jumeily and Hussain [27]	Individualism-Collectivism, Uncertainty Avoidance, Power Distance Perceived usefulness Perceived ease of use	TAM Hofstede cultural dimensions Survey
Al-Gahtani, Hubona and Wang [150]	Hofstede cultural dimensions UTAUT Behavioural intention Use behaviour	UTAUT Hofstede cultural dimensions Survey
Srite and Karahanna [126]	Perceived usefulness Perceived ease of use Subjective norms Behavioural intention Hofstede's cultural dimensions	TAM Hofstede cultural dimensions Questionnaire

The table above shows that the technology acceptance model and the Unified-theory of Acceptance and Use of Technology model is the most used model when studying culture. In addition, the table illustrates that Hofstede's cultural model is the most used cultural model.

3 Conclusion

The research problem that is the nucleus of this paper concerns the oft unrecognized factors that are deterrent to the successful adoption of mobile applications in specific healthcare settings especially among poorer and economically marginalized communities. While the digital divide still prevails in most parts of the word, this paper takes the view that there are, and must be, explanatory responses as to why broadband internet and all its manifest applications are not really advancing us towards the realization of the SDGs.

The chapter introspected the conceptual framework that was posited by Jacobs-Basadien and Pather [8]. We find that there is sufficient evidence that Hofstede's cultural dimensions and the Unified-theory of Acceptance and Use of Technology 2 have appropriate conceptual constructs that allow for an assessment of the role of culture on mobile technology acceptance and use.

The chapter further endorses the theory that individuals' culture persuasions have an influence on diabetic patients' decisions to adopt and use mobile applications for diabetes self-management. We suggest that these findings should be easily transferable into other settings of healthcare instantiations that do indeed rely on mobile applications. The findings are further worthy in that they will assist in promoting a more inter-disciplinary effort in dealing with real-world ICT issues such as healthcare. Finally, we posit that there are other potential areas of ICT4D investigation in which mobile applications are relevant. The notion of culture among target user groups should be kept in mind when planning for the scaling of any mobile application based intervention to ensure maximum uptake, adoption, and eventual social appropriation of the technology.

References

1. Tennant, B., et al.: eHealth literacy and Web 2.0 health information seeking behaviors among baby boomers and older adults. J. Med. Internet Res. **17**, 1–12 (2015)
2. International Telecommunication Union: Statistics. https://www.itu.int/en/ITU-D/Statistics/Pages/stat/default.aspx
3. Statista: Number of internet users worldwide from 2009 to 2021, by region. https://www.statista.com/statistics/265147/number-of-worldwide-internet-users-by-region/
4. Statista: Number of internet users in selected countries in Africa as of January 2022, by country. https://www.statista.com/statistics/505883/number-of-internet-users-in-african-countries/
5. Statistics South Africa: General Household Survey (2021)
6. Presidential Infrastructure Coordinating Commission: A summary of the South African national infrastructure plan (2012)
7. Amante, D., Hogan, T., Pagota, S., English, T., Lapane, K.: Access to care and use of the internet to search for health information: results from the US national health interview survey. J. Med. Internet Res. **17**, 4 (2015)
8. Jacobs-Basadien, M., Pather, S.: The role of culture in user adoption of mobile applications for self-management of health: a conceptual framework. In: Proceedings of the 8th International Conference on Information and Communication Technologies for Ageing Well and e-Health, pp. 37–49. SCITEPRESS - Science and Technology Publications (2022)

9. World Health Organization: mHealth: new horizons for health through mobile technologies. Observatory **3**, 66–71 (2011)
10. Choi, W., Wang, S., Lee, Y., Oh, H., Zheng, Z.: A systematic review of mobile health technologies to support self-management of concurrent diabetes and hypertension. J. Am. Med. Inform. Assoc. **27**(6), 939–945 (2020)
11. International Diabetes Federation: IDF diabetes atlas: 10th edition. https://diabetesatlas.org/
12. World Health Organization: Diabetes
13. Pheiffer, C., Pillay-Van Wyk, V., Joubert, J.D., Levitt, N., Nglazi, M.D., Bradshaw, D.: The prevalence of type 2 diabetes in South Africa: a systematic review protocol. BMJ Open **8**, 2–5 (2018)
14. Statistics South Africa: Mortality and causes of death in South Africa. Pretoria (2016)
15. Erasmus, R.T., et al.: High prevalence of diabetes mellitus and metabolic syndrome in a South African coloured population: baseline data of a study in Bellville, Cape Town. S. Afr. Med. J. **102**, 841 (2012)
16. Erzse, A., Stacey, N., Chola, L., Tugendhaft, A., Freeman, M., Hofman, K.: The direct medical cost of type 2 diabetes mellitus in South Africa: a cost of illness study. Glob. Health Action. **12**, 1636611 (2019)
17. Statistics South Africa: General household survey - statistical release P0318. Pretoria (2019)
18. World Health Organisation: Facts sheet
19. American Association of Diabetes Educators: Self care behaviors. In: Diabetes Self-Management, pp. 1–11 (1997)
20. Zhao, J., Freeman, B., Li, M.: Can mobile phone apps influence people's health behavior change? An evidence review. J. Med. Internet Res. **18**, 1–7 (2016)
21. Dou, K., et al.: Patients' acceptance of smartphone health technology for chronic disease management: a theoretical model and empirical test. JMIR mHealth uHealth **5**, e177 (2017)
22. Khasawneh, A.M.: Concepts and measurements of innovativeness: the case of information and communication technologies. Int. J. Arab Cult. Manag. Sustain. Dev. **1**, 23 (2008)
23. Venkatesh, V., Thong, J.Y.L., Xu, X.: Unified theory of acceptance and use of technology: a synthesis and the road ahead. J. Assoc. Inf. Syst. **17**, 328–376 (2016)
24. Phichitchaisopa, N., Naenna, T.: Factors affecting the adoption of healthcare information technology. Excli. J. **12**, 413–436 (2013)
25. Hoque, R., Sorwar, G.: Understanding factors influencing the adoption of mHealth by the elderly: an extension of the UTAUT model. Int. J. Med. Inform. **101**, 75–84 (2017)
26. Bawack, R.E., Kala Kamdjoug, J.R.: Adequacy of UTAUT in clinician adoption of health information systems in developing countries: the case of Cameroon. Int. J. Med. Inform. **109**, 15–22 (2018)
27. Al-Jumeily, D., Hussain, A.J.: The impact of cultural factors on technology acceptance: a technology acceptance model across Eastern and Western cultures. Int. J. Enhanced Res. Educ. Dev. **2**, 37–62 (2014)
28. Hoque, M.R., Bao, Y.: Cultural influence on adoption and use of e-health: evidence in Bangladesh. Telemed. e-Health **21**, 845–851 (2015)
29. Zayyad, M.A., Toycan, M.: Factors affecting sustainable adoption of e-health technology in developing countries: an exploratory survey of Nigerian hospitals from the perspective of healthcare professionals. PeerJ **6**, 2–15 (2018)
30. Sriwindono, H., Yahya, S.: Toward modeling the effects of cultural dimension on ICT acceptance in Indonesia. Procedia Soc. Behav. Sci. **65**, 833–838 (2012)
31. Hasan, H., Ditsa, G.: The impact of culture on the adoption of IT: an interpretive study. J. Glob. Inf. Manag. **7**, 5–15 (1999)
32. Sun, S., Lee, P., Law, R.: Impact of cultural values on technology acceptance and technology readiness. Int. J. Hosp. Manag. **77**, 89–96 (2019)

33. Zhang, Y., Weng, Q., Zhu, N.: The relationships between electronic banking adoption and its antecedents: a meta-analytic study of the role of national culture. Int. J. Inf. Manag. **40**, 76–87 (2018)
34. Yavwa, Y., Twinomurinzi, H.: Impact of culture on e-government adoption using UTAUT: a case of Zambia. In: 2018 International Conference on eDemocracy and eGovernment (ICEDEG), pp. 356–360. IEEE (2018)
35. Teo, T., Huang, F.: Investigating the influence of individually espoused cultural values on teachers' intentions to use educational technologies in Chinese universities. Interact. Learn. Environ. **27**, 813–829 (2018)
36. Lu, J., Yu, C., Liu, C., Wei, J.: Comparison of mobile shopping continuance intention between China and USA from an espoused cultural perspective. Comput. Hum. Behav. **75**, 130–146 (2017)
37. Beratarrechea, A., Lee, A.G., Willner, J.M., Jahangir, E., Ciapponi, A., Rubinstein, A.: The impact of mobile health interventions on chronic disease outcomes in developing countries: a systematic review. Telemed. e-Health **20**, 75–82 (2014)
38. Martinsons, M.G., Davison, R.M.: Strategic decision making and support systems: comparing American, Japanese and Chinese management. Decis. Support Syst. **43**, 284–300 (2007)
39. World Health Organization: Global Report on Diabetes. Geneva (2016)
40. American Diabetes Association: Improving care and promoting health in populations: standards of medical care in diabetes (2019)
41. Kayyali, R., Peletidi, A., Ismail, M., Hashim, Z., Bandeira, P., Bonnah, J.: Awareness and use of mHealth apps: a study from England. Pharmacy **5**, 33 (2017)
42. Iregbu, S.C., Iregbu, F.U.: A review of self-management of diabetes in Africa. Afr. J. Diabetes Med. **24**, 5–8 (2016)
43. El-Gayar, O., Timsina, P., Nawar, N., Eid, W.: A systematic review of IT for diabetes self-management: are we there yet? Int. J. Med. Inform. **82**, 637–652 (2013)
44. Maniam, A., Dhillon, J.S.: Barriers to the effective use of diabetes self-management applications. In: The 3rd National Graduate Conference (NatGrad2015), pp. 315–320 (2015)
45. Parrinello, C.M., Rastegar, I., Godino, J.G., Miedema, M.D., Matsushita, K., Selvin, E.: Prevalence of and racial disparities in risk factor control in older adults with diabetes: the atherosclerosis risk in communities study. Diabetes Care **38**, 1290–1298 (2015)
46. Mukong, A.K., Van Walbeek, C., Ross, H.: Lifestyle and income-related inequality in health in South Africa. Int. J. Equity Health **16**, 103 (2017)
47. World Health Organization: Diabetes key facts. https://www.who.int/news-room/fact-she ets/detail/diabetes
48. Petersen, F., Jacobs, M., Pather, S.: Barriers for user acceptance of mobile health applications for diabetic patients: applying the UTAUT model. In: Hattingh, M., Matthee, M., Smuts, H., Pappas, I., Dwivedi, Y.K., Mäntymäki, M. (eds.) I3E 2020. LNCS, vol. 12067, pp. 61–72. Springer, Cham (2020). https://doi.org/10.1007/978-3-030-45002-1_6
49. Pheiffer, C., Pillay-Van Wyk, V., Joubert, J.D., Levitt, N., Nglazi, M.D., Bradshaw, D.: The prevalence of type 2 diabetes in South Africa: a systematic review protocol. BMJ Open **8**, 1–4 (2018)
50. Roux, M., le Walsh, C., Reid, M., Raubenheimer, J.: Diabetes-related knowledge, attitude and practices (KAP) of adult patients with type 2 diabetes mellitus in the Free State province, South Africa. S. Afr. J. Clin. Nutr. **32**, 83–90 (2018)
51. Ajzen, I., Joyce, N., Sheikh, S., Cote, N.G.: Knowledge and prediction of behaviour: the role of information accuracy in the theory of planned behaviour. Basic Appl. Psychol. **33**, 101–117 (2011)

52. Kebede, M.M., Pischke, C.R.: Popular diabetes apps and the impact of diabetes app use on self-care behaviour: a survey among the digital community of persons with diabetes on social media. Front. Endocrinol. **10**, 1–14 (2019)
53. Hartz, J., Yingling, L., Powell-Wiley, T.M.: Use of mobile health technology in the prevention and management of diabetes mellitus. Curr. Cardiol. Rep. **18**, 130 (2016)
54. Esposito, M., Minutolo, A., Megna, R., Forastiere, M., Magliulo, M., De Pietro, G.: A smart mobile, self-configuring, context-aware architecture for personal health monitoring. Eng. Appl. Artif. Intell. **67**, 136–156 (2018)
55. Hou, C., Carter, B., Hewitt, J., Francisa, T., Mayor, S.: Do mobile phone applications improve glycemic control (HbA1c) in the self-management of diabetes? A systematic review, meta-analysis, and GRADE of 14 randomized trials. Diabetes Care **39**, 11 (2016)
56. Othman, M., Halil, N.M., Yusof, M.M., Mohamed, R., Abdullah, M.H.A.: Empowering self-management through m-health applications. MATEC Web Conf. **150**, 05018 (2018)
57. Jo, I.-Y., Yoo, S.-H., Lee, D.Y., Park, C.-Y., Kim, E.M.: Diabetes management via a mobile application: a case report. Clin. Nutr. Res. **6**, 61 (2017)
58. Dutta, M.J., Kaur-Gill, S., Tan, N., Lam, C.: mHealth, health, and mobility: a culture-centered interrogation. In: Mobile Communication in Asia: Local Insights, Global Implications, pp. 91–107 (2018)
59. Aminuddin, H.B., Jiao, N., Jiang, Y., Hong, J., Wang, W.: Effectiveness of smartphone-based self-management interventions on self-efficacy, self-care activities, health-related quality of life and clinical outcomes in patients with type 2 diabetes: a systematic review and meta-analysis. Int. J. Nurs. Stud. **116**, 1–10 (2019)
60. Izahar, S., et al.: Content analysis of mobile health applications on diabetes mellitus. Front. Endocrinol. **8**, 1–8 (2017)
61. Istepanian, R.S.H., Al-Anzi, T.M.: m-Health interventions for diabetes remote monitoring and self management: clinical and compliance issues. mHealth **4**, 4 (2018)
62. Deng, Z., Hong, Z., Ren, C., Zhang, W., Xiang, F.: What predicts patients' adoption intention toward mHealth services in China: empirical study. J. Med. Internet Res. **20**, 1–14 (2018)
63. Zhao, Y., Ni, Q., Zhou, R.: What factors influence the mobile health service adoption? A meta-analysis and the moderating role of age. Int. J. Inf. Manag. **43**, 342–350 (2018)
64. Baig, M.M., GholamHosseini, H., Connolly, M.J.: Mobile healthcare applications: system design review, critical issues and challenges. Aust. Phys. Eng. Sci. Med. **38**(1), 23–38 (2014). https://doi.org/10.1007/s13246-014-0315-4
65. Modzelewski, K.L., Stockman, M.C., Steenkamp, D.W.: Rethinking the endpoints of mHealth intervention research in diabetes care. J. Diabetes Sci. Technol. **12**, 389–392 (2018)
66. El-Sappagh, S., Ali, F., El-Masri, S., Kim, K., Ali, A., Kwak, K.-S.: Mobile health technologies for diabetes mellitus: current state and future challenges. IEEE Access **7**, 21917–21947 (2019)
67. Iribarren, S.J., Cato, K., Falzon, L., Stone, P.W.: What is the economic evidence for mHealth? A systematic review of economic evaluations of mHealth solutions. PLoS ONE **12**, 1–20 (2017)
68. Hoque, M.R.: An empirical study of mHealth adoption in a developing country: the moderating effect of gender concern. BMC Med. Inform. Decis. Mak. **16**, 1–10 (2016)
69. A. Khan, R., Qudrat-Ullah, H.: Adoption of LMS in the cultural context of higher educational institutions of the Middle East. In: Adoption of LMS in Higher Educational Institutions of the Middle East. ASTI, pp. 1–5. Springer, Cham (2021). https://doi.org/10.1007/978-3-030-50112-9_1
70. Venkatesh, V., Morris, M.G., Davis, G.B., Davis, F.D.: User acceptance of information technology: toward a unified view. MIS Q. **27**, 425–478 (2003)
71. Venkatesh, V., Thong, J., Xu, X.: Consumer acceptance and use of information technology: extending the unified theory of acceptance and use of technology. MIS Q. **36**, 157 (2012)

72. Dwivedi, Y.K., Shareef, M.A., Simintiras, A.C., Lal, B., Weerakkody, V.: A generalised adoption model for services: a cross-country comparison of mobile health (m-health). Gov. Inf. Q. **33**, 174–187 (2016)
73. Baptista, G., Oliveira, T.: Understanding mobile banking: the unified theory of acceptance and use of technology combined with cultural moderators. Comput. Hum. Behav. **50**, 418–430 (2015)
74. Yuan, S., Ma, W., Kanthawala, S., Peng, W.: Keep using my health apps: discover users' perception of health and fitness apps with the UTAUT2 model. Telemed. e-Health **21**, 735–741 (2015)
75. Tamilmani, K., Rana, N.P., Dwivedi, Y.K.: A systematic review of citations of UTAUT2 article and its usage trends. In: Kar, A.K., et al. (eds.) I3E 2017. LNCS, vol. 10595, pp. 38–49. Springer, Cham (2017). https://doi.org/10.1007/978-3-319-68557-1_5
76. Tamilmani, K., Rana, N.P., Dwivedi, Y.K.: Consumer acceptance and use of information technology: a meta-analytic evaluation of UTAUT2. Inf. Syst. Front. **23**, 987–1005 (2021)
77. Tarhini, A., Hone, K., Liu, X., Tarhini, T.: Examining the moderating effect of individual-level cultural values on users' acceptance of e-learning in developing countries: a structural equation modeling of an extended technology acceptance model. Interact. Learn. Environ. **25**, 306–328 (2017)
78. Masimba, F., Appiah, M., Zuva, T.: A review of cultural influence on technology acceptance. In: 2019 International Multidisciplinary Information Technology and Engineering Conference (IMITEC), pp. 1–7. IEEE (2019)
79. Dehzad, F., Hilhorst, C., de Bie, C., Claassen, E.: Adopting health apps, what's hindering doctors and patients? Health **06**, 2204–2217 (2014)
80. Kroeber, A.L., Kluckhohn, C.: Culture: a critical review of concepts and definitions. Papers. Peabody Museum of Archaeology & Ethnology, Harvard University 47 (1952)
81. Tylor, E.B.: Primitive culture: researches into the development of mythology, philosophy, religion, art, and custom. London (1871)
82. Kluckhohn, F.R., Strodtbeck, F.L.: Variations in value orientations. Row, Peterson., Evanston (1961)
83. Rohner, R.: Toward a conception of culture for cross-cultural psychology. J. Cross-Cult. Psychol. **15**, 111–138 (1984)
84. Hofstede, G.: Culture's Consequences: Comparing Values, Behaviours, Institutions and Organisations Across Nations. Sage, Thousand Oaks, California (1980)
85. Hofstede, G.: Culture's Consequences: Comparing Values, Behaviors, Institutions, and Organizations Across Nations. Sage, Thousand Oaks, California (2001)
86. Hofstede, G., Hofstede, G.J., Minkov, M.: Cultures and Organizations: Software of the Mind. Mac-Graw Hill (2010)
87. Nakata, C.: Beyond Hofstede: Culture Frameworks for Global Marketing and Management. Palgrave Macmillian, New York (2009)
88. Sriwindono, H., Yahya, S.: The influence of cultural dimension on ICT acceptance in Indonesia higher learning institution. Aust. J. Basic Appl. Sci. **8**, 215–225 (2014)
89. Lee, S.G., Trimi, S., Kim, C.: The impact of cultural differences on technology adoption. J. World Bus. **48**, 20–29 (2013)
90. Mutunda, S.: Luvale personal names and naming practices?: A socio-cultural analysis. Int. J. Educ. Cult. Soc. **1**, 75–81 (2017)
91. Tchombe, T.: Handbook of African Educational Theories and Practices a Generative Teacher Education Curriculum (1995)
92. Kanu, M.: The indispensability of the basic social values in African traditions: a philosophical appraisal. New J. Afr. Stud. **7** (2010)
93. Jia, Y., Gao, J., Dai, J., Zheng, P., Fu, H.: Associations between health culture, health behaviors, and health-related outcomes: a cross-sectional study. PLoS ONE **12**, 1–13 (2017)

94. Levesque, A., Li, H.Z.: The relationship between culture, health conceptions, and health practices. J. Cross-Cult. Psychol. **45**, 628–645 (2014)
95. Rebolledo, J.A., Arellano, R.: Cultural differences and considerations when initiating insulin: table 1. Diabetes Spectr. **29**, 185–190 (2016)
96. Barbara, S., Krass, I.: Self management of type 2 diabetes by Maltese immigrants in Australia: can community pharmacies play a supporting role. Int. J. Pharm. Pract. **21**, 305–313 (2013)
97. Tseng, J., Halperin, L., Ritholz, M., Hsu, W.: Perceptions and management of psychosocial factors affecting type 2 diabetes mellitus in Chinese Americans. J. Diabetes Complicat. **27**, 383–390 (2013)
98. Zeng, B., Sun, W., Gary, R., Li, C., Liu, T.: Towards a conceptual model of diabetes self-management among Chinese immigrants in the United States. Int. J. Environ. Health Res. **11**, 6727–6742 (2014)
99. Eh, K., McGill, M., Wong, J., Krass, I.: Cultural issues and other factors that affect self-management of Type 2 diabetes mellitus (T2D) by Chinese immigrants in Australia. Diabetes Res. Clin. Pract. **119**, 97–105 (2016)
100. Kueh, Y.C., Morris, T., Borkoles, E., Shee, H.: Modelling of diabetes knowledge, attitudes, self-management, and quality of life: A cross-sectional study with an Australian sample. Health Qual. Life Outcomes **13**, 129 (2015)
101. Choi, T.S.T., Walker, K.Z., Ralston, R.A., Palermo, C.: Diabetes education needs of Chinese Australians: a qualitative study. Health Educ. J. **74**, 197–208 (2015)
102. Banda, D.: Extract of dissertation on Zambia's culture and cultural identity (2012)
103. Durmaz, Y.: The influence of cultural factors on consumer buying behaviour and an application in Turkey. Glob. J. Manag. Bus. Res. E Mark. **14**, 37–44 (2014)
104. Reid, M., et al.: Development of a health dialogue model for patients with diabetes: a complex intervention in a low-/middle income country. Int. J. Africa Nurs. Sci. **8**, 122–131 (2018)
105. Meier, C., Hartell, C.: Handling cultural diversity in education in South Africa. S. Afr. J. Educ. **6**, 180–192 (2009)
106. Abdulrehman, M.S., Woith, W., Jenkins, S., Kossman, S., Hunter, G.L.: Exploring cultural influences of self-management of diabetes in coastal Kenya. Glob. Qual. Nurs. Res. **3**, 1–13 (2016)
107. Al-Bannay, H., Jarus, T., Jongbloed, L., Yazigi, M., Dean, E.: Culture as a variable in health research: perspectives and caveats. Health Promot. Int. **29**, 549–557 (2014)
108. Müller, A.M.: Behavioural mHealth in developing countries: what about culture? Eur. Health Psychol. **18**, 294–296 (2016)
109. van Hoof, J., Demiris, G., Wouters, E.J.M. (eds.): Handbook of Smart Homes, Health Care and Well-Being. Springer, Cham (2015). https://doi.org/10.1007/978-3-319-01583-5
110. Ayele, K., Tesfa, B., Abebe, L., Tilahun, T., Girma, E.: Self care behavior among patients with diabetes in Harari, Eastern Ethiopia: the health belief model perspective. PLoS ONE **7**, e35515 (2012)
111. Sachdeva, S., Khalique, N., Ansari, M., Khan, Z., Mishra, S., Sharma, G.: Cultural determinants: addressing barriers to holistic diabetes care. J. Soc. Health Diabetes **3**, 33–38 (2015)
112. Matima, R., Murphy, K., Levitt, N.S., BeLue, R., Oni, T.: A qualitative study on the experiences and perspectives of public sector patients in Cape Town in managing the workload of demands of HIV and type 2 diabetes multimorbidity. PLoS ONE **13**, e0194191 (2018)
113. Statistics South Africa: City of Cape Town-2011 Census Suburb Mitchells Plain. Compiled by Strategic Development Information and GIS Department. City of Cape Town (2013)
114. Fritz, H., et al.: Diabetes self-management among Arab Americans: patient and provider perspectives. BMC Int. Health Hum. Rights **16**, 1–7 (2016)

115. Belkhamza, Z., Wafa, S.A.: The role of uncertainty avoidance on e-commerce acceptance across cultures. Int. Bus. Res. **7**, 166–173 (2014)
116. Booysen, B.L., Schlemmer, A.C.: Reasons for diabetes patients attending Bishop Lavis Community Health Centre being non-adherent to diabetes care. S. Afr. Fam. Pract. **57**, 166–171 (2015)
117. Dinbabo, M., et al.: Food choices and Body Mass Index (BMI) in adults and children: evidence from the National Income Dynamics Study (NIDS) and empirical research from Khayelitsha and Mitchells Plain in South Africa (2017)
118. Nilsson, S.: Coloured by Race: A Study About the Making of Coloured Identities in South Africa (2016)
119. Farrar, T.J., Falake, K.A., Mebaley, A., Moya, M.D., Rudolph, I.I.: A mall intercept survey on religion and worldview in the Cape Flats of Cape Town, South Africa. J. Study Relig. **32**, 1–30 (2019)
120. Adejumo, H., et al.: The impact of religion and culture on diabetes care in Nigeria. Afr. J. Diabetes Med. **17**, 17–19 (2015)
121. Behl, A., Pal, A., Tiwari, C.: Analysis of effect of perceived cybercrime risk on mobile app payments. Int. J. Public Sect. Perform. Manag. **5**, 415–432 (2019)
122. Lai, C., Wang, Q., Li, X., Hu, X.: The influence of individual espoused cultural values on self-directed use of technology for language learning beyond the classroom. Comput. Hum. Behav. **62**, 676–688 (2016)
123. Tarhini, A., Hone, K., Liu, X.: A cross-cultural examination of the impact of social, organisational and individual factors on educational technology acceptance between British and Lebanese university students. Br. J. Educ. Technol. **46**, 739–755 (2015)
124. Straub, D., Keil, M., Brenner, W.: Testing the technology acceptance model across cultures: a three country study. Inf. Manag. **33**, 1–11 (1997)
125. Dorfman, P.W., Howell, J.P.: Dimension of national culture and effective leadership patterns: Hofstede revisited. Adv. Int. Comp. Manag. **3**, 127–150 (1988)
126. Srite, S., Karahanna, E.: The role of espoused national cultural values in technology acceptance. MIS Q. **30**, 679 (2006)
127. Davis, F.D.: Perceived ease of use, and user acceptance of information technology. MIS Q. **13**, 319–340 (1989)
128. Lee, I., Choi, B., Kim, J., Hong, S.J.: Culture-technology fit: effects of cultural characteristics on the post-adoption beliefs of mobile internet users. Int. J. Electron. Commer. **11**, 11–51 (2007)
129. Im, I., Hong, S., Kang, M.S.: An international comparison of technology adoption: testing the UTAUT model. Inf. Manag. **48**, 1–8 (2011)
130. Huang, F., Teo, T., Sánchez-Prieto, J.C., García-Peñalvo, F.J., Olmos-Migueláñez, S.: Cultural values and technology adoption: a model comparison with university teachers from China and Spain. Comput. Educ. **133**, 69–81 (2019)
131. Lin, H.-C.: An investigation of the effects of cultural differences on physicians' perceptions of information technology acceptance as they relate to knowledge management systems. Comput. Hum. Behav. **38**, 368–380 (2014)
132. Petersen, F., Pather, S., Tucker, W.D.: User acceptance of ICT for diabetes self-management in the Western Cape, South Africa. In: African Conference of Information Systems and Technology (ACIST), pp. 1–11. Cape Town (2018)
133. Garabedian, L.F., Ross-Degnan, D., LeCates, R.F., Wharam, J.F.: Uptake and use of a diabetes management program with a mobile glucometer. Prim. Care Diabetes **13**, 549–555 (2019)
134. Deacon, A.J., Chee, J.J., Chang, W.J.R., Harbourne, B.A.: Mobile applications for diabetes mellitus self-management: a systematic narrative analysis. In: Successes and Failures in Telehealth Conference Telehealth Conference, pp. 17–30 (2017)

135. Petersen, F., Brown, A., Pather, S., Tucker, W.D.: Challenges for the adoption of ICT for diabetes self-management in South Africa. Electron. J. Inf. Syst. Dev. Ctries. **86**, 1–14 (2019)
136. Anderson, K., Emmerton, L.M.: Contribution of mobile health applications to self-management by consumers: review of published evidence. Aust. Health Rev. **40**, 591–597 (2016)
137. Dao, J., Spooner, C., Lo, W., Harris, M.F.: Factors influencing self-management in patients with type 2 diabetes in general practice: a qualitative study. Aust. J. Prim. Health **25**, 176–184 (2019)
138. American Diabetes Association: Strategies for improving care. Diabetes Care **38**, S5–S7 (2015)
139. McCoy, S., Galleta, D., King, W.K.: Integrating national culture into individual IS research: adoption the need for individual level measures. Commun. Assoc. Inf. Syst. **15**, 12–30 (2005)
140. Srite, M.: Culture as an explanation of technology acceptance differences: an empirical investigation of Chinese and US users. Aust. J. Inf. Syst. **14**, 30–52 (2006)
141. Park, J., Yang, S., Lehto, X.: Adoption of mobile technologies for Chinese consumers. J. Electron. Commer. Res. **8**, 196–206 (2007)
142. Tarhini, A., Hone, K., Liu, X.: The effects of individual differences on e-learning users' behaviour in developing countries: a structural equation model. Comput. Hum. Behav. **41**, 153–163 (2014)
143. Peek, S.T.M., Wouters, E.J.M., van Hoof, J., Luijkx, K.G., Boeije, H.R., Vrijhoef, H.J.M.: Factors influencing acceptance of technology for aging in place: a systematic review. Int. J. Med. Inform. **83**, 235–248 (2014)
144. Hofstede: Country Comparision-Hofstede Insights (2019)
145. Bandyopadhyay, K., Fraccastoro, K.A.: The effect of culture on user acceptance of information technology. Commun. Assoc. Inf. Syst. **19**, 522–543 (2007)
146. Thowfeek, M.H., Jaafar, A.: The influence of cultural factors on the adoption of e-learning: a reference to a public university in Sri Lanka. Appl. Mech. Mater. **263–266**, 3424–3434 (2012)
147. Özbilen, P.: The impact of natural culture on new technology adoption by firms: a country level analysis. Int. J. Innov. Manag. Technol. **8**, 299–305 (2017)
148. Kirsch, C., Chelliah, J., Parry, W.: The impact of cross-cultural dynamics on change management. Cross Cult. Manag. Int. J. **19**, 166–195 (2012)
149. Hoehle, H., Zhang, X., Venkatesh, V.: An espoused cultural perspective to understand continued intention to use mobile applications: a four-country study of mobile social media application usability. Eur. J. Inf. Syst. **24**, 337–359 (2015)
150. Al-Gahtani, S.S., Hubona, G.S., Wang, J.: Information technology (IT) in Saudi Arabia: culture and the acceptance and use of IT. Inf. Manag. **44**, 681–691 (2007)

Design and Initial Evaluation of Technology-Supported Shared Decision Making for Secondary Prevention in Cardiac Patients in the CoroPrevention Project

Wald Habets[1] , Martijn Scherrenberg[2,4] , Cindel Bonneux[1] , Wim Ramakers[1] ,
Dominique Hansen[3,4] , Paul Dendale[2,4] , and Karin Coninx[1(✉)]

[1] HCI and eHealth, Faculty of Sciences, UHasselt, 3590 Diepenbeek, Belgium
karin.coninx@uhasselt.be
[2] Faculty of Medicine and Life Sciences, UHasselt, 3590 Diepenbeek, Belgium
[3] BIOMED/REVAL, Faculty of Rehabilitation Sciences, UHasselt, 3590 Diepenbeek, Belgium
[4] Heart Centre Hasselt, Jessa Hospital, 3500 Hasselt, Belgium

Abstract. Secondary prevention is recommended after a cardiac event to stimulate recovery and reduce the risk of recurrent events. To optimize the results and support the patients to actively play a part in the prevention programme, the European guidelines and EAPC position statements on prevention of cardiovascular diseases suggest a holistic approach and shared decision making (SDM). Up till now, no eHealth solution that offers a holistic approach for secondary prevention that includes SDM has been described. The H2020 project CoroPrevention takes this challenge as one of its research goals, and strives for a technology-supported shared decision making approach for a comprehensive secondary prevention programme for cardiac patients. In this article, we report on the design and initial evaluation of the CoroPrevention-SDM approach. We highlight the stakeholder needs that underpin the design of the technology-supported shared decision making approach, and illustrate the three applications of the CoroPrevention Tool Suite that help patients and the medical staff to bring SDM into practice. How the CoroPrevention-SDM approach and applications underwrite the behavioural goal Medication Adherence, is elaborated as an example. While the overall medical and user experience related benefits can only be assessed in the large scale CoroPrevention randomized clinical trial (RCT), we share the methods and partial results of the initial usability studies and SDM evaluation in this article. In particular, the studies revealed that both patients and caregivers are inclined to use the CoroPrevention-SDM approach to collaboratively set behavioural goals during SDM encounters, and they appreciate the designed supporting applications.

Keywords: Shared decision making · Holistic approach · Secondary prevention · Cardiovascular diseases · Behaviour change · eHealth · Usability evaluation

1 Introduction

Acute coronary revascularizations and the use of efficient short- and long-term secondary prevention have both been linked to a notable decline in cardiovascular morbid-

© The Author(s), under exclusive license to Springer Nature Switzerland AG 2023
L. A. Maciaszek et al. (Eds.): ICT4AWE 2021/2022, CCIS 1856, pp. 362–384, 2023.
https://doi.org/10.1007/978-3-031-37496-8_19

ity and death [6]. Cardiac rehabilitation plays a big role in secondary prevention and multiple studies have shown the beneficial effects of it on recurrence rates and mortality [17]. Therefore, it is a Class IA recommendation to enrol in a cardiac rehabilitation programme [1].

In this article, we extend our previous ICT4AWE publication on the CorePrevention SDM approach [2]. Just as in our previous work, we discuss the need for a guideline-based secondary prevention programme and provide a holistic perspective and its integration of shared decision making into the CoroPrevention project. Contrasting to the initial publication, this article delves deeper into the evaluation of the pre-final applications. In this section, we consider the state of the art for the two identified needs and raise ideas to move beyond the currently implemented clinical practices.

1.1 The Need for a Holistic Approach

State of the Art. International guidelines recommend participation in a comprehensive cardiac rehabilitation programme after a recent cardiovascular event [1,22]. A comprehensive cardiac rehabilitation programme is defined as a programme that contains all core components: parameter monitoring, education, medication, physical activity, nutrition, smoking cessation, and stress management. In the last decades, Digital Health applications have been developed for all these core components separately. The goal of these applications is to increase the participation and duration of secondary prevention programmes. However, the main disadvantages of these applications are twofold: 1) most of these applications are not tailored to the risk profile of a cardiac patient, and 2) to follow a comprehensive, secondary prevention programme, the patient has to use several different applications. Using multiple applications can result in a higher cognitive burden, lower adherence and interference of (or even conflicting) advice offered by different applications.

In scientific literature, numerous studies were published that evaluated eHealth interventions for secondary prevention of cardiovascular diseases [4,10]. A review performed by Brørs et al. [4] concluded that the majority of studies included two or three secondary prevention components, of which education was employed in 21 out of the 24 included studies. To the best of our knowledge, there is no eHealth solution that fully supports a comprehensive, secondary prevention programme, including all key components as defined by Ambrosetti et al. [1] and that was subject to extensive evaluation on medical effectiveness and user experience.

Looking Beyond the State of the Art. The main parameters for follow-up in cardiovascular risk reduction are blood pressure, weight, cholesterol, and glucose levels. For each of these parameters, a target value is defined by the European guidelines and EAPC position statements [1,22] and an outcome goal can be set (i.e. respectively lowering blood pressure, healthy weight, lowering cholesterol, and diabetes management). To improve a parameter value and achieve the associated outcome goal, different strategies can be followed. For example, a healthy weight can be achieved by increasing physical activity, eating healthier, or a combination of both.

It is important that patients understand how they can work on an outcome goal. Setting the goal of losing weight until your body mass index (BMI) is below 25 is too abstract. In the context of behaviour change, people need to set actionable goals that are directly linked to behaviours over which they have direct control [15]. Therefore, we suggest that in a rehabilitation programme the outcome goals for secondary prevention should be linked to behavioural goals. Five such behavioural goals should be considered when aiming at a healthy lifestyle: medication adherence, start moving, healthy nutrition, smoke-free living, and stress relief. For each of these behavioural goals, specific, short-term goals should be set [15]. After defining the behavioural goals for the upcoming period, it is equally important that follow-up is done and that feedback is provided on the progress towards the behavioural goals [19]. Therefore, it is essential that patients can monitor their parameters and caregivers can remotely follow up on these reported values.

1.2   The Need for Shared Decision Making

State of the Art. From a clinical point of view, patients should reduce their cardiovascular disease (CVD) risk as soon as possible, as much as possible. This would require optimizing all outcome goals at the same time, and thus working on multiple behavioural goals simultaneously. After a cardiac incident, some patients want to drastically change their life and are eager to work on multiple or even all behavioural goals at the same time. However, this is not advised, since some behaviour changes oppose each other (e.g. smoking cessation and losing weight) which results in disillusionment for the patient. Furthermore, working on multiple behaviour changes simultaneously is not feasible for everyone. In these cases, a more gradual approach in which patients target one behaviour change at a time works better. Consequently, it has to be decided which behavioural goal is targeted first. There is evidence that some factors (which can be linked to behaviour changes) have a bigger effect on CVD risk than others (SCORE2 working group and ESC Cardiovascular risk collaboration, 2021; SCORE2-OP working group and ESC Cardiovascular risk collaboration, 2021). However, not all patients are willing or able to work on the behaviour change, which complicates to achieve the desired effects. Moreover, there are patients for whom it will be difficult or even impossible to tackle a certain risk factor. E.g., for a person with severe rheumatism, it will be very challenging to achieve the exercise targets but focusing on reducing the other CVD risk factors is still needed.

For this type of situations, where there is no clear best choice and the decision has to be made by balancing the pros and cons of different options (i.e. the behaviour changes), it is recommended to use shared decision making (SDM) [23]. Shared decision making is key for patient-centered care. The European Society of Cardiology also acknowledges that patient engagement (in clinical decision making) is needed to improve cardiovascular care [7, 14]. Shared decision making (SDM) combines the patient's preferences, values, goals, and context with the clinical evidence and caregivers' expertise to make an informed decision [12, 21], i.e. in this case which behavioural goal(s) the patient will work on first. The risk reduction of the different behaviour changes should be balanced with the patient's motivation to work on these behaviour changes. We propose to use digital decision aids or SDM tools in shared decision making encounters with the patient, to support a dialogue about balancing between the patient's motivation for behaviour change and necessary health risk reduction. Decision aids are tools that help patients and caregivers in SDM by making the decision explicit, offering information about the available options (and their advantages and disadvantages), and assisting in clarifying congruence between personal preferences/values and the decision at hand [20].

To actively participate in SDM and become the manager of their own disease, patients need to understand their condition and their own preferences [11]. Therefore, education is an essential component for SDM in the context of secondary prevention. This education can be delivered by caregivers during the encounters using a SDM tool, but also patients can learn on their own using digital resources such as articles, videos, and infographics [18].

Looking Beyond the State of the Art. Bonneux et al. [3] proposed three levels of decision-making in cardiac rehabilitation (CR): (1) the CR programme and its key components to include, (2) details of these key components, and (3) the detailed actions for the key components.

According to Mampuya et al., [13], cardiac rehabilitation is considered as a tool for secondary prevention of cardiovascular disease, which makes us believe that these three decision-making levels are applicable in the context of secondary prevention of CVD as well. Inspiring is also the categorization of different SDM tools at different points in time for these three levels of decision-making as described by Bonneux et al. [3].

The CoroPrevention-SDM approach that we developed takes into account patients' and caregivers' need for a holistic approach and shared decision making in the context of secondary prevention of cardiovascular diseases.

In Sect. 2, we describe the stakeholders' requirements for tools supporting SDM for a comprehensive secondary prevention programme. In Sect. 3, we present our CoroPrevention-SDM approach and highlight how the digital support that was realised in CoroPrevention fulfils patients' and caregivers' needs. The initial evaluation of the approach and tools is described in Sect. 4, Sect. 5 discusses the results of this evaluation and Sect. 6 emphasizes contributions and limitations of the presented research.

2   Stakeholders' Requirements for Shared Decision Making Tools

The CoroPrevention-SDM approach builds on the shared decision making approach of Bonneux et al. [3]. Whereas guidance of the patient is necessary throughout the secondary prevention programme, shared decision making is often facilitated in a discrete way, in a number of (physical) shared decision making encounters. The possibilities of the digital tools supporting the SDM process can be situated with respect to a single SDM encounter, while identifying the following points in time:

1. Preceding to the SDM encounter
2. During the SDM encounter
3. After the SDM encounter

For these three moments in time, we describe in the next sections the goals and needs for both patients and caregivers regarding support for shared decision making.

2.1   The Patient's Perspective

By increasing self-management of the disease by means of shared decision making, the patient becomes an active participant in the SDM process. Throughout this process, patient and caregiver decisions regarding the rehabilitation approach have to be balanced out. The patient's goals and needs that can be supported by digital tools are depicted in Fig. 1.

Before the SDM encounter	During the SDM encounter	After the SDM encounter
Patient goal: become empowered	**Patient goal:** make informed decisions	**Patient goal:** make the behaviour change
Patient needs: • Provide information • Encourage reflection	**Patient needs:** • Facilitate collaborative discussion • Improve understanding	**Patient needs:** • Guide to achieve the goals • Support in turning decisions into practice

Fig. 1. The patient's goals and needs preceding to, during, and after the SDM encounter [2].

Preceding to a SDM encounter, patients can trust on digital tools to become informed about what will happen during the encounter. They should reflect on their preference to be involved in the decision-making process e.g. do they want to take the decision, make a shared decision, or leave the decision to the caregiver. Furthermore, digital tools can support patients in considering their current status, gaining insight into their progress over the last period of time and into the next possible steps. We thus activate and empower the patient to become active participants in the SDM consultation by means of the digital tools.

During the SDM encounter, digital tools can support patients in improving their understanding, reflecting on past behaviour, stating their preferences, and understanding what actions should be taken. The aim is to prepare the patient to make an informed decision together with the caregiver during the SDM consultation and keep the patient motivated to work on the agreed behaviour changes.

After the SDM encounter, patients need to keep on working on the agreed behaviour goals at home. This is where mobile eHealth solutions can contribute to guide the patients in bringing into practice, in their daily life, the decisions made during the encounter. Setback moments in a rehabilitation process are unavoidable, but digital tools can contribute to get back on track. No matter how good the digital SDM aids are designed, their role is restricted to facilitation of the process without ruling out the important interventions of the caregivers.

2.2   The Caregiver's Perspective

From the caregiver's perspective, the digital tools supporting the shared decision making process aim to make guideline-based, to support the patient in search for behaviour changes, and to follow up on the patient's progress for a healthy lifestyle. In the same way as patients do, caregivers have different goals and needs for SDM tools over time (Fig. 2).

Before the SDM encounter	During the SDM encounter	After the SDM encounter
Caregiver goal: be well-prepared for the encounter **Caregiver needs:** • Provide information	**Caregiver goal:** make informed decisions **Caregiver needs:** • Facilitate collaborative discussion • Support education and guidance of the patient	**Caregiver goal:** support the patient in behaviour change **Caregiver needs:** • Follow up on the patient's progress • Intervene when the patient deviates from the plan

Fig. 2. The caregiver's goals and needs preceding to, during, and after the SDM encounter [2].

Preceding to the SDM encounter, the digital tool assists the caregivers' preparation for the upcoming appointment, with special focus on decisions to be made during the encounter. Activities to be supported include reviewing the patient's evolution since last consultation, and looking forward to pending goals and prepare for prescribing guideline-based care to their patients.

During the SDM encounter, digital tool support is very useful for the discussion between the caregiver and the patient regarding the outcome goals that are needed from a clinical point of view (i.e. transferring knowledge to the patient) and for collaboratively setting behavioural goals that are in line with the clinical evidence and the patient's preferences (i.e. facilitating collaborative discussion and motivating the patient). After all, the final aim of the shared decision making approach is to facilitate informed decision making by the patient together with the caregiver during the SDM consultation, and to sustain the patient's motivation for the agreed behaviour changes.

After SDM encounters, caregivers come back to the digital SDM tools to follow up on their patients' progress, though they expect this to be a time-efficient process. Therefore, digital tools, such as dashboard visualizations and alerts, can support caregivers in following up on the patient's progress. Automatic alerts to the caregiver when the patient deviates from the agreed goals and action plans, to keep track of contacting the patient and discussing the situation during the next SDM encounter, contribute to the efficiency of the SDM process.

Figure 1 and Fig. 2 reveal the essentially similar goals and needs of the different stakeholders in the SDM process, while depicting them from the perspective of the different stakeholders. In the next section, we describe the CoroPrevention interpretation of the timeline and digital tools proposed in the categorization of Bonneux et al. [3]. Attention is paid how to satisfy the needs of the different stakeholders (patients and caregivers) in the context of comprehensive, secondary prevention of cardiovascular diseases.

3   CoroPrevention SDM Timeline and Supporting Applications

The CoroPrevention-SDM approach presented in this article is a technology-supported shared decision making approach for a comprehensive secondary prevention programme for cardiac patients, that takes into account the ESC guidelines and EAPC position statements [1,7,22]. This secondary prevention programme adheres to a holistic approach targeting the risk factors for cardiovascular diseases. Shared decision making is incorporated on the process level in the CoroPrevention-SDM approach and on the level of the digital tools of the CoroPrevention Tool Suite. An important design consideration for the Tool Suite was to satisfy all requirements that were stated above (i.e. offering a holistic approach for secondary prevention, supporting shared decision making, and complying with all patient and caregiver needs identified in the previous section). The holistic approach for secondary prevention is reflected in the CoroPrevention Tool Suite - when it reaches the full target implementation - by offering the following 7 modules: parameter monitoring, education, medication, physical activity, healthy nutrition, smoking cessation, and stress management. The modules in the Tool Suite are gradually elaborated further during the project, but one or more versions for their design and specification are already available. Most of these modules can directly be linked to the behavioural goals, i.e. medication adherence, start moving, healthy nutrition, smoke-free living, and stress relief. The two remaining modules, education and parameter monitoring, are essential to support the shared decision making process and remote follow-up by the caregiver.

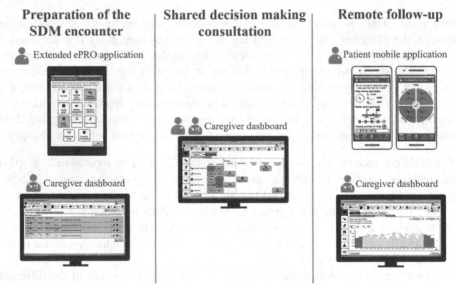

Fig. 3. The timeline and accompanying tools to be used during a single encounter to support shared decision making for a comprehensive secondary prevention program [2].

The CoroPrevention Tool Suite is composed of three digital tools (ePRO, dashboard and mobile application) that support patients and caregivers in shared decision making for the secondary prevention programme during one or more stages of SDM. Figure 3 categorizes the tools according to the three moments in time that were identified before: preceding to the SDM encounter, during the SDM encounter, and after the SDM encounter. In the remainder of this section, we describe these tools and how they are situated with respect to a single SDM encounter. Examples of the tools are given, with specific interest for shared decision making and the Medication module.

3.1 Preparation of an SDM Encounter

Given the short time available for live encounters (with an average of just about 10 min per patient [5]), it is important that both patients and caregivers are well prepared for the encounter.

An extended ePRO application can preserve more time during the encounter by allowing patients to provide a status update about their risk factors and related behavioural goals. In the context of the CoroPrevention Tool Suite, Electronic Patient-reported Outcomes (ePRO) are questionnaires for patients to indicate how they are feeling and what they prefer. In line with the goal to prepare for the encounter, patients use the extended ePRO application on a mobile device (tablet or smartphone) in the waiting room to inform themselves about the SDM process (e.g. an educational video on the shared decision making as such), report on their current status, and state their preferences. These preferences are considered on different levels of abstraction, ranging from high-level goals the patient would like to work to, to very specific preferences on the level of favourite sports activities. The fact that preferences are collected before the encounter and not in front of caregivers relieves feelings of uncertainty patients might have. During the SDM encounter, the collected preferences are depicted on the shared display showing the dashboard, and they can be addressed by the caregiver during the motivational interviewing. Even if patients are reluctant to engage in a conversation on the preferences, the information is available and can be used by the caregiver.

This scenario of use for the ePRO not only saves time during the encounter itself, but the usage of the application also explicitly marks a moment in time that is dedicated for the patient to reflect on their status, behaviour, and preferences.

Figure 4 illustrates the ePRO application with a questionnaire that invites the patients to reflect on their medication adherence in the recent weeks, in preparation for the discussion on Medication as one of the behavioural goals.

Next to patients, caregivers also need to be well-prepared for a SDM encounter. This can be done by checking the patient's file in the caregiver dashboard, the second tool of the CoroPrevention Tool Suite. The patient's performance in the last months for the behavioural goals, and identification of pending goals, are typical preparation activities for the caregiver before the encounter. Furthermore, two clinical decision support systems (CDSS) are integrated in the caregiver dashboard of the CoroPrevention Tool Suite to support caregivers in prescribing guideline-based care to their patients. The EXPERT tool [8,9] provides exercise prescriptions, and a decision support system for medication prescription is available as well. A detailed description of these systems is beyond the scope of this article. It is suggested to use these systems before rather than during a SDM encounter as this is less cumbersome and leaves more time for discussion on SDM-related topics such as the patient's goals and performance during the encounter. Usage of CDSS systems during encounters might also affect the patient's perception of the caregiver's credibility and authority.

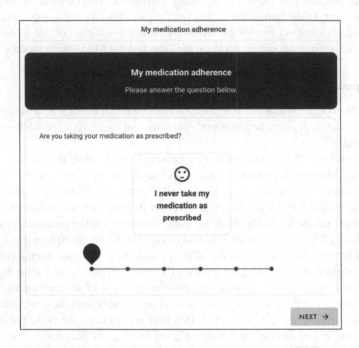

Fig. 4. An example questions of the ePRO asking patients to report medication adherence.

3.2   During an SDM Encounter

The main digital tool of the CoroPrevention Tool Suite during the SDM encounter is the caregiver dashboard. It is intentionally designed not to be a tool for caregivers only, but to function as a tool for both stakeholders of the shared decision making process, patients as well as caregivers. Because the caregiver dashboard is used during a consultation on a shared display to encourage collaboration and spark discussion with the patient, its design took into account the needs of both stakeholder groups. While the interaction with the dashboard is done by the caregiver, the patient needs to be able to interpret the information and specific visualizations albeit guided by the caregiver.

An SDM encounter typically starts by discussing the patient's evolution in the past period and the current status for the behavioural goals and related outcome goals. For the outcome goals (e.g. lowering blood pressure, lowering cholesterol, and healthy weight), shared decision making is not possible in our CoroPrevention approach, as these goals are determined based on clinical guidelines and the caregiver's expertise. Moreover, cholesterol and hypertension are more influenced by medication than by lifestyle changes. Therefore, the caregiver will strongly emphasize the importance of medication adherence to reduce the patient's CVD risk. Medication adherence visualizations in the dashboard support this part of the consultation (Fig. 5 and 7b).

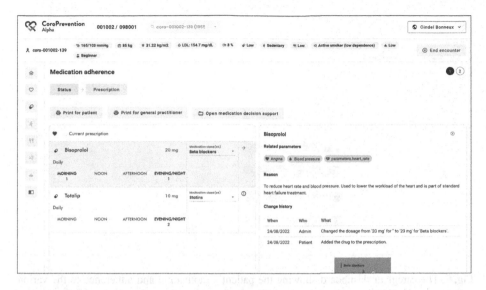

Fig. 5. The caregiver dashboard showing the patient's medication prescription, generated by the CDSS.

It is still important to discuss the patients' outcome goals during the encounters, because behaviour changes such as reducing salt intake, exercising more, and eating healthier can be other ways to work on these outcome goals. So both relevant behavioural goals and outcome goals can be determined and discussed (Fig. 6) This concept builds on the Transtheoretical Model of Health Behavior Change [16].

The dashboard presents the processed results from the ePRO, specifically the patient's motivation to work on the various behavioural goals, with the aim to spark discussion. The levels of (shared) decision making [3] can be recognized during the discussion, depending on the behavioural goals as such: (level 1) the patient and caregiver agree upon one or more feasible behavioural goals for the patient; (level 2 and 3) they discuss and record the plans to achieve the goal. Patient and caregiver follow this process for each behaviour goal that they agreed to include in the secondary prevention programme at that point in time. During this process, the caregiver's role is not only to support the patient in decision-making and achieve a feasible set of goals (Fig. 6), but also to motivate the patient to work on the agreed behavioural goals. The feasible set of goals and - if applicable - the plans to achieve them will guide the patient until the next SDM encounter.

3.3   Remote Follow-Up

The information that results from the SDM encounter is used to configure the third tool of the CoroPrevention Tool Suite: a mobile application that patients use at home to follow up on their behaviour change process and receive support for decision-making in daily life. In the mobile application, patients receive support to make decisions on a daily basis and can follow up on their medication intake (Fig. 7) Furthermore, they can record their progress (e.g. tracking sports activities) and follow up on their journey towards a

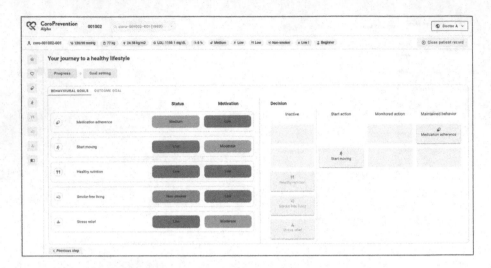

Fig. 6. The caregiver dashboard showing the patient's motivation and adherence to the various behaviour goals (left), as well as the current level of guidance for each module (right).

healthy lifestyle. Based on the patient's progress, the mobile application makes recommendations to increase/decrease the support for the behavioural goals. For example, on the highest level of support, patient will receive reminders for their medication intake and to report this in the app. Once the patient has achieved a high medication adherence for a prolonged period of time, the application will suggest a different level of support, reducing the amount of reminders. Patients can decide themselves whether they accept or decline the recommendation to start or stop working on a behavioural goal. Due to the patient autonomy they make progress in becoming the manager of their own disease. However, there will also be moments when the patient has difficulties. At those moments, the mobile application (and caregivers) will be there to help the patient getting back on track.

In one way the mobile application uses the results from the SDM encounter, in the other way the data that is collected in the mobile application is used as input for the dashboard, both for remote follow-up, and for the next SDM encounter. The caregiver dashboard allows follow up on their patients in various ways, such as monitoring progress, receiving alerts (e.g. when the patient's medication adherence is way too low), and selecting and suggesting educational content that the patient should read.

4   Evaluation of the CoroPrevention-SDM Approach

The impact of the technology-supported shared decision making approach on the medical outcomes and on the patients' motivation to sustain the comprehensive secondary prevention programme, can only be assessed in a longitudinal study. An essential component of the H2020 project CoroPrevention[1] is a large-scale randomized controlled

---

[1] https://www.coroprevention.eu.

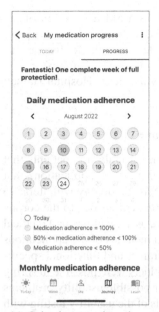

(a) Calendar overview showing medication adherence

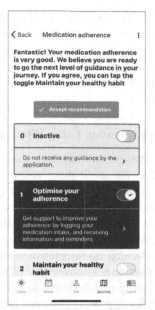

(b) Overview of activated level of guidance for medication adherence

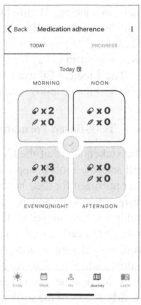

(c) Medication schedule for a single day

Fig. 7. The medication module of the mobile application, through which the patient can report and follow up on their medication adherence.

trial (RCT, https://clinicaltrials.gov/, NCT04433052) that evaluates the medical outcomes as well as the technological support provided in the CoroPrevention Tool Suite. Several hospitals in 6 European countries are involved in the trial. Recruitment starts with screening of 10000 coronary heart disease patients, of which 2000 high-risk patients will be enrolled in the RCT. Over a period of three years, patients and their supporting caregivers will use the CoroPrevention Tool Suite to set personalized goals for the patients and follow up on their progress. Apart from medical outcome and cost-effectiveness analysis, a thorough evaluation of the RCT results is planned from a Human-Computer Interaction perspective, considering a.o. the usability and user experience of the CoroPrevention Tool Suite, patients' motivation for behaviour change, and the contribution of the digital tools in facilitating the CoroPrevention-SDM approach.

To the best of our knowledge, concepts related to shared decision making such as motivational interviewing with support of a digital tool, and collaboratively setting behavioural goals during SDM encounters, have not yet been investigated in the context of secondary prevention of cardiovascular diseases. During the design and development stage of the CoroPrevention Tool Suite, and prior to the start of the RCT, we assessed patients' and caregivers' opinion on our proposed shared decision making approach for secondary prevention in different stages.

In the current article, we share the evaluation methods we used during the design and development of the CoroPrevention Tool Suite with particular interest for shared decision making. Highlights of the findings are reported, as a full description of the analysis results on all modules of the CoroPrevention Tool Suite is beyond the scope of this article. Therefore, the focus is on the Medication module and on the Journey as this last component is key for goal setting and progress follow-up in a SDM context.

The Medical Ethical Committees of Hasselt University and Jessa Hospital Hasselt approved the usability studies.

4.1 Task-Based Formative Evaluation Using Wireframes

The stakeholders of the CoroPrevention Tool Suite, and in particular the patients that will use the mobile application for about three years, benefit from applications that are optimized for their needs. A user-centred design (UCD) methodology with iterative design, prototype and evaluation stages is advisable. The restrictions due to the corona pandemic have inhibited direct contacts with representative users, patients and medical staff, in the early project stages. As a consequence, several modules of the applications were fully designed, and documented via interactive wireframes and functional specifications, when the first live evaluation sessions with stakeholders were possible in spring 2021. Meticulous formative testing was desirable to repair possible usability problems in early stages of the software development. The main goals of the usability testing with the interactive wireframes are (1) to assess the ease of use and understandability of the designs for the CoroPrevention Tool Suite, and prioritize discovered usability issues, and (2) assess the willingness of the stakeholders to use the applications as digital support for the shared decision making process.

Task-based scenarios, covering the most important features of a specific module in the mobile application or the dashboard, were prepared. Ad hoc questionnaires to evaluate the specific modules from the point of view of either a patient or a caregiver were compiled, as well as a general questionnaire to probe for some demographic data and the participants' technology acquaintance.

Depending on the participants' availability, they were invited for 1–2 h to evaluate the wireframes of 1–2 modules of an application. Whereas caregivers evaluated only modules of the dashboard, patients evaluated parts of the mobile app, the dashboard or both. In a real context of use, patients would never use the dashboard on their own but only participate in a SDM encounter with a caregiver. Having patients evaluate the wireframes of the dashboard independently informed the researchers about the understandability of parts of the interface of the dashboard, in particular the visualizations that support the shared decision making process. In this way, a preliminary evaluation by patients in the context of SDM was possible early in the design of the CoroPrevention Tool Suite, when a true SDM setting cannot be organized.

The formative evaluation sessions were guided by a facilitator and an observer. After getting information on the study and signing the informed consent, the participant completed the technology acquaintance questionnaire. The participant was instructed to interact with the interactive wireframe that was shown to the participant and the facilitator on a relatively large display (and to the observer on another display), using the keyboard and mouse/touchscreen. To give an impression about the visual appearance of the wireframes, we refer to Fig. 3 that was constructed using some of the wireframes. The facilitator invited the patient to work through the task list and to think aloud. After evaluating a specific module, the participant completed the corresponding usability questionnaire. All materials used in the usability testing, the interactive wire-frames as well as the questionnaires, were presented in the patients' native language (Dutch).

Twenty-one caregivers, most of them cardiologists in training and physiothera-pists, were recruited in the rehabilitation centre of Jessa Hospital (Hasselt, Belgium), to ensure that each module of the dashboard was evaluated by 7 caregivers. Fifty-six patients were recruited, to end up with 10–11 evaluators for each module in the mobile app and the dashboard. Recruitment happened either in the same rehabilitation centre or via a call in local media. All patients were formerly or actually engaged in a super-vised secondary prevention programme after a cardiac event. The formative evaluation sessions were organized on 19 days in 5 weeks, in March and April 2021.

4.2 Task-Based Evaluation of Pre-final Applications

In the scope of this article, the term "application testing" denotes usability testing by stakeholders of the pre-final mobile and dashboard application, as opposed to wireframe-based evaluation. Obviously, in addition to usability testing, thorough tech-nical, testing including verification, is done by the development company, and accep-tance and readiness for the RCT are evaluated by the involved researchers. Particular attention is given to algorithm validation of the two clinical decision support systems, that have to perform in line with the actual ESC/EAPC guidelines. Till now, the appli-cation testing with stakeholders mainly focused on the Medication module for patients within the mobile app including features such as educational content in the app, and on the Medication module in the dashboard, as well as general features of the dashboard, for patients as well as caregivers.

The main goals of the usability testing with the pre-final applications are to assess (1) whether the overall positive results of the wireframe testing are confirmed, (2) to what extent changes applied to the (wireframe) designs indeed solve previously identi-fied usability issues, and (3) to assemble a first impression on the digital support for the shared decision making process.

The methods used for the mobile application testing with patients are very similar to the above mentioned formative testing techniques applied for wireframe evaluation: task-based testing sessions that are guided by a facilitator and an observer, and during which the participant is invited to think aloud. Additional data collection was done via ad hoc questionnaires, to gather information on technology acquaintance background and about the patients' opinion on the application, and with the standard SUS ques-tionnaire. All materials used in the usability testing, the applications as well as the questionnaires, were presented in the patients' native language (Dutch).

Six patients were recruited in the rehabilitation centre of Jessa Hospital (Hasselt, Belgium), one of which did not show up. The evaluation sessions were organized in August 2022.

To learn about the SDM dynamics and suitability of the dashboard during encoun-ters, two patients were invited for a simulated individual SDM encounter. One of the researchers, a cardiologist in training, took the role of caregiver and engaged in a con-versation with the patient. The caregiver drew the patient's attention to the SDM sup-

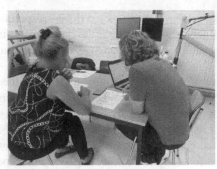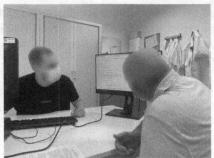

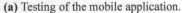

(a) Testing of the mobile application.   (b) A simulated SDM encounter with a caregiver.

Fig. 8. Patient and facilitator during application testing session in the rehabilitation centre.

porting parts of the dashboard (such as medication adherence visualizations), and asked the patient to interpret the information.

The application testing for the mobile app (45–60 min) as well as the simulated SDM encounter (30–45 min) were setup as a single session in a quiet room in the rehabilitation centre (Jessa Hospital, Hasselt, Belgium), without follow-up. This setup is shown in Fig. 8. We avoid calling this summative testing, as usability evaluations will continue to be done in different stages of the CoroPrevention RCT and in parallel research settings.

5   Evaluation Results

5.1   Findings from the Formative Wireframe-Based Evaluation

Analysis of the data collected in the formative evaluation with wireframes should reveal information to steer the next stages of the design and development of the CoroPrevention Tool Suite, and how it supports the CoroPrevention-SDM approach. To this end, the information collected during the observations and the answers on the questionnaires were combined.

Given the relatively large number of participants, the analysis of the observation data took a lot of time but the study revealed useful information. The observation notes per participant and per module were checked by one or two researchers to identify encountered issues. Per module, the issues were clustered and listed for all participants, and possible solutions were added. After discussion between the two involved researchers, a consensus proposal for a priority per clustered issue was formulated. The priorities were coded from 1, very high priority, to 5, very low priority. Issues with priority 1 are major usability issues that could relate to patient safety or seriously block the use of the application. An issue with priority 5 is only discovered for one person, and is not hindering the use of the application. An example of an issue identified in the mobile Medication module with priority level 1, thus possibly related to patient safety, are the Edit and Delete buttons for the medication prescription that are hard to find, which was solved by moving these widgets to the top of the display.

Patient evaluation of the smartphone application (Wire-frame testing)

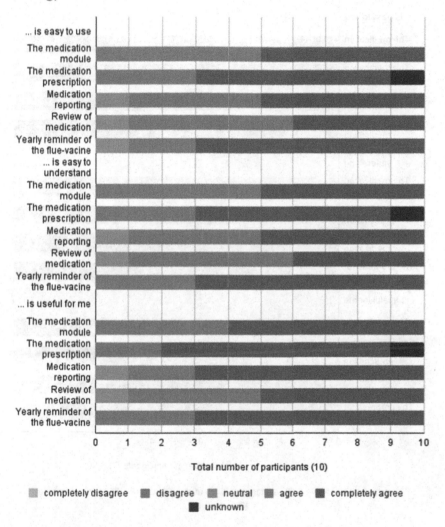

Fig. 9. The patient evaluation of the smartphone application based upon the wireframes. Patients reported on the "ease of use", "ease of understanding" and "usefulness".

Further information on the participants' appreciation of the designs of modules in the different applications, based on the wireframes, is deduced from the questionnaires. To illustrate the type of results that are achieved, we present the patients' rating for the mobile Medication module and the caregivers' rating for the Medication module in the dashboard in Fig. 9 and Fig. 10 respectively.

Caregiver evaluation of the dashboard (Wire-frame testing)

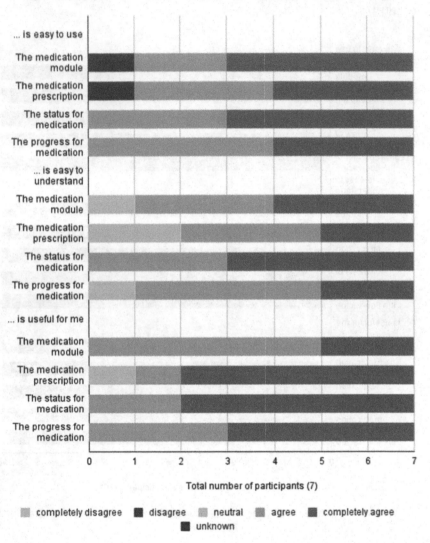

Fig. 10. The caregiver evaluation of the dashboard application based upon the wireframes. Patients reported on the "ease of use", "ease of understanding" and "usefulness".

Caregivers were asked if they were willing to use a caregiver dashboard during their consultations with patients to discuss the patients' progress and set goals for a healthy lifestyle. Similarly, patients were asked if they would be willing to use a caregiver dashboard during a consultation with a caregiver to discuss their progress and set goals for a healthy lifestyle. Furthermore, patients were asked if they would be willing to use a mobile application to follow up at home on their journey towards a healthy lifestyle.

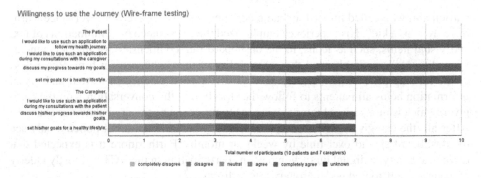

Fig. 11. Patients' and caregivers' willingness to use the digital tools of the CoroPrevention Tool Suite.

The results of our survey are depicted in Fig. 11. All participants (both patients and caregivers) unanimously agreed that they would be willing to use the proposed tools supporting the CoroPrevention-SDM approach. There were a few neutral responses. For the patients that participated in the study, these neutral responses might be due to the fact that the cardiac patients that participated in the usability study already completed cardiac rehabilitation quite a long time ago. Therefore, using these tools might be less relevant for them at this moment.

5.2 Findings from the Evaluation with Pre-final Applications

Due to the small number of patients (5) that tested the pre-final Medication module in the mobile application till date, no firm conclusions can be drawn from either the questionnaire results or the observer notes. Nevertheless, some preliminary findings can be reported, that ask for follow-up in future usability testing (e.g. for next releases of the CoroPrevention Tool Suite that will proceed to the RCT, with additional modules supporting components of the comprehensive secondary prevention programme).

With respect to the task-based mobile application testing of the Medication module by individual patients, we noticed during the observations and partly based on the questionnaires, that the most important issues determined in the formative testing with wireframes have been solved, even if the task-based test scenario during application testing did not cover all individual issues due to time constraints in the test sessions. Considerable redesigns after wireframe-based evaluation were not needed after formative testing, but the issues were solved in the development stage by simple adaptations in the application's design such as added or improved labels for UI widgets, and moving buttons to the top of the screen to make them immediately visible without scrolling.

The simulated SDM encounters showed that the dashboard design facilitates the shared decision making process during the consultation. The navigation structure leads the caregiver through the steps of the SDM encounter, and helps the patient to recognize returning topics of interest during subsequent consultations. Both the structured design of the dashboard and particular visualizations focus the attention on decisions to be taken during the SDM encounter. This is very much illustrated by the remark of one participant, who called himself a "bad reader and writer, slow reader, ever since learning to read as a kid". His experience emphasized the importance of combinations of text and visual items, such as icons, in the dashboard that compensate for the deficiencies in reading skills and enhanced the accessibility of the dashboard for him. Regardless of the reading pace of patients, we noticed that a good balance in textual and visual information helps all patients to follow the storyline in the conversation with the caregiver, which is motivational interviewing to stimulate the necessary behaviour changes. After all, the caregivers will be frequent users of the dashboard, but patients only see the dashboard spread over time by weeks or months. Furthermore it is expected that there is a variety in digital literacy in persons participating in the RCT as mostly elderly persons are confronted with coronary artery disease.

The applied evaluation method with simulated SDM encounters was appreciated a lot by the participants (patients and caregiver) and the involved researchers. Even if the spontaneous course of things during the conversation makes the setting less formal than strictly task-based testing, it comes very close to the realistic "context of use" in the RCT, with guidance of a caregiver.

5.3   Reflections on Formative and Summative Evaluations with Stakeholders

What is impossible to evaluate in a short testing session is the deep influence of the process of shared decision making as such on the (activities towards) behavioural goals of the secondary prevention programme, and fine-grained details in the design of the mobile application and dashboard that facilitate the SDM process. This can only be investigated during and after the longitudinal study in the RCT, and is facilitated by the collection of usage data about the digital tools by all stakeholders, and consequent data analysis. We also have to be aware about the individual experience and influence of the caregiver/case nurse guiding the motivational interviewing with help of the SDM dashboard.

When comparing the preliminary results of the questionnaires of the individual application testing on the Medication module with the results of the formative testing with wireframes, we conclude that overall - as far as we can assume from the low number of participants in the application testing (5) - that the expressed opinions are less positive than after the formative testing. For instance, when probed for the ease of use and ease of understanding the patients replied with 87,5% on average in formative testing with wireframes vs. 70% (ease of use) and 60% (ease of understanding) after application testing. Also, usefulness of the Medication module and its separate components was rated about 90% in formative testing vs. 55% in application testing. We observe the same trend for the opinions on medication prescription and medication reporting.

To some extent, this difference is clarified by some quotes of patients during application testing and formative testing. Some of them are convinced they need a Medication adherence reporting module in an app and appreciate the one they were asked to test, whereas other persons conclude either *"I don't need this to strive for good medication adherence because my memory works just fine"* or *"I prefer the pill box I use already for several years, and I prepare and categorize my medication in the pill box every evening, so I don't want to use an app in addition to that"*.

We hypothesize that the different results in formative and application testing might also be caused by the participants' general stance on, and acquaintance with, technology. As the technology acquaintance background questionnaire was completed by all participating patients and even caregivers, we can compare the patients' answers for participants in the formative vs. application testing. In the formative testing group specifically for the Medication module, 9 out of 10 patients answered "much" or "very much" on a 5-point likert scale, with one patient answering "neutral" to the question "*how much do you like to use technology*"; leading to an average of 3.6 out of 4, or 90%. There is a quite strong contrast with 3 out of 5 participants in application testing stating that they do not like to use technology and the other 2 participants being either in favour of technology use or neutral, thus accumulating in an average of 1.6 out of 4, or 40%. The collected data from the formative testing also show that the distribution of opinions for the Medication module testers is very much in line with the general distribution on technology use for all 56 participating patients in the formative testing with wireframes.

The transformation of the wireframes to the pre-final application designs for the Medication module of the CoroPrevention Tool Suite in the software development stage did not imply major changes; it only solved some issues. As a result, it is not clear whether the difference in results for formative and application testing relate to the artefacts - wireframes vs mobile and dashboard applications - as such, or rather to the coincidental sample of participating testers. We are wondering if participants using wireframes and realizing the formative character of the evaluation stage are more tolerant and thus implicitly expecting improvements in the transformation to final applications, but we are not aware of evidence in literature on this phenomenon. Given the interactive nature of the CoroPrevention wireframes during formative testing, and their similarity with the final application designs, we do not expect this to have a major influence on the results.

6   Contributions and Limitations

The CoroPrevention project investigates the benefits of a comprehensive secondary prevention programme for cardiac patients. With this goal, the project directly adheres to the European guidelines and EAPC position statements [1,7,22] that recommend the holistic approach for cardiac rehabilitation and secondary prevention. In these guidelines, it is also suggested to incorporate shared decision making to sustain the motivation of patients over a long period of time, as typically is needed when striving for and maintaining healthy behaviours. As highlighted in the sections on "state-of-the-art" above, there are examples of technology support for single or limited number of components of secondary prevention programmes. Research initiatives aim to make the programmes and corresponding technology support more and more comprehensive. However, at the time of writing this article, we are not aware of any existing eHealth system that supports the comprehensive approach of the programme while integrating shared decision making for all key components, as well as behavioural and outcome goals.

With the design and realization of the CoroPrevention-SDM approach, and the accompanying CoroPrevention Tool Suite, this research provides an interesting contribution to the realization of a new generation of innovative eHealth systems in the domain of cardiac rehabilitation and beyond. The initial ideas on the key components of the secondary prevention programme as such, the integration of shared decision making in the encounters with the medical staff, and the concepts of the digital tools, were outlined in the paper presented at the ICT4AWE conference in 2022 (ref ICT4AWE). The current article provides the scientific community insights in the evolutions of the research while elaborating the conceptualization of the SDM approach and digital tools. The fine-tuning of both levels, the medical way of working during the encounters and the supporting software applications, goes hand in hand and considers patients and caregivers as stakeholders. The article illustrates how the early designs and wireframes evolved in true digital tools. A major focus is on the evaluation techniques and results, with the evaluation of shared decision making in early stages of design and developments being an important challenge.

Initial results on willingness to be involved in and SDM process, and to use the CoroPrevention Tool Suite were positive. The same applies to initial usability results regarding specific application details. However, we are aware that the presented research methods go along with some intrinsic and practical limitations. Due to the recruitment of patients in the rehabilitation centre and through an open call in local media, there is a possibility for bias in favour of more motivated patients with respect to participating in a secondary prevention programme. One could argue that there also is a bias in favour of persons that are more acquainted with technology or at least more willing to use digital tools for their personal health. Nevertheless, we noticed that the technology acquaintance of the recruited participants is rather diverse, and that the age distribution is representative for persons participating in cardiac rehabilitation programmes. A factor that turned out to have a strong influence on experienced ease of use is the participant's abstraction capability. This was needed to imagine that the data that were shown during the test (medication prescription, blood pressure etc.) were imaginary data and not their own personal health data.

The effect of shared decision making and the value of the CoroPrevention Tool Suite to achieve shared decisions with empowered patients can only be evaluated on the long term. The large-scale CoroPrevention RCT, that starts in the second half of 2022, will allow for more thorough evaluations.

7   Conclusions

One of the challenges tackled by the H2020 project CoroPrevention is to design and develop a holistic approach for a secondary prevention programme for cardiovascular diseases, supported by digital tools. The ESC and EAPC guidelines, that advocate for shared decision making, encouraged the research team to elaborate the CoroPrevention-SDM approach. After identifying the needs for a holistic secondary prevention programme with shared decision making, we reported in this article how these needs drove the requirements for the CoroPrevention Tool Suite. The digital support for the CoroPrevention-SDM approach comprises three applications: 1) an extended ePRO application to collect the patient's status and preferences, 2) a caregiver dashboard with integrated clinical decision support systems and shared decision making support, and 3) a mobile application for the patient that stimulates behaviour change. Both stakeholder groups, patients and caregivers, were kept in mind during the design process, and were involved in the evaluation of the applications. In this article we described the different techniques that were used to evaluate wireframe-based prototypes and the pre-final applications, and we highlighted how we incorporated the evaluation of components of shared decision making. Initial results of the evaluation showed willingness of the stakeholders to use the CoroPrevention-SDM approach and the accompanying Tool Suite, and continue to drive future versions of the digital tools.

Acknowledgements. The research presented in this paper was supported by grants from the Special Research Fund (BOF) of Hasselt University (BOF18DOC26), and from FWO (FWO-ICA project EXPERT network G0F4220N). The CoroPrevention project has received funding from the European Union's Horizon 2020 research and innovation programme under grant agreement No 848056.

References

1. Ambrosetti, M., et al.: Secondary prevention through comprehensive cardiovascular rehabilitation: from knowledge to implementation. 2020 update. A position paper from the Secondary Prevention and Rehabilitation Section of the European Association of Preventive Cardiology. Eur. J. Prev. Cardiol. (2020)
2. Bonneux, C., et al.: The CoroPrevention-SDM approach: a technology-supported shared decision making approach for a comprehensive secondary prevention program for cardiac patients. In: Proceedings of the 8th International Conference on Information and Communication Technologies for Ageing Well and e-Health, pp. 59–69. Scitepress, Digital library (2022). https://doi.org/10.5220/0011042300003188. iCT4AWE - 8th International Conference on Information and Communication Technologies for Ageing Well and e-Health
3. Bonneux, C., Rovelo, G., Dendale, P., Coninx, K.: A comprehensive approach to decision aids supporting shared decision making in cardiac rehabilitation. In: Proceedings of the 13th EAI International Conference on Pervasive Computing Technologies for Healthcare, PervasiveHealth 2019, pp. 389–398. Association for Computing Machinery, New York (2019). https://doi.org/10.1145/3329189.3329241
4. Brørs, G., et al.: Modes of e-Health delivery in secondary prevention programmes for patients with coronary artery disease: a systematic review. BMC Health Serv. Res. **19**(1), 364 (2019)
5. Elmore, N., et al.: Investigating the relationship between consultation length and patient experience: a cross-sectional study in primary care. Br. J. Gen. Pract. **66**(653), e896–e903 (2016)
6. Ford, E.S., et al.: Explaining the decrease in U.S. deaths from coronary disease, 1980–2000. N. Engl. J. Med. **356**(23), 2388–2398 (2007)
7. Graham, I., Filippatos, G., Atar, D., Vardas, P.E., Pinto, F.J., Fitzsimons, D.: Patient engagement. Eur. Heart J. **38**(42), 3114–3115 (2017)
8. Hansen, D., Coninx, K., Dendale, P.: The EAPC EXPERT tool. Eur. Heart J. **38**(30), 2318–2320 (2017)
9. Hansen, D., et al.: The European association of preventive cardiology exercise prescription in everyday practice and rehabilitative training (EXPERT) tool: a digital training and decision support system for optimized exercise prescription in cardiovascular disease. Concept, definitions and construction methodology. Eur. J. Prev. Cardiol. **24**(10), 1017–1031 (2017)
10. Jin, K , et al.: Telehealth interventions for the secondary prevention of coronary heart disease: a systematic review and meta-analysis. Eur. J. Cardiovasc. Nurs. **18**(4), 260–271 (2019)

11. Joseph-Williams, N., Elwyn, G., Edwards, A.: Knowledge is not power for patients: a systematic review and thematic synthesis of patient-reported barriers and facilitators to shared decision making. Patient Educ. Couns. **94**(3), 291–309 (2014)
12. Kon, A.A.: The shared decision-making continuum. JAMA **304**(8), 903–904 (2010)
13. Mampuya, W.M.: Cardiac rehabilitation past, present and future: an overview. Cardiovasc. Diagn. Ther. **2**(1), 38–49 (2012)
14. Institute of Medicine: Crossing the Quality Chasm: A New Health System for the 21st Century. The National Academies Press, Washington, DC (2001). https://doi.org/10.17226/10027. https://nap.nationalacademies.org/catalog/10027/crossing-the-quality-chasm-a-new-health-system-for-the
15. Medynskiy, Y., Yarosh, S., Mynatt, E.: Five strategies for supporting healthy behavior change, pp. 1333–1338 (2011). https://doi.org/10.1145/1979742.1979770
16. Prochaska, J.O., Velicer, W.F.: The transtheoretical model of health behavior change. Am. J. Health Promot. **12**(1), 38–48 (1997)
17. Salzwedel, A., et al.: Effectiveness of comprehensive cardiac rehabilitation in coronary artery disease patients treated according to contemporary evidence based medicine: update of the Cardiac Rehabilitation Outcome Study (CROS-II). Eur. J. Prev. Cardiol. **27**(16), 1756–1774 (2020)
18. Sankaran, S., Bonneux, C., Dendale, P., Coninx, K.: Bridging patients' needs and caregivers' perspectives to tailor information provisioning during cardiac rehabilitation. In: Proceedings of the 32nd International BCS Human Computer Interaction Conference (HCI 2018). The eWiC Series (2018). https://doi.org/10.14236/ewic/HCI2018.49. 2018 British Human Computer Interaction Conference (HCI 2018)
19. Scobbie, L., Dixon, D., Wyke, S.: Goal setting and action planning in the rehabilitation setting: development of a theoretically informed practice framework. Clin. Rehabil. **25**(5), 468–482 (2011)
20. Stacey, D., et al.: Decision aids for people facing health treatment or screening decisions. Cochrane Database Syst. Rev. **4**, CD001431 (2017)
21. Stiggelbout, A.M., et al.: Shared decision making: really putting patients at the centre of healthcare. BMJ **344**, e256 (2012)
22. Visseren, F.L.J., et al.: 2021 ESC Guidelines on cardiovascular disease prevention in clinical practice: developed by the Task Force for cardiovascular disease prevention in clinical practice with representatives of the European Society of Cardiology and 12 medical societies With the special contribution of the European Association of Preventive Cardiology (EAPC). Eur. Heart J. **42**(34), 3227–3337 (2021). https://doi.org/10.1093/eurheartj/ehab484
23. Wennberg, J.E., Fisher, E.S., Skinner, J.S.: Geography and the debate over Medicare reform. Health Aff. (Millwood) Suppl. Web Exclusives 96–114 (2002)

A Personal Health Agent for Decision Support in Arrhythmia Diagnosis

Tezira Wanyana[1,3] ⓘ, Mbithe Nzomo[1,3(✉)] ⓘ, C. Sue Price[2,3] ⓘ,
and Deshendran Moodley[1,3] ⓘ

[1] University of Cape Town (UCT), Cape Town, South Africa
{twanyana,mnzomo,deshen}@cs.uct.ac.za
[2] University of KwaZulu-Natal (UKZN), Durban, South Africa
pricec@ukzn.ac.za
[3] Centre for Artificial Intelligence Research (CAIR), Cape Town, South Africa

Abstract. We propose an architecture for a personal health agent (PHA) that combines machine learning and a Bayesian network (BN) for detecting and diagnosing heart disease, specifically arrhythmia. Machine learning (ML) is used for classifying a patient's ECG signal. Four ML models, i.e. gradient boosting, random forest, multilayer perceptron and support vector machine, are compared and evaluated using a dataset of 5,340 records containing 12-lead ECG signals created from the Chapman-Shaoxing database. Among the four models, the gradient boosting model produces the best accuracy of 82.88% when classifying an ECG signal as either atrial fibrillation, other arrhythmia, or no arrhythmia. The detected pattern is integrated into a BN that captures expert knowledge about the causes of arrhythmia. The BN structure and parameters are informed by expert knowledge from the literature and evaluated using Pitchforth and Mengersen's framework. The agent uses a decision support module to guide the diagnosis process. It suggests what questions to ask to increase certainty of the presence of arrhythmia, and it suggests what arrhythmia causes to follow up. This is achieved using sensitivity analysis and diagnostic Bayesian reasoning respectively. The architecture is evaluated using application use cases.

Keywords: ECG · Arrhythmia · Machine learning · Bayesian networks · Agent architecture

1 Introduction

With the current surge in popularity of wearable devices such as smart watches and bands, many people are becoming increasingly motivated to monitor their health digitally [38]. Such devices contain sensors that can monitor physical activity by providing the heart rate, step count and sleep patterns among others. Some wearable devices, such as Withings Move and Apple Watch, have the ability to monitor the heart rhythm and to provide ECG readings [44]. Data collected by such devices should be presented back to a user in an understandable format that motivates their actions towards improved health [38].

ⓒ The Author(s), under exclusive license to Springer Nature Switzerland AG 2023
L. A. Maciaszek et al. (Eds.): ICT4AWE 2021/2022, CCIS 1856, pp. 385–407, 2023.
https://doi.org/10.1007/978-3-031-37496-8_20

This study explores an architecture for an intelligent personal health agent (PHA) that incorporates both machine learning (ML) and knowledge representation techniques for pattern detection, situation analysis and decision support. The goal of the agent is to retrieve data from a wearable device and assist an individual to understand their heart rhythm. The PHA focuses on electrocardiogram (ECG) readings to determine if arrhythmia is present or not and if present, what its possible causes might be. Arrhythmia is a cardiac condition characterised by heart rhythm irregularities which, if left unattended, may lead to stroke [52]. The most common arrhythmia is atrial fibrillation (AF) [26]. The prevalence of AF has increased by 33% in the past two decades, and this prevalence is expected to increase over the next 30 years. Though this study focuses on arrhythmia, the PHA can be extended to cover additional health conditions.

In previous work [50], we proposed an initial version of the PHA which combined ML and a Bayesian network (BN) to interpret and explain the occurrence of AF in a patient in terms of its risk factors. The architecture consisted of four modules: two exogenous modules, i.e. the AI service and the Domain Expert, which were external to the agent, and two endogenous modules, i.e. the Perception and Deliberation modules. The AI service used an ML model to classify an ECG signal as either *P-wave present* or *P-wave absent*. An absent P-wave is the hallmark characteristic of AF in an ECG signal. In the deliberation module, a BN was used to represent the causal relations between different risk factors that influenced the presence of AF. The probabilities of the ML classification were used as the likelihood values for the evidence captured by the P-wave node. When the detected ECG feature was entered into the P-wave node, and the probabilities were propagated, the probabilities of the states of the AF node changed so that the state that corresponds to the detected ECG feature, "AF present", had a higher probability. The PHA then identified the most probable risk factors of the patient's condition from the BN.

In this paper, we describe an extension and refinement of the ML module, the BN, and the overall agent architecture. In the initial PHA, the user would have had to understand how to use BNs in order to interact with the PHA. The architecture now includes a new decision support module, which allows the agent to offer guidance to the clinician on what questions to ask the patient or what risk factors to follow up. Using the decision support module, the clinician can now easily interact with the BN and the agent. The ML module and the BN previously only detected a single form of arrhythmia, AF, in the ECG signal. Individuals may have other types of arrhythmias beyond AF. The problem is now formulated as multiclass classification of the ECG signal to detect either AF, other arrhythmia, or no arrhythmia (none). The inclusion of the third class (other arrhythmia) increases the generalisability and usability of the ML model, allowing it to detect the presence of not only AF but also other types of arrhythmia and understand its causes. Additionally, we evaluated our architecture on a new dataset. In the original study, a combination of the MIT-BIH Arrhythmia and MIT-BIH AF databases were used to train the ML model. The dataset only represented two rhythm types (AF or none) with 24 ECG records. In this study we use the Chapman-Shaoxing database which contains 5,340 ECG records and 11 types of rhythms.

The deliberation module, which involves obtaining the most probable risk factors of an individual's condition, is carried out using the BN. The scope of the BN has accordingly been extended to cater for three possibilities: AF, other arrhythmia or no arrhythmia. A node (i.e. `ML Prediction: Arrhythmia`) is introduced to form the interface between the ML and the BN. The conditional probability tables (CPTs) of this node are populated using recall values of the applied ML algorithm which is the algorithm with the best accuracy (gradient boosting in this work). In addition, we factor the effect of COVID-19 on cardiac arrhythmia into the design of our BN.

The contribution of this paper is threefold: firstly, an improved PHA agent architecture with comprehensive internal (endogenous) modules including an explicit decision support module; secondly, a multi-class ML model which identifies whether a patient has AF, some other type of arrhythmia, or none, based on an ECG input; and thirdly, an improved prototype arrhythmia BN for interpretation and explanation of the ECG result of a particular patient in terms of arrhythmia risk factors.

The rest of the paper is organised as follows: Sect. 2 discusses related work. Section 3 presents an improved version of the PHA architecture, discussing the essence and relevance of each of the modules. In Sect. 4, details about the dataset used, the model building and the results of the ML experiments are presented. Section 5 discusses in detail how the arrhythmia BN was built and validated. In Sect. 6, we describe the decision support module, and evaluate the PHA with use cases. A detailed discussion is presented in Sect. 7 and we conclude and provide the limitations and future work in Sect. 8.

2 Related Work

2.1 Electrocardiogram Classification

The electrocardiogram (ECG) remains the gold standard in arrhythmia detection [16]. A typical ECG signal consists of P, T and U waves, as well as the QRS complex [51]. ECG is measured using electrodes placed on the skin. A particular arrangement of electrodes gives rise to a lead, with the simplest lead being a pair of electrodes [14]. The most commonly used lead system is the 12-lead ECG. It is derived from 10 electrodes placed on the legs, arms and chest that form 12 leads, namely Leads I, II, III, aVR, aVL, aVF, V1, V2, V3, V4, V5 and V6 [23]. The first six leads are referred to as limb leads, and are derived from electrodes placed on the arms and legs. The latter six leads are referred to as precordial leads and are derived from electrodes placed on the chest [23].

The 12-lead ECG is considered the benchmark because it captures a more complete picture of the heart compared to reduced lead systems. Each lead provides a different angle of the electrical activity in the heart; therefore, with a 12-lead ECG, the same electrical event can be viewed from 12 different angles [20]. Wearable devices for measuring ECG often rely on fewer electrodes and, subsequently, fewer leads. Although more leads currently result in better arrhythmia detection [44], reduced-lead ECGs generated from wearable devices are starting to be viable for detecting arrhythmia and are increasingly showing comparable performance to standard 12-lead ECGs [18,42].

2.2 ECG Classification Using Machine Learning

The classification of ECG data is part of the situation detection module in the PHA. A situation refers to "an external semantic interpretation of sensor data" [54] in an application domain. Example situations from an ECG pattern would be "AF" or "other arrhythmia". Situations are used in the context of the state of monitored features in a physical environment [1]. Situation detection techniques can be categorised as either specification-based or learning-based [54]. Specification-based techniques such as ontologies and evidence theory rely on expert knowledge to model situations and then reason on them with input sensor data. On the other hand, learning-based techniques such as ML uncover patterns or correlations in the data.

ML for arrhythmia classification from ECG signals has gained traction in recent years. Traditional ML algorithms such as tree-based methods and linear models have been widely used and shown to produce good results in ECG analysis, while being simple and computationally inexpensive to train [36]. Popular ML algorithms used in ECG classification include support vector machine (SVM) and ensemble decision trees using techniques such as bagging (e.g. random forest) and boosting (e.g. gradient boosting and adaptive boosting).

2.3 Bayesian Networks

Many systems developed for ECG analysis apply ML techniques [2,27]. These systems have a number of limitations. They are not able to deal efficiently with uncertainty; they are considered black boxes and are hard for domain experts to understand; and they demand large datasets [11]. Also, while these techniques have registered great success in heartbeat recognition, beat segmentation and ECG classification, they have had little success in decision support. BNs have the ability to deal with the uncertainty that is embedded in reasoning in cardiology as well as medical reasoning at large; they are understandable to non-technical users [5] and play a large role in decision support. They have been proposed to support the screening, diagnosis, selection of treatment, prognosis and multimorbidity modelling of different medical conditions e.g. cancer and heart disease [11,21].

BNs describe causal relationships between variables using directed acyclic graphs (DAGs). The variables are represented by nodes. For discrete BNs, each node or variable has a number of exhaustive and non-overlapping states [21]. The interaction between the nodes is specified using conditional probability tables (CPTs) in each node [21], which gives the probability of a certain state occurring, given the state of a parent node. The structure of the BN can be developed by hand or from data. The parameters in the CPTs can be generated from domain experts, data and/or literature [21,40,47], making BNs a flexible modelling tool [15]. The CPT values of input nodes (i.e. those without parents) are usually obtained from a distribution of how the states naturally occur [21]. On compiling the BN, if the user is certain of some information, this information is entered into the BN as evidence [21], and the probability of that state becomes 100%. As a result, the probabilities of each of the nodes in the network are updated using Bayes' rule (Eq. 1 in the Appendix).

Validation of BNs. The structure of a BN is usually validated by experts. The parameters of the BN can be validated by data, if it is available [21]. If not, the framework proposed by Pitchforth and Mengersen [40] can be used to evaluate an expert-elicited BN. This framework addresses seven different types of validity: nomological-, face-, content-, concurrent-, convergent-, discriminant- and predictive validity. One of the tests for assessing predictive validity is sensitivity analysis. This measures how sensitive the network is to changes in input (evidence) and parameter (CPT) values [21]. Measures for analysing sensitivity to evidence, like entropy and mutual information (MI), can be used to determine the degree to which adding evidence about one variable will reduce the uncertainty in our belief of the value of a target variable [21]. Entropy tells us the current uncertainty we have in our belief of the value of some target variable, while MI gives us an indication of the degree to which we can reduce this uncertainty by adding evidence at another variable (see Eqs. 2 and 3 in the Appendix). To gain the largest reduction in uncertainty in the target variable, we should add evidence to the variable with the highest MI value. Thus the MI values can be used to determine a priority ranking in terms of which evidence to gather next. Using this ranking, the PHA can determine which questions should be asked to increase certainty in the target variable.

BNs in Cardiology. BNs were explored as a tool for premature ventricular contraction beat classification based on the ECG features of the sinus rhythm and the shape of the beat waveform [9–11]. Domain knowledge on risk factors that have causal influence on the arrhythmia are not incorporated in the BN.

BNs have been used by a number of authors to model the risk of coronary heart disease (CHD), e.g. [13, 15, 35, 37], cited in Korb & Nicholson [21]. These BNs model the factors that lead to CHD, such as age [13, 35, 37], sex [13, 35], smoking [13, 15, 35, 37], obesity [13, 15, 37], alcohol [15], diabetes [37] and hypertension [13, 15, 37]. The structures of these BNs varied; some BNs modelled some risk factors as influencing others, while some BNs modelled the risk factors as being independent of each other. Only one of these BNs included a node for an ECG and for rapid heartbeats, which are child nodes of the heart disease node [15]. To our knowledge, no BNs in the literature focus on arrhythmia.

2.4   Agent Architecture

The knowledge discovery and evolution (KDE) agent architecture [48] was developed recently for agents that analyse patterns from sensor data in physical systems, and detect, interpret and explain patterns found in this data. The architecture combines "bottom-up" ML techniques for pattern detection with "top-down" knowledge representation and reasoning (KRR) techniques such as BNs for interpreting and explaining these patterns [48, 49]. Although these techniques are rarely combined in agents, there is now a convergence on the fact that purely data driven or knowledge driven systems alone are not sufficient for AI systems and that these systems could benefit from incorporating both techniques [17]. Such systems are known as hybrid systems. In this work, we leverage the strengths of both techniques for the different tasks of the PHA.

3   PHA Architecture

The architecture for the PHA is shown in Fig. 1. The architecture design draws from the KDE architecture [48]. It consists of four modules: the pattern detection module, perception module, deliberation module and the decision support module, that contribute to the various steps of the agent's overall operation. Each module is discussed in the following subsections.

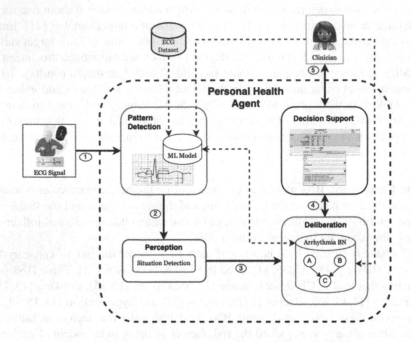

Fig. 1. Agent architecture for a personal health agent (PHA).

The clinician is the domain expert, who plays a key role in different model development activities. These activities are represented by the green dashed arrows. The clinician 1) curates the ECG dataset with labels to train and update the ML model; 2) develops the structure and conditional probability tables of the BN, including how it integrates with the ML model; and 3) continuously updates and refines the models as s/he gains new knowledge. For example, s/he may add new data and retrain the ML model and/or revise the BN.

3.1 Pattern Detection

The first step of the PHA's operational loop is pattern detection. The incoming ECG signal from a wearable device is passed to the pattern detection module (arrow 1). The module uses a pre-trained ML model to classify the ECG signal. The ML model is trained prior to the agent's execution. Details are discussed in Sect. 4. The clinician is responsible for the curation of the ECG dataset.

3.2 Perception

The perception module provides a bridge between the pattern detection module and the deliberation module. It consists of a situation detection module which uses rules, of the form *if* $<pattern>$ *then* $<situation>$, to map patterns detected from the ML model to situations in the BN. For the current version of the PHA agent, the patterns (AF, other arrhythmia and none) can be added directly to the BN as evidence, so these rules are not used.

3.3 Deliberation

The deliberation module focuses on how the PHA arrives at its suggestion for following up a given situation. The main component of the deliberation module is the BN. BNs have been used in other agent architectures in their deliberation processes, e.g. [12,41]. The PHA agent has knowledge that is captured using the BN presented in detail in Sect. 5. The objective of the PHA is to suggest the best way to follow up the observed situation; it does not provide treatment options. For instance, the PHA suggests what further information to find about an individual's lifestyle or what risk factors to check for. On this note, the cost of having false positives is much lower that the cost of having false negatives. The information encoded in the BN can be drawn from expert knowledge or from literature; it can also be designed from data.

Using the BN, prior to deliberation, situation analysis is conducted. The situation obtained in the perception module is mapped onto a corresponding state in the observable node (i.e. ML Prediction: Arrhythmia) in the BN by entering the matching state as evidence. The agent then determines whether a given situation should be followed up or not. A situation where AF or other arrhythmia is suspected to be present needs to be followed up. A normal ECG which indicates that no arrhythmia is present requires no further attention.

In the deliberation module, the agent considers specific evidence of the example form *ML Prediction: Arrhythmia == Atrial fibrillation*. The selected state corresponds to the situation detected during perception. During deliberation, the agent requires context. The agent starts by incorporating context that consists of information about the demographic risk factors, specifically age and sex. The lifestyle risk factors (alcohol abuse, smoking and obesity) also form part of the context, if information about them is available. After all evidence and context has been added to the BN, the belief values of all the disease risk factors (e.g. hypertension) that have causal influence on the arrhythmia node are extracted.

3.4 Decision Support

The decision support module provides an interactive tool which serves as the key interface between the agent and the clinician. The tool allows the clinician to add information about a patient iteratively and to determine the effect of this information on the presence of arrhythmia in the patient. Based on sensitivity analysis of the BN, the agent informs the clinician on the most important information that is required to reduce the uncertainty of the patient having arrhythmia. As more information about the patient is provided, the agent obtains a clearer picture of the patient's situation and is able to determine the risk the patient having arrhythmia or not. In addition, the agent also displays the likelihood of other disease risk factors that the clinician may need to follow up.

4   Machine Learning for Arrhythmia Detection

In this section, we present details about the model building phase of the pattern detection module, which was conducted prior to the agent execution. In this phase, we use a dataset of 5,340 records containing 12-lead ECG signals to train ML models. The full source code for the data preprocessing, hyperparameter tuning and model building is publicly available on GitHub[1].

4.1   Dataset

The Chapman-Shaoxing database [55], a large publicly available ECG database, was used to create the dataset. The database was developed as a result of a collaboration between Chapman University, California and Shaoxing Hospital Zhejiang University School of Medicine, China. It contains 10,646 12-lead ECG records, each from a unique patient, with a duration of 10 s and a frequency 500 Hz. The database contains 11 rhythm categories, with each record belonging to only one: sinus bradycardia, sinus rhythm, atrial fibrillation, sinus tachycardia, atrial flutter, sinus irregularity, supraventricular tachycardia, atrial tachycardia, atrioventricular node reentrant tachycardia, atrioventricular reentrant tachycardia, and sinus atrium to atrial wandering rhythm. The sinus rhythm category denotes a normal rhythm with no arrhythmia, while the sinus irregularity category denotes an unspecified irregular rhythm.

Each signal in the database was filtered using a bandpass Butterworth filter to remove noise. Two demographic features, age and sex, were obtained for each record. Additionally, we computed statistical features from the ECG signals, as proposed in the Physionet/Computing in Cardiology 2020 and 2021 challenges [3,43]. Seven statistical features, i.e. mean, median, standard deviation, variance, skewness, and kurtosis, were calculated for both the R-R intervals and the R-peak values for each of the 12 leads, resulting in 144 statistical features. The R-R intervals and R-peak values were computed using Sznajder and Łukowska's QRS detector [46] based on the Pan-Tomkins algorithm. The root mean square for each lead was also calculated, resulting in another 12 features. Together with age and sex, this resulted in a total of 158 features. The statistical features were then normalised using Scikit-learn's `StandardScaler`, which removes the mean and scales the data to unit variance. The mathematical formula for this is $z = \frac{(x-u)}{s}$, where z is the standard score of a sample x, u is the mean of the samples, and s is the standard deviation of the samples.

There were 1,780 AF records in the database. To ensure a balanced dataset, 1,780 records from each of the other two classes were randomly selected. To determine the effect of the number of classes on the ML model performance, we used a subset of the dataset with two classes, AF and None. Table 1 shows the details of the multiclass and binary datasets, including summary statistics for age and sex. The impact of the number of classes is discussed in Sect. 4.3.

---

[1] https://github.com/mbithenzomo/personal-health-agent-ml.

Table 1. Dataset details.

Dataset	Classes	Records per class	Total records	Sex ratio	Age range	Age percentiles (25th, 50th, 75th)
Multiclass	AF	1780	5340	M: 2,842 F: 2,498	Min: 4 Max: 98	51, 64, 75
	Other	1780				
	None	1780				
Binary	AF	1780	3560	M: 1,826 F: 1,734	Min: 5 Max: 98	53, 67, 77
	None	1780				

4.2 Model Development

Four ML classification algorithms were implemented using Scikit-learn [39]: support vector machine (SVM), random forest, gradient boosted decision trees, and multilayer perceptron (MLP). The first three were selected due to their wide use in the literature for ECG classification, while the MLP was selected as it was the best performing model in our previous work. Hyperparameter tuning for the four algorithms was done using Scikit-learn's `GridSearchCV`, which performs an exhaustive search over specified parameter values and returns the best combination of parameters. The options and selected hyperparameters for each algorithm are shown in the Appendix.

As we did in our previous study [50], we used 10-fold cross-validation to evaluate the performance of the models. Cross-validation has been shown to be effective in accurately assessing the generalisation performance of ML models [19]. A stratified approach was chosen to maintain the distribution of each class in each fold.

4.3 Model Evaluation and Selection

The ML models were evaluated using several metrics, averaged across the test folds during the cross-validation process: overall accuracy, overall confusion matrix, and the precision, recall, and F1-score for each class. Accuracy refers to the percentage of correct predictions for the test data, and is obtained by dividing the number of correct classifications by the total number of both correct and incorrect classifications. The confusion matrix shows the number of correctly classified examples and incorrectly classified examples, with the number of correctly classified examples forming the main diagonal of the matrix.

The precision for a particular class is calculated by dividing the number of correctly classified examples for that class by the total number of examples that were classified as belonging to that class, whether correctly or incorrectly. On the other hand, the recall for a particular class is the number of correctly classified examples for that class, divided by the actual number of examples for that class. The F1 score is a computation of the harmonic mean of the precision and recall. The formulae for these metrics are shown in the Appendix.

Including the demographic features generally resulted in an increase in accuracy for all the models. The impact of data normalisation was most significant in the SVM and MLP models, which performed much better with normalised data. In contrast, the gradient boosting and random forest models were not significantly affected by normalisation. With regards to the number of output classes, the binary classification accuracy was significantly better than the multiclass accuracy. This can be attributed to the fact that many arrhythmias have similar irregularities in the ECG, such as in the R-R interval [7].

Table 2 and Table 3 show the classification results for the multiclass and binary datasets respectively, including the precision, recall and F1-score by class as well as the overall average confusion matrices and accuracy scores. Overall, the best performing model was the gradient boosting model, which achieved an average accuracy of 82.88% for the multiclass dataset and 93.85% for the binary dataset. The 93.85% accuracy achieved for the binary classification is an improvement on the performance of the best performing model in our previous work, which was an MLP that achieved an accuracy of 89.61%.

Table 2. Multiclass classification results (AF, Other and None).

Algorithm	Classes	Precision	Recall	F1-Score	Confusion Matrix			Accuracy
Gradient Boosting	AF	86.24%	89.10%	87.65%	1586	113	81	**82.88%**
	Other	81.48%	76.63%	78.98%	146	1364	270	
	None	80.79%	82.92%	81.84%	107	197	1476	
Random Forest	AF	80.76%	87.02%	83.78%	1549	141	90	78.84 %
	Other	79.79%	68.99%	74.00%	192	1228	360	
	None	76.10%	80.51%	78.24 %	177	170	1433	
MLP	AF	77.04%	79.38%	78.20%	1413	198	169	73.93%
	Other	71.71%	70.51%	71.10%	218	1255	307	
	None	72.89%	71.91%	72.40%	203	297	1280	
SVM	AF	73.82%	81.74%	77.58%	1455	181	144	71.67%
	Other	70.03%	60.39%	64.86%	312	1075	393	
	None	70.72%	72.87%	71.78%	204	279	1297	

Table 3. Binary classification results (AF and None).

Algorithm	Classes	Precision	Recall	F1-Score	Confusion Matrix		Accuracy
Gradient Boosting	AF	92.77%	95.11%	93.93%	1693	87	**93.85%**
	None	94.99%	92.58%	93.77%	132	1648	
Random Forest	AF	88.88%	92.53%	90.67%	1647	133	90.48%
	None	92.21%	88.43%	90.28%	206	1574	
MLP	AF	88.10%	87.75%	87.93%	1562	218	87.95%
	None	87.80%	88.15%	87.97%	211	1569	
SVM	AF	86.09%	89.04%	87.54%	1585	195	87.33%
	None	88.66%	85.62%	87.11%	256	1524	

5   Arrhythmia Bayesian Network

In this section, we describe the development and validation of the BN used in the deliberation module.

5.1 Developing the Bayesian Network

We designed a prototype arrhythmia BN using the Netica GUI[2]. The arrhythmia BN prototype is illustrated in Fig. 2. The aim of the BN is to show factors which could have causal influence on arrhythmia. The structure of the BN was informed by medical idioms for BNs [24]: nodes with prefix "RF" denote risk factors, and the condition (Arrhythmia) is denoted with prefix "C". Other medical idioms [24,33] used in developing the BN were the definitional/synthesis idiom (Lifestyle risk factors summarises the alcohol abuse, smoking and obesity risk factors); and the cause-consequence idiom (Age and Lifestyle risk factors cause the four traditional risk factors of hypertension, ischemic and valvular heart disease and diabetes). CPT values for the nodes were based on literature, including our previous work [50]. Using literature means that models can be created when domain experts are not available [21]. This knowledge has the advantage of having been peer reviewed, compared to eliciting the knowledge directly from domain experts [21].

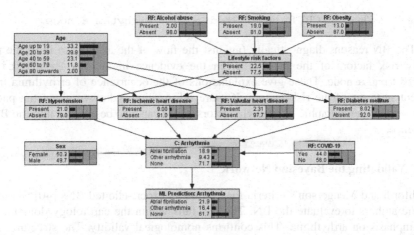

Fig. 2. A prototype BN for explaining the causes of arrhythmia with no evidence added.

There are three lifestyle risk factors in the BN: alcohol abuse, smoking and obesity. Other traditional risk factors are hypertension, ischemic heart disease, valvular heart disease, diabetes mellitus and whether the person had contracted COVID-19 or not. COVID-19 was added to the AF BN [50], since patients who have had COVID-19 developed different types of arrhythmia [29], the most common being AF [8]. Age and sex are demographic factors. Prior probabilities of the age node were obtained from global population percentages [4].

The ML model is applied in the BN in the following way: the chosen ML algorithm is the one with the best accuracy, i.e. gradient boosting (see Table 3). Of special interest is the ML Prediction: Arrhythmia node, which is the node in which the ML prediction is entered as evidence. The CPT values of the ML Prediction: Arrhythmia node contain recall values based on the confusion matrix given in Table 2 for gradient boosting as shown in the example instance below.

---

[2]https://www.norsys.com/download.html.

P(ML Prediction: Arrhythmia == Atrial fibrillation |
C:Arrhythmia == Atrial fibrillation) = recall (Atrial
fibrillation)

These represent the proportion of correctly vs incorrectly classified samples identified by the ML model. These CPT values are defined as the probability of the ML
algorithm detecting a given state given that it is indeed the patient's condition. The
CPT of the ML Prediction: Arrhythmia is shown in Fig. 3. Based on the output of the situation detection module, evidence is entered into one of the states of the
ML Prediction: Arrhythmia node, depending on whether the ML algorithm
identified AF, other arrhythmia or none.

C: Arrhythmia	Atrial fibrillation	Other arrhythmia	None
Atrial fibrillation	89.1	6.35	4.55
Other arrhythmia	8.2	76.63	15.17
None	6.01	11.07	82.92

Fig. 3. The CPT for the ML Prediction: Arrhythmia node.

The BN reasons diagnostically (against the flow of the arrows) to infer the most
likely risk factors of the patient, given the evidence in the ML Prediction:
Arrhythmia node. These give explanations of the occurrence of arrhythmia in the
patient in terms of the risk factors. If more information is known about the patient,
such as their demographic or lifestyle factors, these can also be entered into the BN as
evidence.

5.2 Validating the Bayesian Network

Pitchforth and Mengerson's criteria for evaluating expert-elicited BNs [40] were used
by the authors to evaluate the BN. The BN falls within the cardiology domain, with
an emphasis on arrhythmia. This confirms nomological validity. The structure, node
discretisation and parameters in the BN are what would be expected. This confirms
face validity.

In the prototype arrhythmia BN, the main risk factors for AF match those mentioned
in the literature (e.g. [6,25,34,53]). The risk factors for arrhythmia are similar to those
of AF [28,45], and the most prevalent arrhythmia risk factors found in the literature are
modelled in the BN. The states of the nodes cover the range of values for each node,
with no gaps. The CPTs of input nodes are based on prevalence values from literature.
These evaluations confirm content validity. However, it should be noted that in certain
populations, some risk factors are more prevalent than others. This would also affect
the CPT values of the BN.

Concurrent validity is determined by comparing how the BN and other theoretically similar BNs act. Apart from the AF BN [50], we do not have access to other
working BNs in the cardiology domain. The nodes and discretisation of the prototype
arrhythmia BN are the same as those of the AF BN, apart from the C: Arrhythmia,
COVID-19, ML Prediction: Arrhythmia nodes which are new. In addition,
the discretisation of the Age node changed from four states to five states: an additional
state was added for ages of under 20, since it is possible to experience other types of

arrythmia during these ages. The CPTs of the arrhythmia BN are the same as the AF BN, apart from those of the Age nodes and the four traditional risk factors. Both networks show a similar prior distribution (see Fig. 2). The probability in the AF state increases in both BNs when evidence for the disease risk factors is added, which is as expected. The arrhythmia BN also follows the medical idioms of Kyrimi et al. [24], as outlined in Sect. 5.1.

By comparing the BN to others in the literature, convergent validity could be established. Apart from the AF BN [50], no BNs explaining the causes of arrhythmia were found. The structure of the arrhythmia BN mirrors sub-networks of other cardiology-related BNs, with minor exceptions. For example, in the Busselton BN which modelled the risk of CHD, risk factors such as being overweight, drinking alcohol, smoking, diabetes, age and sex were identified [35]. In this BN, all factors led to the node which predicted a risk of a CHD event in the following 10 years. In another CHD BN [37], age, smoking and obesity led to diabetes, which is similar to the arrhythmia BN. In Ghosh and Valtorta [15], obesity, smoking and alcohol leads to hypertension, and heart disease leads to rapid heartbeats; however, they model hypertension as leading to heart disease, whereas in our BN, these are modelled as two independent risk factors for arrhythmia. A BN modelling cardiovascular risk [13] also identified the factors of weight, smoking, sex and age. Weight could influence hypertension, as in our BN. In their BN though, sex influenced age, and age influenced the smoking habits and weight of the patient. It should be noted, however, that the structure of this cardiovascular risk BN was generated by averaging the structures of 500 different networks whose structure was learned from data. The face validity of the arrhythmia BN was judged to be fair.

Predictive validity is evaluated by assessing the behaviour of the BN when it is executed, the sensitivity of the BN to findings or to parameters, and how the BN behaves for extreme conditions. Evidence was entered into the C: Arrhythmia node's "Atrial fibrillation" state, modelling that a person has AF (see Fig. 4). The inferred values of

Table 4. Comparison of the four traditional risk factor values, given AF, to Nguyen et al. [34].

Node	BN value (Fig. 4)	Min prevalence value in [34]	Max prevalence value in [34]
RF: Hypertension	32.8%	10.3%	71.9%
RF: Ischemic heart disease	16.9%	6.4%	47%
RF: Valvular heart disease	6.02%	5.6%	66%
RF: Diabetes mellitus	11.8%	3.3%	33%

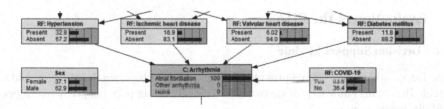

Fig. 4. Extract of the prototype BN showing arrhythmia risk factors, given that AF is present.

these four nodes fall within the ranges outlined in Nguyen et al.'s systematic literature review of the prevalence of AF [34] in developing contexts (see Table 4).

Extreme conditions such as the sex and age of the person were used to evaluate the BN. The BN's results for AF matches the statement of Naccarelli et al. [32] that AF increases with age, and that more men have AF than women, at any age. Adding evidence for lifestyle factors to the BN increased the probability of AF and of other arrhythmia.

The sensitivity of the BN to findings was examined (see Table 5). This table shows what evidence should be sought to increase certainty about the values of the C: Arrhythmia node. Whether the patient has had COVID or not gives the most added certainty, followed by hypertension, the patient's sex, ischemic heart disease, the patient's age, valvular heart disease, diabetes and other lifestyle risk factors.

This ranking reflects the main modifiable risk factors of the most prevalent arrhythmia, AF [22,34]. However, the risk factors may have a larger or smaller effect on arrhythmia, depending on the population being modelled.

Based on the validation, the BN suitably represents factors causing arrhythmia. However, this prototype BN should be tested and evaluated further before it is deployed for real world use.

Table 5. Sensitivity of C: Arrhythmia to findings at other nodes.

Node	Mutual Information	Percent	Variance of Beliefs
C: Arrhythmia	1.11949	100	0.2590261
ML Prediction: Arrhythmia	0.54069	48.3	0.1175418
RF: COVID-19	0.04423	3.95	0.0098642
RF: Hypertension	0.02255	2.01	0.0049399
Sex	0.02009	1.79	0.0045437
RF: Ischemic heart disease	0.01959	1.75	0.0040420
Age	0.01798	1.61	0.0039373
RF: Valvular Heart Disease	0.01517	1.35	0.0025202
RF: Diabetes mellitus	0.00525	0.469	0.0011528
Lifestyle risk factors	0.00029	0.0258	0.0000659
RF: Smoking	0.00006	0.00552	0.0000141
RF: Obesity	0.00004	0.00368	0.0000094
RF: Alcohol Abuse	0.00001	0.000544	0.0000014

6   Evaluation of the PHA

6.1   Decision Support Module

The Decision Support module provides the key interface between the clinician and the agent. The agent is able to provide two types of decision support, i.e. predictive support and diagnostic support.

Predictive Support. The agent assists the clinician to find out the most relevant information that might increase certainty about the presence of arrhythmia in a patient. This is achieved using the sensitivity analysis shown in Table 5. For example, assuming that the ML prediction is already provided: the next most important information is whether the patient has had COVID, and then whether there is hypertension present. At each stage of the process, the system recommends the best questions to ask based on the previous answers given and it updates its conclusions. A screenshot of the dashboard obtained using AutoNetica[3] is shown in Fig. 5. It provides an ordered set of the most important questions, based on the MI scores, that would increase the certainty in the C: Arrhythmia node. In this way the clinician is guided through a set of questions. As the answers are provided, the posterior probabilities (at the bottom of the screen) of the different arrhythmia states are updated.

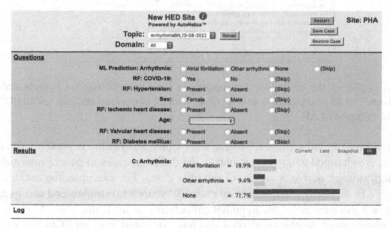

Fig. 5. A display of the of the most relevant questions to ask (using Autonetica).

Diagnostic Support. The agent also provides a diagnostic support interface to the clinician. Assuming that the clinician believes that a patient has Arrhythmia, then the agent is able to advise the clinician of the most likely underlying diseases that may have caused the arrhythmia in this patient. The diagnostic support interface is shown in Fig. 6. The clinician supplies demographic information and lifestyle risk factors for the patient, if this is available. Based on the supplied information, the PHA displays the probabilities of the patient having traditional risk factors that should be followed up (see bottom of Fig. 6). At the top of this interface is a link to the predictive decision support described above. The interface is implemented in NeticaJ[4], the Java version of the Netica API.

6.2 PHA Evaluation

To evaluate the PHA, we apply case-based evaluation [21] on a set of application use cases. Cases are generated to test different situations i.e., a situation where atrial fib-

[3]https://www.norsys.com/WebHelp/NETICA/X_AutoNetica.htm.
[4]https://www.norsys.com/netica-j.html#download.

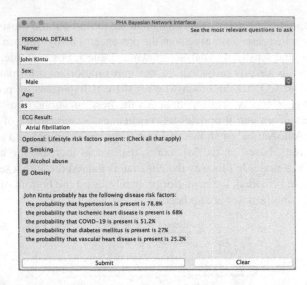

Fig. 6. A display of the traditional risk factors and their probabilities for hypothetical patient "John Kintu": an 85 year old male who is obese, smokes, abuses alcohol and has an ECG which shows the presence of AF.

rillation is present and a situation where some other arrhythmia is present. The context variables are changed to extreme values in the different cases to ensure reasonable network performance across a variety of possible cases. For example, the extreme upper case would be an obese male individual above 80 years who smokes and abuses alcohol.

The first use case is for the hypothetical patient, "John Kintu", an 85 year old male who is obese, smokes, abuses alcohol and has presented with an ECG that shows the presence of AF. Figure 7 shows the BN with the same information about the hypothetical patient, "John Kintu" as shown in Fig. 6 entered as evidence. The agent suggests that for John's demographic factors and his lifestyle risk factors (obesity, smoking and alcohol abuse), he would have 78.8% chance of having hypertension and 68% chance

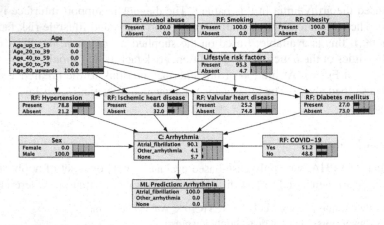

Fig. 7. BN for hypothetical patient "John Kintu" with evidence entered, generated in Java using NeticaJ.

of ischemic heart disease. He would therefore have to confirm using medical tests if these conditions are indeed present and manage them.

For the second use case, let us consider another hypothetical individual who is a 25 year old female with two lifestyle risk factors, alcohol abuse and smoking. Assuming that from her ECG, the predicted situation is "other arrhythmia", this is captured as evidence in the ML prediction: Arrhythmia node. The patient's age and sex as well as lifestyle risk factors are also captured. As shown in Fig. 8, the chances that indeed, the patient has "other arrhythmia" is 33.7%. This patient has a 16.4% probability of having hypertension and 12% probability of having ischemic heart disease. The low probabilities of the traditional risk factors can be attributed to the fact that the patient is young.

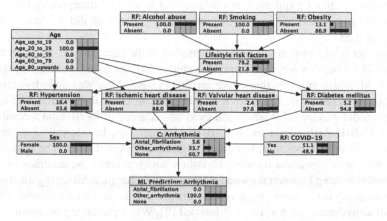

Fig. 8. The BN with evidence for a hypothetical 25 year old female with two lifestyle risk factors: alcohol abuse and smoking. The situation detected is that she has "other arrhythmia".

It is important to note that the agent does not suggest with full certainty that someone has AF, other arrhythmia or none. The moment the agent predicts that the patient has AF or other arrhythmia, the clinician should consider confirming the condition using a medical test.

7 Discussion and Conclusions

In this paper, we have described an architecture for a personal health agent (PHA) to support situation detection, situation analysis and decision support for diagnosing arrhythmia. The PHA is based on an agent architecture that incorporates an ML model for detecting irregular patterns and situations in a patient's ECG signal, a BN for capturing expert knowledge about the causes of arrhythmia, and a decision support module which guides the diagnosis process. The architecture combines an ML model, a BN and a decision support module to detect the presence of arrhythmia in a patient and to determine its likely causes. The ML model takes in an ECG signal and detects whether arrhythmia is present in the patient. The BN, which captures expert knowledge from the literature contains an ML prediction node. This is used to integrate the ML model predictions into the inference process. Once evidence is entered in the ML prediction node, together with the demographic, lifestyle and disease risk factors of the patient, the probability of the patient having arrhythmia is determined using Bayesian inferencing.

We introduced a decision support module that provides specific support for clinical decision making. The module supports both predictive and diagnostic reasoning. It uses sensitivity analysis and predictive reasoning to identify the most relevant questions for the clinician to ask the patient to determine whether arrhythmia is present or not. It uses diagnostic reasoning to determine the possible causes of a patient's arrhythmia given the information that is currently available for the patient. The decision support module provides interactive user interfaces which guides the clinician through the diagnosis process without requiring knowledge about using and interpreting BNs. This is an improvement on the previous PHA architecture [50] which did not have a decision support module.

The other key extension was the augmentation of the agent to cater for other arrhythmia conditions besides AF. In our previous study [50], the focus was on distinguishing between AF and normal rhythms from an ECG signal. This was done by training an ML model to classify an ECG pattern based on the absence of a P-wave. The best performing model was an MLP which achieved an accuracy of 89.61% on a combination of the MIT-BIH Arrhythmia and MIT-BIH AF databases. In this study, we include a third class for other types of arrhythmia and use a different dataset. The best performing model is now a gradient boosting classifier, which achieves an accuracy of 82.88% when distinguishing between the three classes on the Chapman-Shaoxing database. The drop in accuracy is not surprising given the similarities in certain ECG characteristics in different arrhythmias, such as the R-R interval [7]. When evaluating the gradient boosting classifier on the binary problem (AF or normal) the model achieves an accuracy of 93.85%, which is an improvement on our previous work.

Like the ML model, the BN was extended to accommodate AF, other arrhythmia and none. In our previous BN, the Age node only catered for patients 20 years old and over. AF is typically not experienced in younger people, but other types of arrhythmia can be. An additional state in the Age node was added to cater for under 20 year olds. As a result, the CPT values of the traditional risk factors were updated. In the current BN and PHA, there is a stronger interface between the ML model and the BN since we added a node (the ML Prediction: Arrhythmia node) for which the CPT is obtained from the recall values of the ML classifier. This allows the BN to account for the false positives of the ML classifier, such that a prediction of arrhythmia by the ML classifier does not provide a definitive diagnosis of the presence of arrhythmia.

A key aspect of this architecture is the integration of ML and BNs to support situation detection, situation analysis and decision-making. Some architectures that incorporate BNs for decision support have been proposed previously [12,30,31,41]. Similar to these architectures, our architecture incorporates a BN in deliberation and decision support. However, these architectures did not incorporate ML into the BN inference process and did not provide an interactive decision making module.

8   Limitations and Future Work

The PHA has some limitations. Firstly, the ML model was trained using a 12-lead dataset. This dataset was selected due to its large size, expert annotation, inclusion of demographic information, and that it incorporated various types of arrhythmia. To our knowledge, there is no equivalent publicly available dataset for wearables. As part of our ongoing work, we will evaluate our architecture on ECG datasets from wearable devices as these become available. Additionally, the feature extraction in this study focused on the R-R interval and R-peak of the ECG signal. The use of additional features, such ventricular rate, atrial rate and characteristics of the QRS complex may result in better differentiation between AF and other arrhythmias. The need for manual feature extraction can be eliminated by deep learning, which will be explored in future work.

In the current arrhythmia BN, we modelled only the key risk factors for arrhythmia. The BN can be extended to incorporate other risk factors associated with arrhythmia. While the BN was evaluated using Pitchforth and Mengersen's framework based on expert findings from the literature, we did not consult any experts to verify the BN. We acknowledge that this should be done before it can be deployed for real world use. Furthermore, the CPT values for the BN may differ, and should be customised for the population where it will be used.

Acknowledgements. This work was financially supported by the Hasso Plattner Institute for Digital Engineering through the HPI Research School at UCT.

Appendix

Bayes' Rule

$$Pr(A|B) = \frac{Pr(B|A)Pr(A)}{Pr(B)} \tag{1}$$

where Pr(A|B) is the posterior probability of A given B; Pr(B|A) is the posterior probability of B given A; and Pr(A) and Pr(B) are prior probabilities of A and B respectively.

Entropy and Mutual Information

$$ENT(X) = -\sum P(x)logP(x) \tag{2}$$

$$MI(X|Y) = ENT(X) - ENT(X|Y) \tag{3}$$

Hyperparameter Selection Table

Algorithm	Hyperparameter	Options	Selected Options
Gradient Boosting	n_estimators	300, 500, 800	800
	criterion	friedman_mse, squared_error, mse	friedman_mse
	loss	log_loss, exponential	log_loss
	max_depth	1, 3, 10	3
Random Forest	n_estimators	300, 500, 800	800
	criterion	gini, entropy, log_loss	entropy
	max_depth	50, 100, None	None
	max_features	sqrt, log2, None	sqrt
SVM	C	0.5, 1, 1.5	1.5
	kernel	poly, rbf, sigmoid	rbf
	gamma	scale, auto	auto
	decision_function_shape	ovo, ovr	ovo
MLP	hidden_layer_sizes	N/A	(158, 100, 50)
	activation	identity, logistic, tanh, relu	tanh
	batch_size	auto, 64, 100	auto
	solver	lbfgs, sgd, adam	adam
	learning_rate	constant, invscaling, adaptive	adaptive
	max_iter	200, 500, 1000, 2000	500

ML Metrics: Accuracy, Precision, Recall, F1-Score

$$Accuracy = \frac{TP + TN}{TP + TN + FP + FN} \tag{4}$$

$$Precision = \frac{TP}{TP + FP} \tag{5}$$

$$Recall = \frac{TP}{TP + FN} \tag{6}$$

$$F1Score = 2 * \frac{Precision * Recall}{Precision + Recall} \tag{7}$$

References

1. Adeleke, J.A., Moodley, D., Rens, G., Adewumi, A.O.: Integrating statistical machine learning in a semantic sensor web for proactive monitoring and control. Sensors **17**(4), 807 (2017). https://doi.org/10.3390/s17040807
2. Al Rahhal, M.M., Bazi, Y., Al Zuair, M., Othman, E., BenJdira, B.: Convolutional neural networks for electrocardiogram classification. J. Med. Biol. Eng. **38**(6), 1014–1025 (2018). https://doi.org/10.1007/s40846-018-0389-7
3. Alday, E.A.P., et al.: Classification of 12-lead ECGs: the PhysioNet/Computing in Cardiology Challenge 2020. Physiol. Measur. **41**(12), 124003 (2020). https://doi.org/10.1088/1361-6579/abc960

4. Ang, C.: Visualizing the world's population by age group (2021). https://www.visualcapitalist.com/the-worlds-population-2020-by-age/. Accessed 12 Aug 2022
5. Chen, S.H., Pollino, C.A.: Good practice in Bayesian network modelling. Environ. Model. Softw. **37**, 134–145 (2012). https://doi.org/10.1016/j.envsoft.2012.03.012
6. Chung, M.K., et al.: Lifestyle and risk factor modification for reduction of atrial fibrillation: a scientific statement from the American Heart Association. Circulation **141**(16), e750–e772 (2020). https://doi.org/10.1161/CIR.0000000000000748
7. Clifford, G.D., et al.: AF classification from a short single lead ECG recording: the PhysioNet/Computing in Cardiology Challenge 2017. In: 2017 Computing in Cardiology (CinC), pp. 1–4. IEEE (2017). https://doi.org/10.22489/CinC.2017.065-469
8. Coromilas, E.J., et al.: Worldwide survey of COVID-19-associated arrhythmias. Circ.: Arrhythmia Electrophysiol. **14**(3), e009458 (2021). https://doi.org/10.1161/CIRCEP.120.009458
9. De Oliveira, L.S., Andreão, R.V., Sarcinelli-Filho, M.: Detection of premature ventricular beats in ECG records using Bayesian networks involving the P-wave and fusion of results. In: 2010 Annual International Conference of the IEEE Engineering in Medicine and Biology, pp. 1131–1134. IEEE (2010). https://doi.org/10.1109/IEMBS.2010.5627116
10. De Oliveira, L.S., Andreão, R.V., Sarcinelli-Filho, M.: Premature ventricular beat classification using a dynamic Bayesian network. In: 2011 Annual International Conference of the IEEE Engineering in Medicine and Biology Society, pp. 4984–4987. IEEE (2011). https://doi.org/10.1109/IEMBS.2011.6091235
11. De Oliveira, L.S.C., Andreão, R.V., Sarcinelli-Filho, M.: The use of Bayesian networks for heart beat classification. In: Hussain, A., Aleksander, I., Smith, L., Barros, A., Chrisley, R., Cutsuridis, V. (eds.) Brain Inspired Cognitive Systems 2008. AEMB, vol. 657, pp. 217–231. Springer, Cham (2010). https://doi.org/10.1007/978-0-387-79100-5_12
12. Drake, R., Moodley, D.: INVEST: ontology driven Bayesian Networks for investment decision making on the JSE. In: Second Southern African Conference for Artificial Intelligence Research, pp. 252–273 (2022)
13. Fuster-Parra, P., Tauler, P., Bennasar-Veny, M., Ligeza, A., Lopez-Gonzalez, A., Aguiló, A.: Bayesian network modeling: a case study of an epidemiologic system analysis of cardiovascular risk. Comput. Methods Programs Biomed. **126**, 128–142 (2016). https://doi.org/10.1016/j.cmpb.2015.12.010
14. Geselowitz, D.B.: On the theory of the electrocardiogram. Proc. IEEE **77**(6), 857–876 (1989). https://doi.org/10.1109/5.29327
15. Ghosh, J.K., Valtorta, M.: Building a Bayesian network model of heart disease. In: 38th Annual on Southeast Regional Conference (ACM-SE 38), pp. 239–240 (2000). https://doi.org/10.1145/1127716.1127770
16. Hagiwara, Y., et al.: Computer-aided diagnosis of atrial fibrillation based on ECG signals: a review. Inf. Sci. **467**, 99–114 (2018). https://doi.org/10.1016/j.ins.2018.07.063
17. Harmelen, F.: Preface: the 3rd AI wave is coming, and it needs a theory. In: Neuro-Symbolic Artificial Intelligence: The State of the Art, pp. V–VII. IOS Press BV (2022). https://doi.org/10.3233/FAIA210347-fm
18. Hartikainen, S., et al.: Effectiveness of the chest strap electrocardiogram to detect atrial fibrillation. Am. J. Cardiol. **123**(10), 1643–1648 (2019). https://doi.org/10.1016/j.amjcard.2019.02.028
19. Hastie, T., Tibshirani, R., Friedman, J.: Model assessment and selection. In: Hastie, T., Tibshirani, R., Friedman, J. (eds.) The Elements of Statistical Learning: Data Mining, Inference, and Prediction, 2nd edn., pp. 219–259. Springer, New York (2009). https://doi.org/10.1007/978-0-387-84858-7_7
20. Klabunde, R.E.: Cardiac electrophysiology: normal and ischemic ionic currents and the ECG. Adv. Physiol. Educ. **41**(1), 29–37 (2017). https://doi.org/10.1152/advan.00105.2016

21. Korb, K.B., Nicholson, A.E.: Bayesian Artificial Intelligence. CRC Press (2011)
22. Kornej, J., Börschel, C.S., Benjamin, E.J., Schnabel, R.B.: Epidemiology of atrial fibrillation in the 21st century: novel methods and new insights. Circ. Res. **127**(1), 4–20 (2020). https://doi.org/10.1001/jama.2019.18058
23. Kusumoto, F.M.: ECG Interpretation: From Pathophysiology to Clinical Application. Springer, Boston (2009). https://doi.org/10.1007/978-0-387-88880-4
24. Kyrimi, E., Neves, M.R., McLachlan, S., Neil, M., Marsh, W., Fenton, N.: Medical idioms for clinical Bayesian network development. J. Biomed. Inform. **108**, 103495 (2020). https://doi.org/10.1016/j.jbi.2020.103495
25. Lau, D.H., Nattel, S., Kalman, J.M., Sanders, P.: Modifiable risk factors and atrial fibrillation. Circulation **136**(6), 583–596 (2017). https://doi.org/10.1161/CIRCULATIONAHA.116.023163
26. Lippi, G., Sanchis-Gomar, F., Cervellin, G.: Global epidemiology of atrial fibrillation: an increasing epidemic and public health challenge. Int. J. Stroke **16**(2), 217–221 (2021). https://doi.org/10.1177/1747493019897870
27. Lu, J., et al.: Efficient hardware architecture of convolutional neural network for ECG classification in wearable healthcare device. IEEE Trans. Circuits Syst. I Regul. Pap. **68**(7), 2976–2985 (2021). https://doi.org/10.1109/TCSI.2021.3072622
28. Mayo Clinic: Heart arrhythmia (2022). https://www.mayoclinic.org/diseases-conditions/heart-arrhythmia/symptoms-causes/syc-20350668. Accessed 13 July 2022
29. Mohammad, M., Emin, M., Bhutta, A., Gul, E.H., Voorhees, E., Afzal, M.R.: Cardiac arrhythmias associated with COVID-19 infection: state of the art review. Expert Rev. Cardiovasc. Ther. **19**(10), 881–889 (2021). https://doi.org/10.1080/14779072.2021.1997589
30. Moodley, D., Simonis, I.: A new architecture for the sensor web: the SWAP framework. In: ISWC 2006: 5th International Semantic Web Conference (2006)
31. Moodley, D., Simonis, I., Tapamo, J.R.: An architecture for managing knowledge and system dynamism in the worldwide sensor web. Int. J. Semant. Web Inf. Syst. (IJSWIS) **8**(1), 64–88 (2012). https://doi.org/10.4018/jswis.2012010104
32. Naccarelli, G.V., Varker, H., Lin, J., Schulman, K.L.: Increasing prevalence of atrial fibrillation and flutter in the United States. Am. J. Cardiol. **104**(11), 1534–1539 (2009). https://doi.org/10.1016/j.amjcard.2009.07.022
33. Neil, M., Fenton, N., Nielson, L.: Building large-scale Bayesian networks. Knowl. Eng. Rev. **15**(3), 257–284 (2000). https://doi.org/10.1017/S0269888900003039
34. Nguyen, T.N., Hilmer, S.N., Cumming, R.G.: Review of epidemiology and management of atrial fibrillation in developing countries. Int. J. Cardiol. **167**(6), 2412–2420 (2013). https://doi.org/10.1016/j.ijcard.2013.01.184
35. Nicholson, A.E., Twardy, C.R., Korb, K.B., Hope, L.R.: Decision support for clinical cardiovascular risk assessment. In: Pourret, O., Naim, P., Marcot, B. (eds.) Bayesian Networks: A Practical Guide to Applications, pp. 33–52. Wiley, Chichester (2008). https://doi.org/10.1002/9780470994559.ch3
36. Olier, I., Ortega-Martorell, S., Pieroni, M., Lip, G.Y.: How machine learning is impacting research in atrial fibrillation: implications for risk prediction and future management. Cardiovasc. Res. **117**(7), 1700–1717 (2021). https://doi.org/10.1093/cvr/cvab169
37. Orphanou, K., Stassopoulou, A., Keravnou, E.: DBN-extended: a dynamic Bayesian network model extended with temporal abstractions for coronary heart disease prognosis. IEEE J. Biomed. Health Inform. **20**(3), 944–952 (2015). https://doi.org/10.1109/JBHI.2015.2420534
38. Patel, M.S., Asch, D.A., Volpp, K.G.: Wearable devices as facilitators, not drivers, of health behavior change. JAMA **313**(5), 459–460 (2015). https://doi.org/10.1001/jama.2014.14781
39. Pedregosa, F., Varoquaux, G., Gramfort, A., Michel, V., Thirion, B., Grisel, O., et al.: Scikit-learn: machine learning in Python. J. Mach. Learn. Res. **12**, 2825–2830 (2011)

40. Pitchforth, J., Mengersen, K.: A proposed validation framework for expert elicited Bayesian networks. Expert Syst. Appl. **40**(1), 162–167 (2013). https://doi.org/10.1016/j.eswa.2012.07.026

41. Price, C.S., Moodley, D., Pillay, A.W., Rens, G.B.: An adaptive probabilistic agent architecture for modelling sugarcane growers' decision-making. S. Afr. Comput. J. **34**(1), 152–191 (2022). https://doi.org/10.18489/sacj.v34i1.857

42. Rajakariar, K., Koshy, A.N., Sajeev, J.K., Nair, S., Roberts, L., Teh, A.W.: Accuracy of a smartwatch based single-lead electrocardiogram device in detection of atrial fibrillation. Heart **106**(9), 665–670 (2020). https://doi.org/10.1136/heartjnl-2019-316004

43. Reyna, M.A., Sadr, N., Alday, E.A.P., Gu, A., Shah, A.J., Robichaux, C.: Will two do? Varying dimensions in electrocardiography: The PhysioNet/Computing in Cardiology Challenge 2021. In: 2021 Computing in Cardiology (CinC), pp. 1–4. IEEE (2021). https://doi.org/10.23919/CinC53138.2021.9662687

44. Scholten, J., et al.: Six-lead device superior to single-lead smartwatch ECG in atrial fibrillation detection. Am. Heart J. **253**, 53–58 (2022). https://doi.org/10.1016/j.ahj.2022.06.010

45. Scripps: Top 10 things you should know about heart rhythm (2015). https://www.scripps.org/sparkle-assets/documents/heart_rhythm_facts.pdf. Accessed 09 July 2022

46. Sznajder, M., Łukowska, M.: Python online and offline ECG QRS detector based on the Pan-Tomkins algorithm (2017). https://zenodo.org/record/591747. Accessed 22 July 2022

47. Uusitalo, L.: Advantages and challenges of Bayesian networks in environmental modelling. Ecol. Model. **203**(3–4), 312–318 (2007). https://doi.org/10.1016/j.ecolmodel.2006.11.033

48. Wanyana, T., Moodley, D.: An agent architecture for knowledge discovery and evolution. In: Edelkamp, S., Möller, R., Rueckert, E. (eds.) KI 2021. LNCS (LNAI), vol. 12873, pp. 241–256. Springer, Cham (2021). https://doi.org/10.1007/978-3-030-87626-5_18

49. Wanyana, T., Moodley, D., Meyer, T.: An ontology for supporting knowledge discovery and evolution. In: Gerber, A. (ed.) Southern African Conference for Artificial Intelligence Research (SACAIR), pp. 206–221 (2020)

50. Wanyana, T., Nzomo, M., Price, C.S., Moodley, D.: Combining machine learning and Bayesian networks for ECG interpretation and explanation. In: 8th International Conference on Information and Communication Technologies for Ageing Well and e-Health (ICT4AWE), pp. 81–92. INSTICC, SciTePress (2022). https://doi.org/10.5220/0011046100003188

51. Wasilewski, J., Polonski, L.: An introduction to ECG interpretation. In: Gacek, A., Pedrycz, W. (eds.) ECG Signal Processing, Classification and Interpretation: A Comprehensive Framework of Computational Intelligence, pp. 1–20. Springer, Cham (2012). https://doi.org/10.1007/978-0-85729-868-3_1

52. Weimann, K., Conrad, T.O.F.: Transfer learning for ECG classification. Sci. Rep. **11**(1), 1–12 (2021). https://doi.org/10.1038/s41598-021-84374-8

53. Williams, B.A., Chamberlain, A.M., Blankenship, J.C., Hylek, E.M., Voyce, S.: Trends in atrial fibrillation incidence rates within an integrated health care delivery system, 2006 to 2018. JAMA Netw. Open **3**(8), e2014874–e2014874 (2020). https://doi.org/10.1001/jamanetworkopen.2020.14874

54. Ye, J., Dobson, S., McKeever, S.: Situation identification techniques in pervasive computing: a review. Pervasive Mob. Comput. **8**(1), 36–66 (2012). https://doi.org/10.1016/j.pmcj.2011.01.004

55. Zheng, J., Zhang, J., Danioko, S., Yao, H., Guo, H., Rakovski, C.: A 12-lead electrocardiogram database for arrhythmia research covering more than 10,000 patients. Sci. Data **7**(1), 1–8 (2020). https://doi.org/10.1038/s41597-020-0386-x

The SMART BEAR Project: An Overview of Its Infrastructure

Qiqi Su[1]([✉]), Vadim Peretokin[2], Ioannis Basdekis[3], Ioannis Kouris[4],
Jonatan Maggesi[5], Mario Sicuranza[6], Alberto Acebes[7], Anca Bucur[2],
Vinod Jaswanth Roy Mukkala[5], Konstantin Pozdniakov[1], Christos Kloukinas[1],
Dimitrios D. Koutsouris[4], Elefteria Iliadou[8], Ioannis Leontsinis[9], Luigi Gallo[6],
Giuseppe De Pietro[6], and George Spanoudakis[3]

[1] Department of Computer Science, City, University of London, London, UK
{Qiqi.Su,Konstantin.Pozdniakov,C.Kloukinas}@city.ac.uk
[2] Philips Research, Eindhoven, The Netherlands
{vadim.peretokin,anca.bucur}@philips.com
[3] SPHYNX Technology Solutions AG, Zug, Switzerland
[4] Biomedical Engineering Laboratory, School of Electrical and Computer Engineering, National Technical University of Athens, Athens, Greece
[5] Computer Science Department, Università degli Studi di Milano, Milan, Italy
maggesi@di.unimi.it, vinod.mukkala@unimi.it
[6] Institute for High-Performance Computing and Networking, National Research Council of Italy, ICAR - CNR, Naples, Italy
{mario.sicuranza,luigi.gallo,giuseppe.depietro}@icar.cnr.it
[7] Atos Research and Innovation, Madrid, Spain
[8] 1st Otolaryngology University Department, National and Kapodistrian University of Athens, Athens, Greece
[9] 1st Cardiology Clinic, Medical School, National and Kapodistrian University of Athens, Athens, Greece

Abstract. The paper describes a cloud-based platform that utilizes Artificial Intelligence (AI) and Explainable AI techniques to deliver evidence-based, personalized interventions to individuals over 65 suffering or at risk of hearing loss, cardiovascular disease, cognitive impairments, balance disorders, or mental health issues, while supporting efficient remote monitoring and clinician-driven guidance. As part of the SMART BEAR integrated project, this platform has been developed to support its large-scale clinical trials. The platform consists of a standards-based data harmonization and management layer, as well as a security component, a Big Data Analytics system, a Clinical Decision Support system, and a dashboard component to facilitate efficient data collection across pilot sites.

Keywords: Cloud · AI · Semantic interoperability · HL7 FHIR · Healthcare · GDPR · Evidence-based · Ageing · Hearing loss · Cardiovascular disease · Balance disorder

© The Author(s), under exclusive license to Springer Nature Switzerland AG 2023
L. A. Maciaszek et al. (Eds.): ICT4AWE 2021/2022, CCIS 1856, pp. 408–425, 2023.
https://doi.org/10.1007/978-3-031-37496-8_21

1 Introduction

The EU-funded SMART BEAR project[1] develops an integrated platform to provide evidence-based personalized support for several pressing healthcare issues faced by the aging EU societies, including hearing loss, cardiovascular disease, cognitive disease, and balance disorders. Providing support for these health-related issues to the ageing population, in order to promote healthy and independent living, is particularly important in the EU societies since ageing can have a significant social and financial impact due to a higher incidence of these issues.

In SMART BEAR, continuously collected data from a variety of sensors, assistive medical and mobile devices will be harmonized and analyzed in order to provide effective recommendations and personalized interventions. The developed SMART BEAR platform will be tested with five thousand elderly participants from six EU countries: France, Greece, Italy, Romania, Portugal, and Spain. The large-scaled project is scheduled to commence in autumn 2022 and run for 24 months. Prior to this, a smaller-scaled pilot study, named Pilot-of-Pilots (PoP), with 100 participants is already underway in the island of Madeira, Portugal since June 2022.

There has been an increased interest in e-health monitoring systems situated at homes in recent years, leading to the creation of Health Smart Homes. Such technologies can facilitate monitoring patients' activities, in order to improve the quality of care for the elderly and increase their well-being in a non-obtrusive way. Health Smart Homes can also enable efficient and decentralized healthcare services at home, which allows for greater independence and empowerment, preventing social isolation for the individuals, and maintaining good health longer. Furthermore, elderly individuals can avoid being placed in institutions such as nursing homes and hospitals for as long as possible, thus reducing the burden on the healthcare system (Mshali et al., 2018).

Health Smart Homes are powered by the Internet of Things (IoT), and more specifically, Medical IoT, which refers to the increasing range of applications of IoT in the medical domain (Akyildiz et al., 2015). Major advancements in wireless technology and computing power have enabled the current wide use of IoT and has led to the proliferation of specialized and diverse Medical IoT devices that can generate and transmit data through an open protocol, which can then be analyzed subsequently. Among the benefits of Medical IoT are ease of service delivery, early diagnosis, improved patient management, and reduced manual errors (Adhikary et al., 2020).

The growth of Medical IoT monitoring devices for medical and well-being measurements is not the only factor that is changing the landscape in consumer health and personalized medicine. Through a connected infrastructure of medical devices, software applications, health systems and services, as well as the data generated at an accelerated rate, are transforming the delivery of healthcare. Today, e-health systems equipped with Big Data Analytics (BDA) capabilities enable the provision of high-quality decision support, thus improving the quality of care. Information exchange and data reusability, combined with the application of data mining and machine learning (ML) analytics, can facilitate the conversion of information into knowledge (Dash et al., 2019).

---

[1] https://www.smart-bear.eu/.

Despite significant progress in this domain, challenges remain. As the scientific community does not have a commonly accepted method of systematically evaluating the captured information and derived knowledge, the challenge remains in determining how these resources can be utilized productively without being exploited commercially. A well-known specification for the representation of clinical data is the HL7 (Health Level Seven) FHIR (Fast Healthcare Interoperability Resources) standard – and we use it as the underlying basis for our data harmonization solution. HL7 FHIR also incorporates a well-defined semantics which is captured using widely accepted ontologies such as LOINC[2] and SNOMED-CT[3]. Standardizing the data representations will facilitate the development of analytics and decision models, with the potential to provide accurate, personalized interventions.

Data protection must also be adequately addressed in addition to knowledge production. All applicable legal requirements and privacy obligations must be met when processing sensitive personal data, including those imposed by the General Data Protection Regulation (GDPR), which is an EU legal framework that fundamentally changed how personal data is managed lawfully in the European Union. In this context, it is not sufficient just to have implemented organizational procedures and IT-enabled processes for exercising certain GDPR rights. Vulnerabilities do occur even in the most well-designed and well-coded IT applications. Furthermore, 82% of the healthcare providers have reported to experience attacks against their Medical IoT according to the Health Insurance Portability and Accountability Act statistics[4]. Therefore, continuous security and privacy assurance measures must be implemented, to ensure the security and privacy of the stored data, as well as the integrity of any platform on which they are stored and managed (integrity, confidentiality, and availability of data at rest, in transit, and during processing for data flows). In light of the legal obligations imposed by the GDPR and the state-of-the-art guidelines, such as the NIST encryption guidelines[5], data minimization, pseudo-anonymization, transparency in the processing of personal data, and audit support are among the appropriate technical (and organizational) measures that need to be considered, preferably at an early stage, to ensure that all legal requirements are met.

Last but not least, BDA systems for healthcare decision-making must not only focus on the production of ML knowledge but also convey it in an easy-to-use way. Currently, e-health systems do not appear to be rated satisfactorily in terms of their usability (Basdekis et al., 2012), while understanding ML models still remains an open question (Liao et al., 2020). Furthermore, the integration of ML models in the healthcare field continues to be criticized for not adhering to high standards of accountability, reliability, and transparency (Anderson, 2018). These limitations can be addressed by utilizing Explainable Artificial Intelligence (XAI) techniques, which aims to make ML results more understandable to humans, to increase the trust of end-users in the ML algorithms that produced them, and eventually their confidence in applying ML algorithms in sensitive domains. These systems, in particular, are being used within a high-stress

---

[2] https://loinc.org/.

[3] https://www.snomed.org/.

[4] https://www.hipaajournal.com/82-of-healthcare-organizations-have-experienced-a-cybera ttack-on-their-iot-devices/.

[5] https://csrc.nist.gov/Projects/cryptographic-standards-and-guidelines.

environment, by non-technical end-users, and perhaps with time constraints that made the situation even worse. Thus, the acceptance and usability by the involved end-users of such functionality is a critical factor for its success and a key requirement in the SMART BEAR project.

The presented paper is an extended version of an earlier research paper (Peretokin et al., 2022). The discussion of the components in the SMART BEAR infrastructure has been greatly expanded here.

2   The SMART BEAR Architecture

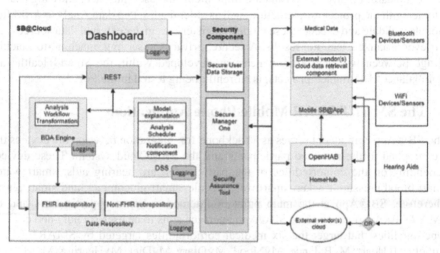

Fig. 1. The SMART BEAR Architecture (Peretokin et al., 2022).

There are three main systems in the SMART BEAR architecture as shown in Fig. 1, namely the mobile phone application (SB@App), the SMART BEAR Home Hub (Home-Hub), and the SMART BEAR Cloud (SB@Cloud). Data are continuously collected from all linked portable devices via the Mobile SB@App (e.g., hearing aid program, steps measurement, and blood pressure), and through the Mobile SB@App itself (e.g., questionaries about the diet, mood, sleep quality, or medication adherence). The HomeHub then accumulates data from different home-based sensors, such as movement sensors and weight scales. Finally, SB@Cloud is the core system that is responsible for the secure storage and model-driven big data analysis of the collected data, as well as personalized decision-making. There are several components within SB@Cloud, namely the BDA Engine, the Data Repository and its underlying Information Model, the Synthetic Data Generator, Decision Support System (DSS), and the Dashboard.

SB@Cloud interacts with the SB@App and the HomeHub, as well as the external medical system and device vendor clouds through Representational State Transfer (RESTful) interfaces. All collected data from the SB@App and the HomeHub reaching the SB@Cloud are already anonymized before the transmission and are then stored in the Data Repository in compliance with the GDPR rules.

All components inside the SB@Cloud are also interconnected with the RESTful interfaces. The REST layer in the SB@Cloud is used for retrieving, saving, or analyzing the data that are store in the database, as well as provides the interfaces to both the Dashboard and external components to SB@Cloud. The REST services also allow interactions between the BDA Engine and the Data Repository, so that the end-users can perform a data analytics workflow with multiple tasks to the BDA Engine for analysis. Communications between components, as well as authentication at the Dashboard, are secured according to GDPR through the security component, which also ensures all security mechanisms are functioning correctly. Moreover, the security component facilitates interoperability with external platforms that represent medical/usage data using the FHIR standard. Finally, the Dashboard implements the user interface, allowing users to interact with the project infrastructure such as enter data, set up data Analysis Workflow models, validate and execute these models, register/unregister external data sources, and retrieve/visualize execution results. A secure, privacy-preserving, machine-to-machine bridge between two platforms, which was developed within the Smart4Health[6] and Holobalance[7] EU-funded projects, is currently being tested in the PoP.

3   The SMART BEAR Mobile Phone Applications

The SB@App component serves as a backbone for integration between the devices that are supplied to the recruited participants and the SB@Cloud system. These devices, depending on the comorbidities of the participants, are hearing aids, smart watch, smart blood pressure tracker, smart weight scale, smart glucometer, and smart phone. Therefore, SB@App is the main point of interaction between participants and the SMART BEAR platform. The SB@App interface aims to be user-friendly and contains functionalities that target the six medical comorbidities targeted by SMART BEAR, namely MyHeart, MyBalance, MyMood, MyDiary, MyDiet, MyHearing, MyMemory, MyMedication, MySmartBear and MyAppointments.

SB@App is responsible for sending all collected data to SB@Cloud, as well as receiving informational material and data analysis results performed by the platform. Furthermore, the functionalities of SB@App also include notifications/alerts management, calendar-based appointment setup with clinicians, questionnaire and surveys, and reporting on participants' interaction with the SMART BEART platform. SB@App connects to the available devices using either their Application Programming Interface (API) or their respective Software Development Kit, depending on what is available for each.

4   The SMART BEAR Home Hub

The SMART BEAR HomeHub component is based on the openHAB platform[8] – an open-source implementation towards a common approach in addressing security/software development and protocol connectivity concerns of Smart IoT. In SMART

---

[6] Smart4Health: Citizen-centered EU-HER exchange for personalized health. https://smart4health.eu/.

[7] Holobalance: Holograms for personalized virtual coaching and motivation in an ageing population with balance disorders. https://holobalance.eu/.

[8] https://www.openhab.org/.

BEAR, the HomeHub monitors the use of light sources, temperature, humidity, and movement inside a patient's home. Another reason why openHAB was chosen as the HomeHub solution is because it allows sensors or devices from different vendors to be integrated in a single solution.

5   The SMART BEAR Cloud Components

A detailed discussion of each SB@Cloud component is presented in this section to allow a fuller picture of their utility and how they fit to the overall architecture.

5.1   Data Repository

Database Implementation. The data repository component of SB@Cloud contains a combination of FHIR-compliant and non-FHIR databases. The FHIR database stores those data that represent medical entities, whereas the non-FHIR database stores data related to non-medical entities. The non-FHIR database contains data that are not mapped to FHIR models, such as dashboard user settings or intermediate results of the analytics models when these are applied to FHIR data. Data transmitted by the HomeHub can also be stored in the non-FHIR database. Finally, intervention, notifications, and alerts generated by the DSS are also stored in the non-FHIR database.

Data Model Specification Compliant with FHIR. HL7 FHIR is the latest standard from HL7, an international standards development organization that has been publishing healthcare interoperability standards since 1989. The FHIR standard incorporates the best of and builds upon the lessons learned from the different approaches taken previously by HL V2 and HL7 V3, while simultaneously using well-known, modern technologies such as REST and JSON. In addition to providing out-of-the-box tooling, the standard is published for free and is open source. Therefore, FHIR was chosen to be used within SMART BEAR as the standard for clinical data for its speed and ease of implementation, as well as the fact that REST and JSON are an especially good fit for mobile applications, which the project makes use of.

The FHIR standard is also used by a number of leading international organizations that provide solutions to specific healthcare problems. Among these organizations is Integrating the Healthcare Enterprise (IHE)[9], which is an initiative by healthcare professionals and industry to improve the way computer systems share health information, as well as the Personal Connected Health Alliance (PCHA)[10], which is a membership-based Healthcare Information and Management Systems Society Innovation Company that develops the Continua Design Guidelines (CDG) in order to advance patient-centered health, wellness, and disease prevention. IHE and PCHA are updating their technical specifications to incorporate FHIR. Furthermore, FHIR is also used nationally in The Netherlands as part of the MedMij project[11], and is implemented in Estonia's national

---

[9] https://www.ihe.net/.
[10] https://www.pchalliance.org/.
[11] https://medmij.nl/en/home/.

electronic health record system as well. Several countries, including the Netherlands, Switzerland, and Belgium, have established national core profiles for FHIR that standardize clinical information relevant to the respective countries. A standard that is gaining such strong acceptance in Europe will make it easier to support future needs in data exchange.

Due to the nature of the data treated in the project, and in accordance with the FHIR standard, an Implementation Guide (IG) was required. For this reason, an analysis of the IGs published on the FHIR registries was carried out. Among these, particular attention was paid the Personal Health Device (PHD)[12] and International Patient Summary (IPS)[13] IGs.

The PHD IG adapts FHIR resources to transmit measurements and supporting data from PHDs to different types of systems, such as electronic medical records and clinical decision support platforms. This IG is of particular interest due to the fact that it is based on the CDG as well as the ISO/IEEE 11073 PHD Domain Information Model (Huang et al., 2020). In spite of this, given that many health data gathered in SMART BEAR are questionnaires rather than PHDs, this IG was not considered appropriate for the SMART BEAR project.

The IPS IG defines the rules to produce a document containing the essential healthcare information about a subject of care. IPS is designed for, but not limited to, supporting unplanned, cross-border care. Although this IG provides an important contribution to identify a minimal, specialty-agnostic, condition-independent, clinically relevant dataset for a patient, it was also not considered relevant for the SMART BEAR project.

For these reasons, the project defined a dedicated SMART BEAR IG in compliance with the FHIR standard and in line with the choices adopted in many European projects. A set of identified FHIR resources is used to profile the SMART BEAR IG, along with the terminologies individuated from the international standard code systems, as well as internal value sets. The tool chosen for modelling the FHIR information model is SUSHI[14], considering that it integrates well with the IG publisher which is an official tool provided by HL7. Currently, the published IG consists of 84 profiles (of type Observation, Condition, Questionnaires, Bundle, Patient, DeviceUseStatement, FamilyMemberHistory, MedicationStatement, ResearchSubject), 2 extensions, 33 value Sets, and 133 examples.

The Clinical Data Repository
The SMART-BEAR Clinical Data Repository (CDR) is based on the Health Data Hub, which is built around the HL7 FHIR standard. The CDR is also able to structure and dispose of clinical information using the FHIR standard as the specification. Thus, SMART BEAR CDR is capable of storing and serving clinical information in a secure, scalable, and HL7 standardized manner. Furthermore, this allows the BDA and DSS developers to focus on developing algorithms and applications appropriate to the requirements of the SMART BEAR pilot program, enabling them to create a common set of products

[12] http://hl7.org/fhir/uv/phd/.
[13] https://hl7.org/fhir/uv/ips/.
[14] https://fshschool.org.

and solutions that are seamlessly connected using standardized information. SNOMED-CT will be used to annotate medical terminology that is not fully covered by FHIR. By adapting the Atos Terminology Server (ATS), some of the different clinical terminologies commonly used across the healthcare industry, such as ICD9 and LOINC, will become interoperable. The implementation and customization of the ATS will occur in the second phase after the finalization of the PoP, and a RESTful API will also be provided. As a result of this API, clinical information may be accessed safely through interaction with the FHIR database for terminology purposes.

5.2 Synthetic Data Generator

In order to ensure fitness for purpose of a system of such complexity during its development, it is essential to test it with realistic data and use this information to guide its design and development. Therefore, we have adopted Synthea[15], a synthetic patient generator that generates realistic patient records pertaining to the entire life of a patient, including condition onset, encounters with physicians, observations, and prescriptions.

5.3 Security

Data protection is considered a critical issue, especially when dealing with special categories of personal data (Article 9, GDPR). In this context, SB@Cloud, by virtue of its design, supports privacy. In particular, the Security Component provides mechanisms that handle data minimization, authentication, and other security and privacy aspects through pseudonymization and resource identifier reassociation (Basdekis et al., 2019). In order to protect the transmission of any (sensitive or not) data, this component supports Role-based Access Control authentication and authorization of all RESTful API endpoints and introduces services for the management of privacy-related requests in order to demonstrate compliance with GDPR. More specifically, the RESTful API implements token-based access via encrypted HTTPS connections. Due to the fact that the data is stored in two separate repositories, where pseudonymized medical and usage data are stored in the CDR and personal data and Personalized Identifiable Information are stored in a separate encrypted repository, it is possible to continue analyzing fully anonymized data after the project has concluded, provided all personal information has been deleted. Therefore, after the completion of the SB project, the Security Component data will no longer be needed for research purposes (e.g., analytics and interventions) and will be disposed of.

In parallel, The Security Component is also responsible for monitoring, testing, and assessing the security and privacy of all platform operations. A comprehensive audit of key infrastructure components and processes will also be performed, as well as leveraging monitoring mechanisms developed in the context of the project to provide an evidence-based, certifiable assessment of the platform's security posture, along with accountability provisions for changes in the security posture and analyses of the cascading effects of those changes. In addition to several built-in security assessments addressing Confidentiality, Integrity, and Availability principles, custom metrics related to the platform's

---

[15] https://synthea.mitre.org/.

components will be used, utilizing an evidence-based approach to provide security and privacy assurance assessments with certifiable results.

5.4 Information Model

As described above, data is partitioned across two databases in SMART BEAR – clinical data in the FHIR database, and non-clinical or private information that is not exposed to analytics in a non-FHIR one.

Due to the fact that FHIR is a platform specification meant to be confined to a specific use case, we have profiled various resources in the FHIR database according to our requirements (Fig. 2). Basic demographic information such as name, age, and ethnicity are stored in the Patient resource, whereas most of the clinical information is stored in Conditions and Observations, which are tied to the Encounter resource.

Each assessment is represented by an Encounter resource instance, since patient assessments are performed by clinicians in SMART BEAR. This Encounter resource is central to the information model, as all other resources either link to or from it, creating a graph in which all relevant nodes (resources) can be reached. The Conditions resource records any clinical issues that were noted during an assessment. FHIR Observations contain issues of lesser importance, as well as 'negations' - issues that a clinician has determined that the patient does not have. As a result of this fine but important distinction between a lack of data (unknown value) and a refuting observation (known negative), we can develop more accurate analytics algorithms. Furthermore, a significant part of the data acquired by the clinical assessments comes in a form of over 20 Questionnaires; these are internationally recognized; standard data collection points whose outcome scores will be used for analytical purposes.

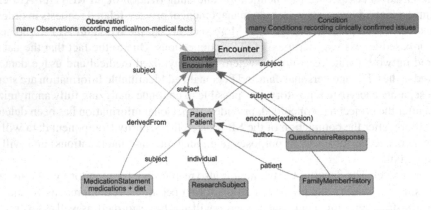

Fig. 2. Information Model of FHIR Resources in Use (Peretokin et al., 2022).

Most Observations follow a simple 'key-value' pattern, where Observation.code identifies the type of measurement, or type of condition in case of Conditions, and Observation.value[x] records the measurement value. As an example, in case of the patient having anxiety, Condition.code will be populated with "197480006 |Anxiety disorderl" from SNOMED. Should they not be affected by anxiety, Observation.code will have the same terminology code but Observation.valueCodeableConcept will be populated with "260385009 INegativel".

FHIR Vital Signs standard profiles is also adhered to where possible. For example, in the case of blood pressure, the Observation.component is utilized to record systolic/diastolic measurements, BodySite for the left or right arm, and LOINC codes are used to indicate the patient's standing/supine position. SMART BEAR IG contains a wealth of Conditions, as well as positive and negative Observation examples to assist users in understanding the FHIR database.

Furthermore, specialized resources are used where appropriate. FamilyMemberHistory for example is used to record the family history of hearing loss and ResearchSubject is used to record the source of referral to our clinical study. MedicationStatement records both the list of medications the patient is taking using the Anatomic Therapeutic Chemical value set endorsed by the World Health Organization (WHO), and the diet they are prescribed.

Previously mentioned Conditions and Observations relied on over 120 terminology mappings, with most codes coming from SNOMED, to link the semantic meaning within. Codes from LOINC and MeSH[16] complement the rest of the mappings. In order to prevent the development of new medical knowledge, the creation of custom codes was avoided as much as possible. Only four new codes have been introduced in SMART BEAR, which have no equivalents in any of the searched code systems. Several food/diet-related concepts that are not available in the SNOMED international core, but are available in the Australian edition, were used for this reason. We have verified that this does not impose any additional licensing constraints on SNOMED.

To adhere to the principle that introducing new codes should be avoided as much as possible, two SNOMED post-coordinated expressions were crafted to accurately represent very specific concepts: "number of non-scheduled visits due to volume overload in subjects with heart failure" as:

4525004 lemergency department patient visitl :362981000 lqualifier valuel = 260299005 lnumberl, 42752001 ldue tol = 21639008 lhypervolemial

and "number of Visits to the Emergency Room due to Hypertension peak" as:

4525004 lemergency department patient visitl :362981000 lqualifier valuel = 260299005 lnumberl, 42752001 ldue tol = 38341003 lhypertensionl

We chose to re-use the FHIR extension and value set published by the German Corona Consensus Data Set project (Sass et al., 2020), which is partially based on WHO ISARIC eCRF value set when it came to recording the patient's ethnicity. As a result of the reuse of existing knowledge, long-term interoperability is enhanced.

Analytics are a crucial aspect of the system, as it provides the necessary intelligence for the task at hand. They are driven by the BDA Engine, which has several requirements placed upon it – raw data processing, incremental updates, and scalability. Clinical data are stored in the system in a FHIR repository, as previously mentioned. Despite its

---

[16] https://www.nlm.nih.gov/mesh/meshhome.html.

advantages as an excellent interface for clinical data, FHIR interfaces make compromises when processing bulk data. It is for this reason that the BDA engine requires the capability of converting and flattening the hierarchical format of FHIR into a relational format that is more appropriate for bulk data processing. In order to run analytics continuously, this conversion should be possible to do incrementally as new data is received in the clinical repository, as well as being able to scale to large data volumes.

5.5 BDA Engine

The BDA Engine mainly addresses the functionalities required for processing Data Analysis Workflows, as well as providing and storing the execution results. A set of APIs is provided to perform analysis on raw data. In terms of ML, a preliminary extraction of data analytics - which will be carried out on the pre-processed datasets - are going to indicate variables or combinations of variables for the feature selection approach. It is important to note that all ML methods and techniques are data-driven, and the "best" method will be determined after its application. A longer, more detailed, discussion of how the BDA component's AI & XAI capabilities are planned to be used, in particular in the setting of the Hearing Loss comorbidity, is presented elsewhere (Iliadou et al., 2022).

The preliminary extraction of data analytics is performed by the following subcomponents featured in the BDA Engine architecture: Delta Lake[17], Spark[18], Trino[19], and Airflow[20]. A bottom-up approach will be used to describe the components, with the layers at the bottom being closest to the data repositories. Figure 3 illustrates its architecture, which is an expanded version of the architecture presented in (Anisetti et al., 2021).

A cloud object store, Delta Lake, provides ACID[21] table storage and is the closest component to the data repositories. With Delta Lake, a Lakehouse Architecture can be built using existing storage systems, including Amazon S3, Azure Data Lake Storage, Google Cloud Storage, and Hadoop Distributed File System (HDFS)[22] (Armbrust et al., 2020). The Lakehouse Architecture also enables Business Intelligence and ML analysis on all data. In the case of SMART BEAR, the adopted standard is HDFS.

On the third layer from the bottom, Spark and Trino are collocated together, providing the capability to access data and perform queries on those datasets. Spark is a multi-language engine supporting data engineering, data science, and ML on both single-node machines and clusters. Spark was chosen due to its capabilities of processing tasks encompassing custom analytics on large data volumes, as well as the fact that it features many bindings with other commonly used Data Science and ML libraries. Additionally, Spark is capable of handling batch and streaming data. Trino on the other hand provides

---

[17] https://delta.io/.
[18] https://spark.apache.org/.
[19] https://trino.io/.
[20] https://airflow.apache.org/.
[21] ACID is an acronym refers the four properties that define a transaction: Atomicity, Consistency, Isolation, and Durability.
[22] https://hadoop.apache.org/docs/r1.2.1/hdfs_design.html.

the capability of accessing and processing data from multiple systems in a highly parallel and distributed manner. In addition to supporting HDFS data, Trino also provides the BDA Engine with the ability to manage On-Line Analytical Processing queries and data warehousing tasks.

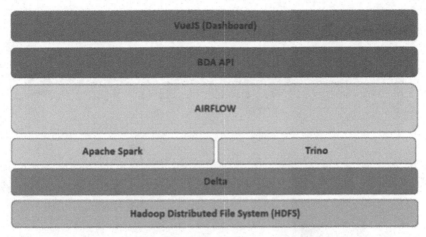

Fig. 3. The BDA Architecture (Peretokin et al., 2022).

Airflow is located on the fourth layer from the bottom and allows programmatic authoring, scheduling, and monitoring of workflows written in Python.

5.6 Decision Support System

The DSS is intended to aid clinicians in assessing every patient in terms of the optimal assessments that must be completed to assess the patient, and to provide them with the optimal combination of devices to monitor their health during the pilot study. As a result of the continuous collection and analysis of data that will be digested into the platform, this component is designed to evolve throughout the project. Initially, the DSS available for the PoP was developed in accordance with the rules and medical guidelines provided by the clinicians so as to establish a ground truth system that is based on the most current medical knowledge. For each of the monitoring conditions of the SMART BEAR project (Hearing Loss, Cardiovascular Diseases, Mild Cognitive Impairment, Mild Depression, Balance Disorders, and Frailty), the medical teams provide the rules-based scenarios and relevant interventions that should be administered to the participants. Rules-based algorithms take into account the personalized thresholds that are set for each patient individually. Cardiovascular Diseases, for example, have optimal and extreme cut-off values for blood pressure, which trigger notifications and alerts to the patient and clinical care team.

Data collected at the PoP will be used to develop BDA engine models, and the output from the analytics will be analyzed in conjunction with the measured parameters in order to determine the extent to which patients are satisfied and what adjustments need to be made to the personalized thresholds. It is possible for the DSS to be extended to support all the new interventions that will be provided by clinicians if the results of the analytics provide insights that lead to new interventions. It must be noted that any new intervention must first be validated by the clinicians before it is included in the interventions provided to the patient.

5.7 Dashboard

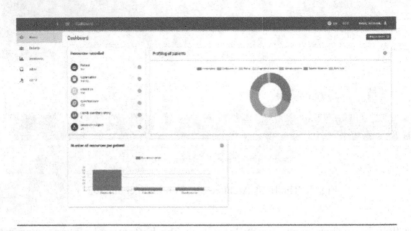

Fig. 4. Dashboard Homepage (Peretokin et al., 2022).

The SMART BEAR Dashboard is a component aimed at providing clinicians with a user-friendly graphical user interface. The Dashboard home page is shown in Fig. 4. Clinicians can utilize the Dashboard to create and manage patients, taking into account their devices and medications, conducting first visits and check-ups, performing analytics on data, and developing interventions. All collected data are stored in FHIR and non-FHIR repositories depending on their clinical value: the first collection takes place during the Baseline Assessment of a patient, which includes medical history, physical examinations, and questionnaire responses. By analyzing the information provided, the dashboard visualizes suggestions about the eligibility of prospective participants for the SMART BEAR pilot studies. According to the conditions detected, the profiling functionality suggests specific tabs and questionnaires that should be activated by the clinician. Although the patient's profile is ultimately selected by a clinician, the profiling functionality redirects users to the clinical tools and devices that are required to match a patient's profile consistently with the SMART BEAR protocol, regardless of which clinical tool is chosen. Upon creation and eligibility determination of a patient, the Dashboard displays specific tabs that enable patient management and provide information regarding demographics, such as living situation and ethnicity, participation in synergies, and type and status of devices provided.

As shown in Fig. 5, the patient management tab is another featured functionality that allows users to visualize the delivered notifications. Currently, the analytics and intervention mechanism are still in the development phase. These mechanisms aim to assist the clinicians to perform analytics on the collected data either targeting all patients or only a specific subgroup defined by certain parameters, in order to monitor the patients in the future with a determined condition. Based on the outcome of the analytics and with support from the DSS, the Dashboard visualizes suggestions for clinicians on the interventions to be delivered. The final choice of the intervention is still to be made by clinicians, and they will also be able to monitor the intervention outcome. Examples of analytics to be made available in the Dashboard are discussed in (Bellandi et al., 2021).

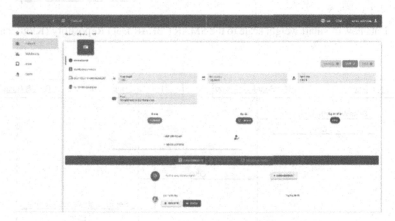

Fig. 5. Patient Management Page (Peretokin et al., 2022).

6 Interaction Specifications

Having introduced each component in the SMART BEAR architecture, this section presents an example of how these cooperate, though some interaction specification diagrams. These diagrams are representative of the main data flows in SMART BEAR (Kloukinas et al., 2020). The example described here is the MyDiet functionality of the SB@App.

In order for the MyDiet functionality to suggest appropriate dietary recommendations to a participant, their current weight needs to be collected first by using the smart weight scale. If the vendor of the smart weight scale has its own mobile application, then this vendor-provided application will be available to the participant and will transfer the new measurements to the vendor cloud, from where the Data Repository of SB@Cloud will retrieve this information periodically. This smart weight scale – vendor application – vendor cloud – Data Repository data flow is shown in Fig. 6.

In the case the vendor of the smart weight scale does not have its own mobile application, Fig. 7 shows the alternative data flow where the new weight measurements will be collected by the SB@App and transmit them to the HomeHub, which then transmits them to the Data Repository.

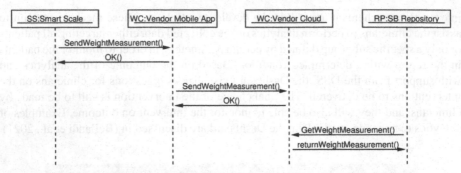

Fig. 6. Data flow of smart weight scale to the SMART BEAR Data Repository (Kloukinas et al., 2020).

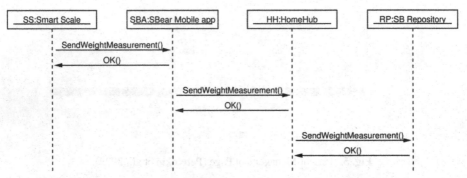

Fig. 7. Alternative data flow of smart weight scale to the SMART BEAR Data Repository – in the case of absence of vendor-provided mobile application (Kloukinas et al., 2020).

Figure 8 shows an alternative data flow of Fig. 7 if the HomeHub is not available. In this case, SB@App anonymizes its own data and connects directly to the SB@Cloud to in order to transfer the data to the Data Repository.

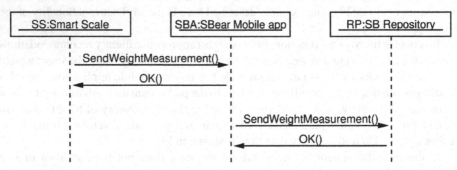

Fig. 8. Alternative data flow of smart weight scale to the SMART BEAR Data Repository – in the case of absence of the HomeHub (Kloukinas et al., 2020).

Finally, Fig. 9 shows how the DSS takes into account the measurements stored in the Data Repository, along with other data such as particular dietary requirements from the participant's profile, to form a set of recommended recipes for the participant. This recommendation is then transmitted to the SB@App and notes the choices made by the participant through the MyDiet functionality. The choice is then transmitted back to the Data Repository to allow future analysis of appropriate recipes and uptake of the suggestions of the MyDiet functionality.

7 Future Work

In order to demonstrate the efficacy, extensibility, sustainability, and cost-effectiveness of SB@Cloud, it will operate for at least three years where its solution will be tested and validated through five large-scale pilots involving 5000 elderly individuals living at home in Greece, Italy, France, Spain-Portugal, and Romania. It is expected to generate useful evidence during this period, such as metrics and observational evidence base, from analysis of the collected data that is driven by high-level BDA and decision models for offering personalized healthcare and medicine solutions in clinical practice. Since the pseudonymization mechanism is in place, SMART BEAR intends to develop a data sharing and valorization model (DSVM) that will support further analysis using anonymous data even after the lifecycle of the project. Through the integration of new data providers and open sources, the DSVM will identify methods for extending the data collected by SMART BEAR on both a technical and organizational level. Using the outcomes of data analysis, we will be able to enhance the platform's performance, personalize its relationship with its end-users further, develop new services, and monetize data-intensive services.

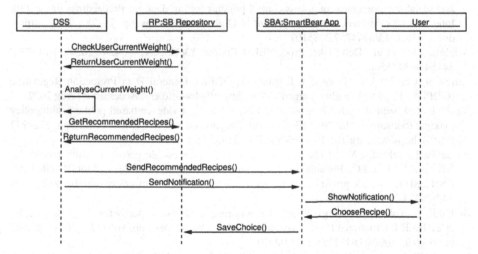

Fig. 9. DSS to MyDiet recommendation use case.

8 Conclusion

This paper provides an overview of the cloud-enabled, standards-based integrated system developed by the SMART BEAR project. This system allows for recording assessments and monitoring, as well as delivering clinician-vetted interventions to facilitate monitoring, empowering, and promoting healthy living at home for senior citizens. Based on widely accepted standards such as HL7 FHIR and advanced analytics, the system is supported by an underlying semantic interoperability solution. It is intended to leverage the platform during the SMART BEAR PoP, and further refine it to support the planned large-scale pilots in all participating countries.

Acknowledgement. This work was supported by the European Commission's Horizon 2020 research and innovation program under the SMART-BEAR project, grant agreement No 857172.

References

Adhikary, T., Jana, A.D., Chakrabarty, A., Jana, S.K.: The internet of things (IoT) augmentation in healthcare: an application analytics. In: Gunjan, V.K., Garcia Diaz, V., Cardona, M., Solanki, V.K., Sunitha, K.V.N. (eds.) ICICCT 2019, pp. 576–583. Springer, Singapore (2020). https://doi.org/10.1007/978-981-13-8461-5_66

Akyildiz, I., Pierobon, M., Balasubramaniam, S., Koucheryavy, Y.: The internet of Bio-Nano things. IEEE Commun. Mag. **53**(3), 32–40 (2015). https://doi.org/10.1109/MCOM.2015.706 0516

Anderson, C.: Ready for prime time?: AI influencing precision medicine but may not match the hype. Clin. OMICs **5**(3), 44–46 (2018). https://doi.org/10.1089/clinomi.05.03.26

Anisetti, M., Ardagna, C.A., Braghin, C., Damiani, E., Polimeno, A., Balestrucci, A.: Dynamic and scalable enforcement of access control policies for big data. In: Proceedings of the 13th International Conference on Management of Digital EcoSystems, pp. 71–78 (2021). https://doi.org/10.1145/3444757.3485107

Armbrust, M., et al.: Delta lake. Proc. VLDB Endow. **13**(12), 3411–3424 (2020). 10.14778/3415478.3415560

Article 9, General Data Protection Regulation (GDPR). General Data Protection Regulation (GDPR) – Final text neatly arranged (2018). https://gdpr-info.eu/. Accessed 20 Aug 2022

Basdekis, I., Pozdniakov, K., Prasinos, M., Koloutsou, K.: Evidence based public health policy making: tool support. In: 2019 IEEE World Congress on Services (SERVICES), pp. 272–277 (2019). https://doi.org/10.1109/SERVICES.2019.00080

Basdekis, I., Sakkalis, V., Stephanidis, C.: Towards an accessible personal health record. In: Nikita, K.S., Lin, J.C., Fotiadis, D.I., Arredondo Waldmeyer, M.-T. (eds.) MobiHealth 2011. LNICSSITE, vol. 83, pp. 61–68. Springer, Heidelberg (2012). https://doi.org/10.1007/978-3-642-29734-2_9

Bellandi, V., et al.: Engineering continuous monitoring of intrinsic capacity for elderly people. In: 2021 IEEE International Conference on Digital Health (ICDH), pp. 166–171 (2021). https://doi.org/10.1109/ICDH52753.2021.00030

Dash, S., Shakyawar, S.K., Sharma, M., Kaushik, S.: Big data in healthcare: management, analysis and future prospects. J. Big Data **6**(1), 1–25 (2019). https://doi.org/10.1186/s40537-019-0217-0

Huang, Z.Y., Wang, Y., Wang, L.: ISO/IEEE 11073 treadmill interoperability framework and its test method: design and implementation. JMIR Med. Inform. **8**(12), e22000 (2020). https://doi.org/10.2196/22000

Iliadou, E., Su, Q., Kikidis, D., Bibas, T., Kloukinas, C.: Profiling hearing aid users through big data explainable artificial intelligence techniques. Front. Neurol. (2022)

Kloukinas, C., et al.: Smart Big Data Platform to Offer Evidence-based Personalised Support for Healthy and Independent Living at Home. Deliverable to the SMART BEAR (857172) Project funded by the European Union D6 – SMART BEAR Architecture (Public), City, University of London, UK (2020). https://www.smart-bear.eu/wp-content/uploads/2021/06/D6-D2.2.pdf. Accessed 21 Aug 2022

Liao, Q.V., Gruen, D., Miller, S.: Questioning the AI: informing design practices for explainable AI user experiences. In: Proceedings of the 2020 CHI Conference on Human Factors in Computing Systems, pp. 1–15 (2020). https://doi.org/10.1145/3313831.3376590

Mshali, H., Lemlouma, T., Moloney, M., Magoni, D.: A survey on health monitoring systems for health smart homes. Int. J. Ind. Ergon. **66**, 26–56 (2018). https://doi.org/10.1016/j.ergon.2018.02.002

Peretokin, V., et al.: Overview of the SMART-BEAR technical infrastructure. In: Proceedings of the 8th International Conference on Information and Communication Technologies for Ageing Well and E-Health, pp. 117–125 (2022). https://doi.org/10.5220/0011082700003188

Sass, J., et al.: The German corona consensus dataset (GECCO): a standardized dataset for COVID-19 research in university medicine and beyond. BMC Med. Inform. Decis. Mak. **20**(1), 341 (2020). https://doi.org/10.1186/s12911-020-01374-w

Author Index

Printed in the United States
by Baker & Taylor Publisher Services